STARTING YOUR OWN PRACTICE FROM SCRATCH

Medicare Part B, G-Codes, PQRS and ICD-10

Caroline Joy Co, PT, DPT, CHT, CSFA

DEDICATION

Dedicated to my family

Papa, Mama, Achi, Ching and Ivo

Starting your Own Practice from Scratch
Medicare Part B, G-Codes, PQRS and ICD-10

Rehabsurge, Inc.'s mission is to support healthcare and education professionals to continue their educational and professional development. Rehabsurge is committed to identifying, promoting, and implementing innovative continuing education activities that can increase and impart professional knowledge and skills through books, audiobooks, or digital e-books based on sound scientific and clinically derived research. The first Rehabsurge continuing education book was published in July 2009.

As a sponsor of Continuing Education (CE) seminars and workshops, we enable professionals to enhance their skills, pursue professional interests, and redefine their specialties within their respective disciplines while earning CEUs, CE credits, or Contact Hours. Offerings include CE books, audiobooks, and digital e-books, all of which are focused on the latest treatment and assessment approaches and include discussions of alternative and state-of-the art therapies.

DISABILITY POLICY:

Rehabsurge seeks to ensure that all students have access to its activities. To that end, it is committed to providing support services and assistance for equal access for learners with disabilities. Rehabsurge has a firm commitment to meeting the guidelines of the Americans with Disabilities Act and Section 504 of the Rehabilitation Act of 1973. Rehabsurge will provide support services and assistance for students with disabilities, including reasonable accommodations, modifications, and appropriate services to all learners with documented disabilities.

ISBN: 1450596398
EAN-13: 9781450596398

Printed in the United States of America

Disclaimer:

This book is intended for informational and educational purposes only. It is not meant to provide any medical advice. Many of the product names referred to herein are trademarks or registered trademarks of their respective owners. Care has been taken to confirm the accuracy of the information presented and to describe generally accepted practices. However, the authors, editors, and publisher are not responsible for errors or omissions or for any consequences from application of the information in this book and make no warranty, expressed or implied, with respect to the currency, completeness, or accuracy of the contents of the publication. Application of this information in a particular situation remains the professional responsibility of the practitioner.

For permissions and additional information, contact us:

Rehabsurge, Inc.
Phone: +1 (516) 515-1267
PO Box 287
Baldwin, NY 11510.
Email: ceu@rehabsurge.com

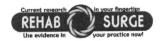

ABOUT THE AUTHOR

Caroline Joy Co, PT, DPT, CHT, CSFA, is a licensed physical therapist and certified hand therapist whose clinical experience includes acute, subacute, home health, and outpatient settings. Her background includes Community-Based Therapy that is designed to help people with disabilities access therapy in their communities. She is the President and CEO of PTSponsor.com, an online resource for U.S. hospitals and clinics that seek to sponsor and hire foreign-trained rehabilitation therapists. She specializes in hand therapy through an integrated approach that includes education, counsel, and exercise. She is also certified in functional assessment for work hardening and work conditioning.

Co is also the President of Rehabsurge, a continuing education company and a contracting agency. Her past affiliations include Long Beach Medical Center, Horizon Health and Subacute Center, and Grandell Therapy and Nursing Center.

Co was a professional speaker for Summit Professional Education, Cross Country Education and Dogwood Institute. She received her transitional doctorate from A.T. Still University and her BS in Physical Therapy from University of the Philippines College of Allied Medical Professions. She is licensed in California, Nevada, and New York.

FULL DISCLOSURE

To comply with professional boards/associations standards, all planners, speakers, and reviewers involved in the development of continuing education content are required to disclose their relevant financial relationships. An individual has a relevant financial relationship if he or she has a financial relationship in any amount occurring in the last 12 months, with any commercial interest whose products or services are discussed in their presentation content over which the individual has control. Relevant financial relationships must be disclosed to the audience.

As part of its accreditation with boards/associations, Rehabsurge, Inc. is required to "resolve" any reported conflicts of interest prior to the educational activity. The presentation will be scientifically balanced and free of commercial bias or influence.

To comply with professional boards/associations standards:

I declare that neither I nor my family has any financial relationship in any amount occurring in the last 12 months, with a commercial interest whose products or services are discussed in my presentation. Additionally, all planners involved do not have any financial relationship.

Caroline Joy Co, PT, DPT, CHT, CSFA

CONTENTS

Course Description

The primary goal of this course is to provide you with a step-by-step guide to build your very own practice from scratch. As such, this course is dedicated to helping you put up your very own health facility where you can readily offer your professional therapeutic services to the people in your area. From beginning to end, its content will give you step-by-step guidelines. If you put your heart and mind to the task, then you will surely succeed in establishing your own health facility.

Physical therapy is one of the most challenging fields in the health care industry to run. In an ever-changing and fast-paced healthcare industry, rules and regulations about coding and billing affect physical therapy practice. Over the years, patients who are the primary payers of health care have become more meticulous in scrutinizing the manner in which care is provided for them (Forbes, 2014). Such attitude has risen among patients because of cases where there have been overpayments of medical bills where a request for refund has to be made when a case of overpayment is detected. The focus of this book is to enhance the skills of the physical therapist in practically solving challenges associated with coding and billing in order to make a profit from the care rendered to patients (American Physical Therapy Association, 2014).

Physical therapy is now a health care service for which practitioners can bill their patients separately. In the past, physical therapy services were usually billed as part of the hospital charges. However, because more and more patients are availing themselves of physical therapy on an outpatient basis for a variety of reasons, there is a need for both the physical therapists and the billers of their services to know how billing and coding impact payments for care rendered. This improvement in terms of billing and financial remuneration for physical therapy is one step towards the recognition of physical therapy as one of the most important components of health care provision and a profession distinct in itself. (APTA, 2014; CMS, 2014).

While it is positive that physical therapy services can be billed separately, problems usually arise when patients pay through various modes such as their HMOs (health maintenance organizations), Medicare, Medicaid and other pre-paid health insurance service. Commonly, physical therapists are underpaid, receive late payments or, in worse cases, are not even paid for the services they rendered. With this problem in the forefront, Medicare Part B steps in to give a solution, albeit a challenging one. The challenging part of this solution lies in the fact that billers need to have operating knowledge of codes and coding guidelines, types of health care insurance coverage plans and providers and their respective guidelines, record management systems, and other technical and non-technical concepts related to physical therapy service provision.

This book is therefore conceptualized and designed to help the independent physical therapy practitioner and biller understand the most important things to know about Medicare Part B guidelines and how to bill and get paid for the services they render. Understanding records management systems and how claims can be facilitated through different health care insurance providers will help billers and independent physical therapy practitioners efficiently collect payments for services rendered.

In addition, this book discusses documentation and billing strategies that can help physical therapists understand Medicare standards for outpatient programs. Appropriate billing and documentation should be present in the medical record, because Medicare is increasingly reviewing therapy claims to ensure that the therapy provided did require the skills of a therapist. The book explains establishing medical necessity, providing safety, and supervising assistive personnel, along with denial and appeal management, regulatory guidelines for insurers, and improving cash flow with denial management strategies. The extensive overview of CPT codes and ICD-10 codes provided, as well as a description of the PQRS and functional limitation guidelines implemented by Medicare, will help the physical therapist provide Medicare patients with the most thorough documentation to support the need for services rendered. Proper coding and documentation ensure that facilities will keep their money upon a post-payment medical record audit.

The information provided here in no way represents a guarantee of payment. Benefits for all claims will be based on the patient's eligibility, provisions of the law, and regulations and instructions from the Centers for Medicare & Medicaid Services (CMS). It is the responsibility of each provider or practitioner submitting claims to become familiar with Medicare coverage and its requirements.

Topics such as choosing the right business structure, defining your specialty, and determining if your business would be viable are written for quick and easy comprehension while conveying numerous applicable instructions and related guidelines. Surely, this book will be helpful once you decide to found your very own healthcare establishment. Take advantage of this book's guidance and instructions, and make your dreams of owning your own healthcare facility a reality!

Course Objectives

1. To define a practice that will separate you from competition

2. To identify if there is a market for your practice in your target geographical location

3. To choose the right business structure, right slogan and right branding

4. To decide which payment options you will accept-- No fault, worker's comp, third party payers or cash

5. To device a marketing and business plan

6. To choose the best billing and accounting system for your facility

7. To prepare for a grand opening day

INTRODUCTION

A few hours ago, you had your annual performance review. You can still hear the voice of your boss; "You were late 15 times last year. You called in sick 10 times, what can you contribute to our organization?" It annoys you. You work so hard every single day. You have enough savings. You know that you are skilled and talented. Your patients tell you, "You are amazing!" Now you wonder, can I be my own boss? Is it time?

The primary goal of this course is to provide you with a step-by-step guide to build your very own practice from scratch. As such, this course is dedicated to helping you put up your very own healthcare facility where you can readily offer your professional therapeutic services to the people in your area. From beginning to end, its content will give you step-by-step guidelines and useful information. If you put your heart and mind to the task, then, you will surely succeed in establishing your own health facility.

Topics such as choosing the right business structure, defining your specialty and determining if your business would be viable are written for quick and easy comprehension while conveying numerous applicable instructions and related guidelines. Surely, this book will be helpful once you decide to found your very own healthcare establishment. Take advantage of this book's guidance and instructions, and make your dreams of owning your own healthcare facility a reality!

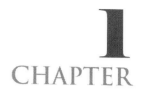

CHAPTER

DEFINING YOUR PRACTICE

There is an important concept only a few know regarding establishing a place of business. It is so important that the very success and ultimate the survival of your business literally depend on it. What am I talking about? Let us discuss it through a brief story and see if you can guess what it is before the end of this chapter.

Mr. Hubbard had some savings he had set aside from his years as a physical therapist in his town's outpatient physical therapy clinic. He had always dreamed about putting up his very own outpatient clinic and, therefore, he was determined to start one in his neighborhood. As a good physical therapist himself, he fully confident he would be swimming in riches after building his own physical therapy and wellness center.

He had planned everything—from buying the right equipment, getting the right location, renovating designs for the building he planned to lease—and after all that, he truly believed that there was no way his business would fail. Mr. Hubbard presented his business plan to SCORE (Service Corps of Retired Executives). Bill from SCORE asked him, "Is there another physical therapy center in the area?" Based on the services you proposed, it seems that your services also compete with gyms and health spas. Who is your target population? Why would people choose you over the other physical therapy centers?

This has surprised Mr. Hubbard. He clearly has not thought about this. Bill said, "It seems to me that you have not defined your practice. If you have not found your target market yet, your business is bound to fail."

If you had paid close attention, you would be able to observe that Mr. Hubbard had decided on what kind of business he had first, built it, and then assumed that clients would flock to it. He neglected to perform one important step in establishing a business, and that was to identify his niche market and then see to it that that market exists in his area. In other words, one must determine what consumers need before determining what to sell. If you determine first what you want to offer (products or services) and then wait around for customers to just come into your business establishment, then you are in for trouble.

Mr. Hubbard's Story

Let us first define what a niche market is. To be brief, it is the business principle that requires you to concentrate on a specific market segment (Van Der Hope, 2008). A niche market is akin to setting your eyes on a target and aiming before pulling the trigger of your gun. The logic behind this is that all giant businesses can never truly be able to supply all the services and products that all consumers want and need. This only means that a relatively small and new business out there has a chance to succeed once its owner can identify that part of the market that must be sought out so that the small business can meet its needs that are not being met by the bigger businesses in the area.

Mr. Hubbard has to take the time to stop, think, and identify his niche market. The same applies to you, whether you are a physical therapist, occupational therapist, or a chiropractor. Your niche market is important to you as the lifeblood of your planned or operating business. Here are some helpful methods you can utilize to identify your niche.

You have to be the only one, or at least one of the very few businesses, that is able to provide this certain service or product. To do this, examine and study very well your place of market and identify that certain service or product that no one supplying. This only means that if the area where you plan to set up business is already saturated with physical therapists, etc., then it might be a good idea to look somewhere else for another location that is much more feasible based on this method (Falkenstein, 2000).

For example, if you think about fast food, McDonald's, Subway, and Taco Bell come to mind. McDonald's target markets are those who love the burgers, fries and the popular kid's meal. Subway sells sandwiches and focuses on health. Taco Bell sells Mexican-style food. If you decide to sell fast food in this area, you should not sell burgers, fries, sandwiches, or tacos. Hypothetically, you should probably choose to be a Chinese fast food place who sell "kung pao" chicken and pork fried rice, these would products or service that is relatively unique in the area and that cannot be found at other fast food chains.

As a practitioner, you should find something that will make you unique. Price is usually a battle you cannot win. Here are some ideas:

1. Offer hydrotherapy by having a pool in your clinic

2. Have the latest laser or traction machine

3. Be open on holidays and weekends

4. Focus on specialties such as pediatric, hands, sports, women's health, or wound care

5. Offer weight loss programs and beauty regimens

6. Sell vitamins

7. Offer yoga or pilates

You must only provide a service if you think that a market actually exists for it. A small group of loyal patrons is enough to secure your investment as a viable one (Falkenstein, 2000). If you remember, *Seinfeld*, Jerry told the Babu Bhatt to open a restaurant truly dedicated to serving Pakistani food. If the restaurant owner first identified how many people in his area are interested in Pakistani food, he would know that it is too little to sustain his business. As a practitioner, if you intend to focus on sports, you should check if there are athletes (professional or student) in your area. If there aren't, then, it might not be a good idea.

You must promote and sell your business expansively. It is imperative that you continually do so, because information about your available services needs to reach the ears of potential clients. In your case, your possible prospects would most probably be overworked laborers, people with disabilities or injuries, or maybe just people who work with extremely high levels of pressure in their environment and need to rethink their tiresome, unhealthy lifestyle in order for them not to suffer a severe mental as well as physical breakdown (Falkenstein, 2000).

You might choose to work with the upper middle class with health insurance. You should identify the size of your market and promote your business.

You might also choose to work with cash clients. This is something you have to define right from the beginning. As your professional services will advertise, you will address their complaints regarding the alleviation of work-related injuries or discomfort, such as lower back pain, shoulder pain, and upper trapezius pain. Even aches and difficulties resulting from non-work activities, disabilities, and injuries are included in the kinds of problems you will be dealing with when it comes to your patients.

As part of defining your niche, it is suggested that at this point, you must engage the services of reliable marketers and have them mass produce high-quality business cards (around 5,000 pieces will do, in full color), 1,000 letterheads, 1,000 envelopes, and 1,000 brochures on the kinds of therapy you will offer. Do this with a minimum budget of roughly $500.00.

You can have these items done through online customization stores that do printing such as Gotprint. com and Overnightprints.com. Gotprint requires at least 500 count per order, while Overnightprint has a lower minimum (about 100 count per order). ClickPrint.com also has interesting discount packages and can provide you with printed items that have a raised ink design. My personal favorite is Printing4less.com in terms of mass mailing. They will get you discount postage rates, mail the brochures for you and remove the duplicates on your mailing list. They also allow you to mail an odd number count. They will allow you mail 1,432 cards or 453 brochures. Most companies will require you to mail in multiple of 500 or 1000.

The brochure must contain something about you, your educational background and experience in your profession, a map of the facility's location, and a list of the techniques and services that you offer along with the corresponding prices.

As a business principle, make target-marketing work for you. Take time to define with care what your chosen niche market is, if it exists in the area, and then carefully determine whether the marketplace where you are planning to set up business will be able to sustain your practice. Doing so will help prevent you from wasting your precious time, effort, and money. Once you have a specific market segment singled out and verified, then by all means, begin establishing your health facility.

Naming Your Health Facility

Once you have determined your niche market and its positive presence in your locale, the next step is to name your new health facility. It may initially sound like a trivial task, but it is actually one of the biggest factors that determine the success of any business establishment. Indeed, business owners at this point should definitely pay attention to the simple question: What's in a name? This is simply because that by choosing the right name, you will ultimately raise the chances of success of your establishment, thus saving you much time and money in the long run. The first thing your potential clients are going to notice, whether in your brochures, your business cards, or on your website, is the name of your business. In this sense and context, the name of your facility is even more important than your sales pitch or even the specific names of your offered services. Your facility may be the best in town, but if customers are going somewhere else because your competitors sound more attractive or easier to remember by name than you do, then all your efforts in promoting your establishment will go to waste (Kishel, 2005).

Consider the name of your business as the "entry point" or, from the outside, the only seeming differentiator that sets you apart from your business rivals. With this in mind, be warned that potential clients have the tendency to make instantaneous judgments based on your facility's name. This helps customers decide just where they want to spend their hard-earned money. It is therefore imperative— absolutely essential—that you strike the right "tone" with your potential clients using your business name (Kishel, 2005).

It would be most ideal for business names to be original, upbeat, and instantly informative with regards to what your establishment does. If you want to attract the right clientele, you must envision a name that stands out from the crowd. It must also be easy to recall. However, the name must also be one the public will find trustworthy as well as professional sounding.

To start the process of naming your business establishment, you must bear in mind three key things regarding the name:

It should be original.

It should be legally available.

It should represent you and your profession for many years to come.

It must be easy to recall.

Other Tips

When brainstorming your facility's name, try to avoid one that will put limits on your business. Think ahead into the future. What if you will have to sell your facility? Naming your business after yourself may sound like a great idea, but if you plan to sell it down the road, it is more advisable to choose a more generic name. This does not mean your business will inevitably fail. On the contrary, your business might be so successful that another company may want to go into business with you and perhaps even buy your share of the proprietorship. Picking a name that will not limit your business will therefore be beneficial in both cases.

Another reason a generic-sounding name is preferable is that the services you might be offering for the first year may end up as something different or more varied in the long run. For example, if you name your facility with something like "_____ Physical Therapy Center" but then enter a partnership with a chiropractor after a year or two, you would have to adjust the name to help promote both you and your partner's services. That would mean having to legally register it again with the local authorities, which is another hassle on your part.

It is highly recommended that the name you choose must emphasize qualities that you wish to promote. However, keep in mind that a health facility requires a name that is appropriate, so also take note of the circumstances when formulating the name of your business. Appropriateness must be considered at all times.

It is also sound advice to formulate a business name that is relatively easy to pronounce and spell. The reason behind this is quite simple. Should somebody hear the name of your business on the local radio or from someone on the street, they should be able to Google the name of your business to easily locate you. A name that is easy to spell thus avoids confusion and frustration in these searches.

It is important for you to Google the name and trademark search the name you are planning to use as well. If that particular name brings up too many listings on the search engines, you may have a tough time attracting customers. List all the names of your competitors. If your name sounds too similar with that of a rival facility, there will definitely be legal battles on the way (Attorney, 2007). Remember, originality matters when it comes to choosing a suitable name for your health facility, or any other business for that matter.

Once you have brood over all the appropriate and clever words and ideas that you can think of, jot down all possible names on a whiteboard. Then, narrow the list to the most suitable choices. Have your colleagues, friends, and even family look at the list. Their opinions will definitely help you arrive at a good decision.

Don't forget about a slogan. If you hear "Just Do It", you think of Nike. If you hear "Melts in Your Mouth, Not in Your Hand", you think of M&Ms. Let us take for example a health establishment by the name of Wagner Wellness Center. Possible slogans could include:

Promoting wellness through the science, art, and philosophy of healing

Get on the wagon to health and wellness Relieve pain, correct subluxation, and maintain optimal health

The function of the slogan is to emphasize what your business stands for. Clientele like to know what they are getting into, so show them your values and mission. Be as creative as you can with your slogans without sounding like you are doing what is called a "hard sell." Remember that people get turned off by too much sales talk since it may come off as superficial and too ambitious. Keep things real, but show them that you are committed in providing them the right service. Here are examples of bad slogans:

Virgin Trains "Business Brains take Virgin Trains"

Ferrero Rocher "A sign of good taste"

Kentucky Fried Chicken "The Secret's in the taste" ("Finger Lickin' Good!" was the better slogan.)

If you wish to incorporate, choosing its name is a formal procedure since it has to be legally registered with the secretary of state's office or the proper authorities involved. The name of the corporation must be unique because in the event that the name is already in use or is reserved, then the application for registration of your corporation's name will be bluntly rejected. The words "incorporated," "corporation," "company," "limited" or the letters "Inc.", or "Corp." must be included in the name.

Whether it is better to go into a partnership or opt to join a corporation, the choice is up to you, based on your financial standing, the people you plan to deal with, and the viability of your establishment.

You must know the importance of feeling secure in your business's future stability, even if at first you feel as though you don't have enough start-up capital. It is a wise move to evaluate your financial situation and foresee all that could possibly happen in the months to come when your health facility is still trying to take off. You should carefully plan for weathering these first few months after your opening.

The first several months are always critical in the sense that since you are starting out, you still have to earn back all that you used as start-up capital before you can really say that your health facility has really started to bring in profits. In line with this, you might want to consider joining a corporation or perhaps engage in a partnership with a trusted colleague (Kishel, 2005).

Let us first dissect the definitions of the significant terminology in this chapter: sole proprietorship, partnership, and corporation. Listed are some definitions in order for you to understand the distinctions among the three business structures.

A sole proprietorship is when a business establishment is owned by a single entity. Given that the owner is actually an individual, he or she is the only one personally liable for all the debts that might be incurred by the business.

A partnership is when a business establishment is owned by one or more individuals or corporations.

This can also be in any combination. Within the bounds of a partnership, each of the two partners will be held liable for all debts incurred within the duration of the partnership.

A corporation is the most common form of business organization, and one, which is chartered by a state and given many legal rights as an entity separate from its owners. Since a corporation has a distinct legal existence from its directors and shareholders, the directors and shareholders are not personally liable for any debts incurred by the corporation outside of the amount that these individuals contributed. Even though the shareholders are actually the ones who "own" a corporation, the ones who really manage the daily operations are called "directors."

The biggest differences among these three are the legal distinctions they have from one another. Legal differences may be especially complicated to comprehend for someone who is not familiar with the law. So, it is highly advisable that before making a final decision about business structure to adopt, one should first consult with his or her lawyer and accountant.   At this junction, you will notice that the main difference between all three is liability. In a corporation, each one of its members is protected since personal risk is limited by the member's investment. If, for example, a corporation fails and is sued in court, the people who invested in the corporation will enjoy a certain level of protection. Lawsuits will generally be directed at the assets of the corporation rather than personal assets.

A partnership does not offer that limited liability protection. The simplified definition is that two people equally own the business and are therefore equally responsible for whatever happens to it. If their business establishment is sued, all of the partners share equal, undivided responsibility. In the event that their joint venture succeeds, however, the partners share the resulting wealth equally.

Sole proprietorship also does not offer limited liability protection. It simply means that as the only owner of the establishment, all of the control, responsibility, liabilities, and profit are those of the sole proprietor alone.

Business experts recommend what is called a corporate shield. This protects your personal assets so that creditors will not be able to harass you at home.

The cost to incorporate involves investing a few hundred dollars and additional money for maintaining corporate books and records. The average processing time is at least 45 days. Opting to become a part of a big corporation will shield you from being harassed when creditors want their money back, should your healthcare facility incur financial problems.

In order to be considered as having a valid corporation, you must comply with the following requirements:

Observe organizational meetings

Record the minutes of every meeting

Formulate and adhere to a set of bylaws

Submit licenses and permits

Include Inc. or Corp. in business name

Include statement of purpose

Include statement of location

Have 200 shares no par value, with payment of a minimum of $10.00 tax

Include a biennial statement (a reporting requirement in certain states) during the anniversary month of the incorporation. Your registered agent service provider will notify and instruct you on how to file your biennial statement.

A requirement of the IRS for corporations that wish to hire employees or open a bank account is an EIN (Employer Identification Number). To acquire an EIN, submit a valid individual tax identification number (ITIN) or US Social Security Number (SSN). You have to fill out Form SS-4 to get an EIN, and you can submit this form online.

As mentioned previously, before deciding which business structure to adopt, you should duly consult your personal lawyer. Coordinate with your attorney to pick the business structure that best fits your financial standing as well as the kind of business you are establishing (which in this case is a health facility where you will practice your healing profession).

Also, be sure that if you choose to incorporate, do adequate research on the corporation you are planning to invest in. It is not uncommon that people in business are hoodwinked by scammers who pose as legitimate corporations. The same goes for a partnership. Make sure that the people you are entrusting part of your establishment to be sincere, responsible professionals who will aid you in making your planned health facility a success. You must share a healthy rapport with your partner/s, so look for a partner with whom you can get along well.

Overall, the choice as to what form of business structure you wish to take on rests on your judgment. Each of the three kinds of business structures has its pros and cons. Base your choice on sound advice and sufficient research, and you will definitely arrive at a good decision.

Here are some websites that might help you incorporate cheaply:

- legalzoom.com

- mycorporation.com

- incorporate.com

As a healthcare provider, you are tasked with helping those in need of treatment for bodily pains. You should provide therapy and sound advice on how to optimize their daily lives, whether at work or at home. You must bear in mind that your plan to enter into a business venture must involve defining the kind of practice that you wish your clientele to avail of. Be straight to the point in making the boundaries of what your facility can and cannot provide. This will avoid confusion among the general public who will want to take advantage of your services.

Let us say that the reasonable amount for you to be able to start your healthcare facility is approximately $50,000.00. In the event that you decide to enter into a partnership for whatever reason, a good idea would be for you to be partners with those who have a different field of specialty than you. For example, if you are a physical therapist, opt for a chiropractor or an occupational therapist as a partner or have them both as partners. This will broaden the range of services that you may offer your clientele. This can also help you raise sufficient capital. Also, it might help you avoid "anti-kickback laws" because you are referring within your facility. Check with your lawyer for details.

The benefits of a partnership, aside from the legal advantages, include helping your facility gain better authority as a group of professionals who are licensed practitioners in their respective fields. If you partnered with a chiropractor and you are a physical therapist, you may go about advertising your health facility by means of a comprehensive catchphrase about the services that you offer such as: **"Highly specialized physical therapy and chiropractic care helping people remain at their optimal level of function."** or **"Our advanced techniques, programs, and equipment will promote a fast recovery and a return to high level of performance."**

Location

Another aspect of defining your practice is your facility's location. Location is more than simply going out and choosing a particular building. Being at the right place at the right time gives any business an added boost. Take into consideration the following aspects:

The State and City where you set up your business. Since sales and income taxes vary from one state to another, opt for a location that is business-friendly. Also, check the regulatory requirements of the state you are in. Research on the government economic incentives, taxes, regulations, rent, etc., in the city you are in. After gathering information, evaluate whether it would be in your best interest to move to another state or city that would be more suitable for your facility. Also, in terms of scope of practice, are you allowed to see patients without a referral? Which body parts or conditions can you treat?

Accessibility with regards to parking areas, streets, and other establishments. As much as possible, be in a neighborhood that is in the vicinity of businesses that attract similar clients. Try to be in a location where parking is readily available. Pick a place that can be easily reached on foot. Also, the facility should be clearly visible from the street.

Think of making things convenient for your clientele when they want to locate your business. Also, don't forget to consider your circumstances. It would be costly to have a far commute from your residence to your facility. Seek a location that is not too far from where you live to save on gas or fares.

Safety. If the crime rate in the area is high, choose a different location. Otherwise, you will need to spend extra on security alarms, surveillance videos, and cleaning up vandalism.

Zoning. Check with the zoning requirements in your area since you have to be sure whether a healthcare facility such as yours is actually allowed in the locale. If you are considering converting a house into an office, depending on the state, only a small portion of the house can be converted. Check this with the local government or your local housing/zoning authority for details.

Size of the facility. For a healthcare facility, you will require a minimum space ranging approximately from 1,500–2,000 sq. ft. A facility that is cramped will not attract customers. Space contributes to proper ventilation. A small office and facility can make your clients feel smothered. Also, a location that is too spacious will result in increased maintenance costs.

After settling on your location, be sure to acknowledge the name of the community in your ads, brochures, flyers, banners, etc. Do not hesitate to let the location name of your facility help define your practice.

Study Your Competition

Part of any business strategy is the study of your competition. In fact, it is one of the most vital aspects of business success. Any establishment that wishes to earn a good profit and continue to thrive must get to know its competition. You can definitely expect that you will not be the only service provider of your kind in your area, especially if your clinic is located in the middle of a major city. Your competition is composed of other medical practitioners who have set up office within a ten-mile radius of your health facility.

These other health facilities compete with you to get a larger share of the clientele who are looking for the kind of products and services that you all similarly sell. To succeed in outselling your rival medical professionals, you must get to know their medical practices individually, analyze the information you have gathered about them, and then use what you have learned to your advantage.

Some of the other good reasons why one should study their competition include:

To improve your products and services and make them more superior than that of your competition's

To discover your competition's points of weakness and then exploit them to your advantage

To learn the way your competition operates so that you can always stay several steps ahead of them

To formulate your own improved marketing ideas for your health facility

Business is about conquering one's market and winning the customer. It is your competition that determines your prices, how you charge your fees, your levels of profitability, and the consistency with which you earn them. All your marketing endeavors, and even your business plan, must be prepared according to your existing or potential competition as well as their possible reactions to your progress. Anticipating your rivals' responses is also a wise tactic.

Basically speaking, studying your competition is all about getting to know what they are doing and what they are not doing. Ask yourself the following questions when trying to study your competition:

- What would happen if you modified your offerings in such a way that you targeted a different set of clientele from that of your competition?

- Why do your potential customers buy from your competitors? What advantages do they perceive?

- What are your competition's primary strengths?

- What are their areas of specialization, differentiation, segmentation, and concentration?

- What does your competition have that you do not?

- What does your competition offer that you do not?

- How can you emphasize this advantage in your sales and marketing efforts?

- What is your competition doing more of or better than you?

- What is your competition's unique advertising proposition?

- What are your competition's weaknesses?

- How can you exploit these weaknesses?

- What do you do better than your competition?

- In what ways are your products or services superior to your competition's offerings?

- In what areas do you have a distinct advantage over your competition?

- What can you do to counterbalance your competition's strengths and maximize your advantages?

- How can you better position yourself against your competitors in a tough market?

- How could you modify or adjust your marketing strategy in such a manner that you could accomplish dominance in a specific area, with a particular customer or market segment?

The best approach to beat your competition is to study their programs and determine where you can improve. Do not commit the common mistake of dismissing their major competition. Ignoring your rivals simply will not serve you well. Criticizing and belittling the competition is also ineffective.

Those who erroneously neglect to study their competition fail to scrutinize and find out how to outdo their rivals in tough markets. Instead, one should have respect for the successful competitors in their field. Value what they are doing competently and seek out ways to improve upon their best features. Doing so will help you offset your competition's advantages over you.

The first step in studying your competition is to make a list of all other health facilities that offer services and products similar to your own. Enumerate those that are within a ten-mile radius of your health facility to have a larger scope. Make use of the Internet when doing your research. Gather their addresses and contact details and visit each of their websites to see what are the services and products that they offer, their working days and working hours, their promotional gimmicks, if any, etc.

Treat the study of your competition as a learning endeavor that will help you grow professionally. There is plenty to learn from other health establishments' methods. All you have to do is open your eyes and study them very well while also being analytical.

Office Hours

You should think about the number of hours you want to put into a specified number of workdays. For the first three months, you should count on working 8 hours a day, 3 days per week, for a total of 24 working hours in a week. One schedule could be like the one below:

Office hours: Mondays, Wednesdays, Fridays: 9:00 A.M.–1:00 P.M., 3:00 P.M.–7:00 P.M.

With this set up, you can make use of Tuesdays, Thursdays, and Saturdays for marketing or for engaging in a part-time job. If you have a partner, you can alternate the days, so that you can make good use of the office space.

Payment Options

Determining the types of payment accepted at your healthcare facility is another important step. Do you accept only cash, take checks, or include payments via credit or debit card?

If you will accept credit or debit cards, then you have to spend money on a credit card machine as well as pay for a monthly credit card processing fee. Each method of payment has advantages and disadvantages, but remember that the more convenient a client finds paying you, the greater the chance that that client will pay for your services. A customer-friendly business is a great way to earn referrals.

Lastly, do not forget to determine services offered and the price point. Nothing can be as annoying as being kept in the dark about payments for any kind of service, so do not make things inconvenient for your customers. Have a menu board printed on sturdy paper in clear, easy-to-read writing. One format for this list would be to make a table indicating services offered, fees for payments not collected at the time of service (insurance, cash, and credit), and fees for payment at the time of service.

This will also be a good time to create a business plan, which will help you project if your prices are reasonable and if your business will survive. We advise that you purchase business plan software to help you create a business plan and calculate costs, overhead, and projections.

Example: Income for 1 month:

Estimate: 2 new patients per week; each patient will be seen for 12 visits.

4 weeks total: 8 new patients; 96 visits (8 patients x 12 visits)

Assuming you charge: Initial evaluation: $200; Visit: $40.

4 weeks total:

Initial evaluation= $200.00	8 patients	1,600.00
Visits = $40.00	96 visits	3,840.00
	4 weeks total	5,440.00
	Year's total (4 weeks x 13)	70,720.00

Then, you calculate your overhead expenses. Think about your salary, employees, rent, and utilities. If your overhead is significantly more, you can consider:

1. Increasing the number of new patients by intensifying marketing;

2. Increasing the number of patient visits;

3. Selling exercise aides, booklets, vitamins, and power drinks;

4. Decreasing your overhead;

5. Increasing your fees; or

6. Incorporating wellness into your practice.

Check out Palo Alto's "business plan pro" to help you create a business plan. This way, you can find out if your business will be viable.

Building Your Identity

Your health facility's identity is one of the basic aspects that set you apart from the competition. Unless you wish to fall into anonymity, building your identity as the expert health provider in your community will have to take first priority at this point in your preparations.

Branding is not limited to simply just making announcements that your establishment is now open to serve the people in the area. It goes much deeper than that, because branding is a continuous process that does not stop at a simple banner that says "Now Open to Serve You." It refers to the relationship shared by your health facility and other aspects of the business (i.e., clientele, investors, distributors, media, as well as your very own employees at the facility). Creating your business identity through brand building can either make or break your health facility's future success. It is imperative that you give due recognition in the importance of branding with regards to sales and marketing.

Brand building can be defined as an ongoing relationship between your business and the most significant people in it, such as your customers, the media, your investors, the people who work for you, your family, your suppliers, etc. Similar to any newly developing relationship, the process of making people become aware of your identity and then trust your establishment takes time. As your business moves forward, you can engage in better, broader strategies and methods to facilitate improvements in your marketing. This means to say that you have to take things one step at a time, since not all brand building techniques are easy to afford and effortless to execute.

So what exactly are the things that create identity? Focus on a single concept to be included in all your marketing materials. For example, "We respect your time; you will wait 15 minutes or less."

Here are some ideas that are simple enough and reasonably affordable to start off with:

Your outside sign. You can budget $2,000.00 for this. That is but a small price to help ensure that your establishment gets noticed. People who walk by your facility will likely notice the design of the outside sign first. The way your facility's name is written, the materials used, and the color combinations involved all will create a lasting impression on passersby.

Your objective is to make the sign look as professional as possible. Think over the entire design many times, taking into consideration the style of the building itself, the surrounding structures, and, of course, your own personal taste. You may want to also incorporate awnings and canopies, use custom dimensional lettering (available at OfficeSignStore.com), or install dramatic lighting for maximum effect. For this endeavor, engage the services of a professional sign store.

Online exposure. It is understandable why many would want to concentrate heavily on offline branding and think that online promotion can wait for a few months. This is a big mistake. Given the widespread accessibility of the Internet, more and more American consumers are going online to search for consumer advice and products. For approximately $20.00, you can have your own website via small-business Web hosting from the likes of big-time companies such as Microsoft. Do not hesitate to take advantage of the Internet trend in building your company's identity. You can also hire freelancers to design your website. Check out sites like www.upwork.com or www.elance.com. You can hire a designer to create corporate identity kits, websites, and brochures at a very low price.

Spend a reasonably big amount on a single great ad. The trick here is to have an attractively written and clever ad and then have it used repetitively. Small space ads can attract more if printed several times through several issues of a popular newspaper in the locality. Consider this as a good investment if you are hesitant about the fees.

Benefit from a Blog. In relation to online branding, you can take advantage of a blog. When written in the right way, blogs let you get close to potential customers and encourages greater visibility for your services. They serve as a way of letting people see you as an expert in your personally chosen industry.

Promotional materials are important. Do not disregard the value of basic promotional materials. Invest in refined business cards, customized stationery, and a logo. Doing so will boost your reputation as a player in the industry that you work in. With regards to a logo, employ the services of a professional graphic designer. You should also make the designer come up with a business identity package for your facility or even assist you in planning out the design of your marketing plan. Check out websites like www.thelogocompany.net and www.logoworks.com.

Make voicemail work for you. Customers will likely easily forget your bland voicemail if you merely state your name and cell phone number. Add something to facilitate instant recall, such as a useful professional tip or a statistic. List several of these so that you can alternate your voicemail message without much effort. Keep the theme of your message consistent and fresh.

Brand building through wearable items. Make use of clothing that has your brand logo emblazoned on it as generous giveaways to loyal clients and employees. Presenting items such as T-shirts, baseball caps, and scarves give the recipients the feeling of being special. When worn outside your facility, it gives your brand name more exposure. Engage the services of marketers who can custom print logos onto clothing, such as Zazzle.com.

Remember customer details. Make it a point to keep track of your clients. A software program that can readily keep a list of all your clients (even potential ones), and their personal information (i.e., birthdays, anniversaries) would be a good investment if it means helping you maintain positive customer relationships. Make use of e-mails by sending personalized messages on special occasions to your clients or keeping them posted on special offers. These small things help establish lasting customer relations. My favorite program is schedulicity.com. It is an online appointment scheduler software but also tracks client information. It charges as low as $19.95/month for a single user and $39.95/month for multi-user.

Postcards. Have attractive postcards printed that have carefully thought out messages with subjects such as "back care," "freedom from pain," "CPR class," "free blood pressure screenings," "Thank you for your referral," "discount for cash patients," "Happy Birthday," "Happy Holidays," etc. Know when and to whom to hand these postcards. Think of them as an extension of your gratitude and effort to let clients know they are valued.

Posters. Have several posters made in unique, attractive, and informative. You may have one design that advertises discounts for patients who pay with cash instead of credit cards or checks. Put these posters inside and outside your facility. Make sure to put your health facility's contact details along with the address.

Menu board, brochures, or pamphlets. Essential to your front desk is the menu board which consists of the list of services offered by your facility and the corresponding prices. Informative and convincing brochures or pamphlets are also a must.

You may visit Gotprint.com to get your money's worth on high quality, full color, and glossy brochures, catalogs, business cards, flyers, and even post cards. For around $160.00, you may get one thousand brochures. For chiropractors, go to www.patientmedia.com to take advantage of their 18-title starter package consisting of the most popular conceptual principles and symptomatic concerns of chiropractic care. Packages of 50 for each of the 18 titles may be purchased for $275.00. These prices were quoted at the time of writing.

Patient education presentation via DVD. Still available from www.patientmedia.com is a 4-in-One DVD that contains videos on patient education you can present to your patients in the consultation and/or report room. This is another form of brand building, establishing your desire to be of help to your patients by thoughtfully giving them an audio/visual presentation of their choices in staying well.

Make use of these helpful methods to build your identity as a reliable service provider in your community. As of now, these are the most affordable and least difficult ones to you since you are only starting out.

They are cost-effective and can reach out to many people. You cannot afford to lose to competition by neglecting to build your identity.

As previously mentioned, developing trust and rapport with your clients takes time and the process is continuous. You simply do not stop building your establishment's identity or reaching out to more people to attract more clientele. Investing time and money on reasonable ways to build a brand can help establish your health facility as a respectable business.

Before deciding on the specific range of treatments you will offer at your health facility, it may be helpful to first make a list of the kinds of complaints and common problems that patients seek help for.

Suggestions on Services Offered

One may advertise that you can provide treatment for the following:

Ankle sprain

Ankle strain

Arthritis

Back and neck pain or stiffness

Bursitis

Cardiopulmonary diseases

Carpal Tunnel Syndrome

Degenerative disc and joint disease

Fibromyalgia

Foot or knee pain

Frozen shoulder

Golfer's elbow

Headaches

Herniated "slipped" discs

Joint strains

Nerve pain, sciatica

Neurological and muscular illness

Optimal wellness

Osteoarthritis

Poor posture

Rib pain or injury

Scoliosis or spinal curvature

Shoulder pain, rotator cuff injuries

Spina bifida

Sports injuries

Stress related conditions

Tailbone pain or injury

Tendinitis

Tennis elbow

Tension headaches

TMJ (temporomandibular joint) issues

Whiplash injury (car, bike accidents, falls)

You may also categorize your services into the following:

Prevention advice. This refers to suggestions on methods of carrying out one's daily tasks that may help a patient retain his or her independence.

Rehabilitation advice. This refers to recommendations for convalescing patients to help them recover faster.

Providing daily living equipment. This refers to the selling items that help individuals retain their independence.

Adaptation techniques. This refers to helpful ways of modifying a patient's home environment when he or she is afflicted with a lasting or chronic disability or illness.

These lists contain ideas to help you decide on what services to offer and what patient conditions you will be willing to take on at your practice. Below are a number of suggestions about pricing some commonly offered therapeutic services in many healthcare facilities. (Costhelper, 2009).

Name of Service	Service Fee (your facility)	Service Fee
Chiropractic Evaluation		$220.00
Chiropractic Adjustment		$45.00
PT Evaluation		$110.00
Chiropractic Report of Findings		$45.00
Chiropractic Re-eval		$150.00
Joint Mob, Trigger Point, and Other Manual Therapy		$25.00

(Continued)

Name of Service	Service Fee (your facility)	Service Fee
Stretching, Exercise and Other Therapy		$25.00
Strengthening and Other Neuromuscular Re-ed		$25.00
Traction		$25.00
Iontophoresis		$25.00
Modalities		
Hot Packs/Cold Packs/TENS		$25.00
Ultrasound		$25.00
Laser Treatment		$25.00

Insurance and Necessary Legal Concerns

Our world has evolved into one where insurance policies have gained such importance that they are integral parts of people's lives. We cannot deny the fact that the practicality of insurance is what people find so appealing. Insurance is protection; it shields us from the possible financial losses that we may incur should we have the misfortune of experiencing unforeseen accidents, failures, thefts, and other tragedies.

You will never be able to totally control or eliminate all risks in life. Your health facility will be an important investment and source of income for you. You should not take any chances or ignore possible complications. Business insurance will be able to provide your health facility with the protection it needs to safeguard it from these risks.

When insuring your business, think about the kind of insurance package that would most likely be able to fulfill most of your business needs as well as provide the level of protection you would most prefer. The two types of business insurance starting businesses need are **Property and Liability Insurance**.

Property Insurance provides protection against damage. It covers the assets that your business has in its possession. This includes the building you are using as well as all business equipment. Related to property insurance is **Contents Insurance**, which protects your business equipment against theft, flood, or fire. In order to find out how much insurance you will need under property or contents insurance, make a list of your business' assets with corresponding specific dollar values for each item.

Once you have this list, you can decide which of your assets needs to be insured and for what amount. Calculating this will help establish the insurance premium. Some items may not need insurance since doing so would not justify the cost of the insurance premium. Before deciding to insure a certain item, ask yourself whether you can readily afford that piece of equipment if it were stolen or destroyed. If the answer is no, then you definitely should have that item insured.

Liability Insurance, on the other hand, provides protection for your company from being sued in a court of law. It protects your establishment from liability resulting from negligence that may inflict injury on other individuals, like a client or an employee. In addition, liability insurance shields your business if a person is injured as a consequence of using your service.

Lawsuits are extremely expensive, considering all the legal expenses involved and the price of settlement, all of which could push your business into a state of bankruptcy in no time. Liability insurance is therefore definitely a good investment.

Since you are a medical professional, the specific kind of liability insurance that you will need is called **Malpractice Insurance**, which falls under Professional Liability Insurance. Those in healing professions should carry malpractice insurance. It is mandatory in some parts of the country (Halley, 2008).

Concerning the legal concerns of your health business, you must meet the requirements of the various authorities in order to have smooth business transactions later on. These include the federal government, the state authorities, the county authorities, and the city government (SBA.gov, 2007).

With the federal government, you must seek an application in order to obtain your **EIN or Employer Identification Number**. You must also acquire from them a compliance poster, and then research all you need to know about minimum wage, the **Family and Medical Leave Act (FMLA)**, and other employer-employee issues so as to comply with these. Go to the official websites of the United States Department of Labor (US DOL) as well as the Occupational Safety and Health Administration (OSHA) (SBA.gov, 2007).

With the state authorities, you must comply with unemployment insurance tax, sales tax, compliance poster, worker's compensation, and new hire reporting.

Meanwhile, the county authorities will ask you to process your business name filing. You should also apply for a business license, have a fire inspection done at your health facility, and get a certificate of occupancy. Have proof that you already have business insurance and send a legal notification to the local County Assessor (SBA.gov, 2007).

Lastly, the City authorities will ask for your building or construction permit. Part of their assessment will include your facility's plumbing and electrical fixtures to determine if your facility is safe for clients. Make sure you have an illegal entry alarm to fend off burglars. The local police department will take it as a positive reason to let you operate (SBA.gov, 2007). Never neglect your legal responsibilities with regards to your health facility, both now and in the future. If you fail to comply with the requirements of the authorities, then you may run into problems. Take our advice and see to it that you comply with all legal requirements, from the safety needs of your facility to the legal rights and benefits of your employees.

Payment

As with any business establishment, when it comes to billing your clients, you must be clear on what methods of payment you will accept from your clientele. Although it is highly desirable that your patients will immediately pay through ready money after consultation and/or treatment, you must face the reality that not all of your patients will have cash on hand. They may find it more convenient to pay with a check or credit card.

You must also consider that despite the generally expensive fees that accrue after several hours of treatment at your health facility; your clients may still be reluctant to bring large amounts of cash for security reasons. Hence, customers may prefer credit card or check payments.

Accepting multiple forms of payment will attract clients. The majority of customers will choose businesses that provide more convenience in all transactions, especially regarding payment (Kishel, 2005). Even though offering this convenience may be overwhelming at first, you must acknowledge its advantages in attracting and keeping customers.

To encourage patients to pay with cash, you can offer a discount for bills paid with cash. (This does not apply to patients under worker's compensation and no fault).

Setting Up Your Billing System

Once you have determined the prices of all your services offered at your health facility, you must then set up your billing system in such a manner that all payment transactions will go smoothly. To help you comply with the government standard, organize your billing by consulting the Healthcare Common Procedure Coding System (HCPCS).

The HCPCS was created in 1978 as a standardized means to categorize medical services, supplies, and equipment. Initially, the utilization of HCPCS codes by medical practitioners was voluntary. In 1996, the Health Insurance Portability and Accountability Act (HIPAA) was passed by the U.S. Congress, which required the Center for Medicare and Medicaid Services (CMS) to implement a standard system for reporting and billing transactions in health care (Halley, 2008).

These HCPCS codes, or Healthcare Common Procedure Coding System, are specifically utilized to catalog each and every service a medical practitioner may offer to a Medicare patient. This includes all services that are either surgical or diagnostic. The system allows Medicare, a federally administered system of health insurance, to monitor all transactions in an organized manner, saving Medicare much time and effort and ensuring optimum service for all clients (Straube, 2010). Adopting the Healthcare

Common Procedure Coding System would go a long way in providing your Medicare patients with appealing convenience.

Having such a set of standardized codes that are used by all medical practitioners and establishments across the country allows for uniformity, ensuring that doctors and other health providers are being paid the same amount for a particular medical procedure with respect to geographic region (Straube, 2010). For example, no matter where a doctor is located who administers an allergy shot (code 95115) to a Medicare patient is, he or she will still receive the same payment from Medicare as any other doctor would receive in the same Medicare region.

Healthcare Common Procedure Coding System numbers are divided into two sets. The first set of codes, called Level I, is a five-digit numeric code established by the American Medical Association. The CPT is made up of identifying codes and descriptive terms whose primary purpose is for billing transactions between patients and their attending physicians.

The second code set, Level II, is used for those medical services outside of Level I. These include prosthetics, orthotics, medical equipment, and supplies. Level II codes are alphanumeric, meaning they start off with a single letter, like an AE@ or AK@ used for durable medical equipment, followed by four numbers.

The following are more specific ranges of Level II codes and their corresponding medical services.

- E0100–E1830: durable medical equipment
- G0001–G0148: temporary procedures/professional services
- K0001–K0530: prosthetics, orthotics, supplies and dressings
- L0100–L4398: orthotic procedures

Modifiers refer to two-digit numeric or alphanumeric characters that are attached to Level I and HCPCS Level II codes. They indicate a service or procedure was changed by particular conditions. Because of modifiers, the definition of the code remains unchanged despite the added meanings.

Over the years, more and more practitioners have engaged themselves in the use of electronic health records systems. Physical therapists are no exception to this, and more and more practitioners, assistants and billers for physical therapy services are engaged in the use of electronic health records systems in their respective clinics or facilities. Despite its growing use, clinicians sometimes find it difficult to understand the intricacies related to documenting patients' records electronically, thereby reflecting problems in evaluating the use of electronic records systems.

At the onset of 2015, Medicare implemented its Meaningful Use Program. This requires physicians and other health care providers included in the same program meet the required *meaningful use* or else sanctions are to be taken for those who do not comply with the adoption of the EHR in practice.

Technically, this matter is not fully a source of concern for physical therapists because they are not yet required by Medicare to do so. However, since other allied health care professions with whom care will be coordinated are using the system, physical therapists should be familiar with the system to be used to better coordinate care. In 2015, eligible providers will be penalized for not using Medicare's Meaningful Use program, so they expect physical therapists treating their patients to be using compatible electronic health records (APTA 2015).

According to the CMS website, more than 447,000 health care providers received payment for participating in the Medicare and Medicaid Electronic Health Record (EHR) Incentive Programs as of March 2015. In May 2013, CMS declared more than half of all eligible health care providers had been paid under the Medicare and Medicaid EHR Incentive Programs. More than $20.2 billion in Medicare EHR Incentive Program payments have been made to providers between May 2011 and March 2015 (CMS 2015).

As a response to the need for having patients' records stored and managed electronically, various EHR companies have been accredited by Medicare to assist practitioners in storage of health records and setting up a system to ensure that retrieval, storage and manipulation of these records comply with the requirements needed for coding, billing and making payment claims for Medicare Part B coverage.

This chapter provides a comprehensive list of some of the EHR companies, which have been accredited and certified by the CMS to be contracted by practitioners and facilities to provide services towards the implementation of their own electronic health records. These companies provide software that can be used for outpatient physical therapy.

The most cost efficient way to make things simple and quick with regards to managing your payment system is through obtaining practice management software for billing such as File-mate 1500 available at http://www.formmagic.com/file-mate1500.html. It costs only $119.00 (one-time payment).

It breaks the HCFA / CMS 1500 form into logical sections and guides you through each screen, making it easy to complete medical claim form and get paid faster. It lets you use your laser and ink jet printer with either plain paper or preprinted HCFA / CMS 1500 forms. You can produce print image files to quickly send medical reimbursement information to most online Clearing Houses. You can create your own library of CPT / HCPCS and ICD-9 codes for quick data entry.

You can also use VisionShare to make billing and payment easier. This service enables you to use your existing broadband Internet connection to grant you speedy, economical access to your Medicare Administrative Contractor (MAC). For $29.95 per month, VisionShare will allow you to send claim files, receive remittance advice, determine patient eligibility, obtain reports, and request status of sent claims.

For electronic billing purposes, you may use the PC-ACE Pro32 software, which is downloadable via the Internet free of charge. It is supported by the Electronic Data Interchange Support Services (EDISS).

The most popular electronic health records software are listed below:

WebPT

This provider charges an average range of $49- $99.50 per month per physical therapist. WebPT usually charge $49 monthly per practitioner and this fee includes unlimited technical support for documentation, faxing and emailing options, and integrated reporting of functional limitation. Also, the monthly fee includes assistance in documenting and creating SOAP files. Other services that WebPT provides with the monthly rate are:

a. Reporting regarding how the practice is managed;

b. Modules specific for each practice specialty;

g. Code selector that includes both CPT and ICD coding;

h. Built-in edits in terms of CCI;

i. Outcome measurement tools auto-scoring system;

j. Tracking of therapy caps;

k. Information about discounts on the supplies of clinics; and

l. Alerts and monitoring system following the 8-minute rule.

The provider also has another system that can be used by staff members who do not provide actual care for patients. This function is charged $29 per month. Providers who want to avail of the services of WebPT need to pay a one-time set up fee of $495 for the first facility under the system and an additional cost of $249 for every additional clinic or office within the same facility. If, however, the provider does not wish to avail of the full services offered by WebPT, the provider can opt to choose a structured service cluster depending on personalized needs. These services include:

Front Office Package. This package costs $99 per month for the first clinic or facility to be set-up and an additional $49 for annexed or extension clinics. Under the Front Office packages, the following are included as part of the service:

1. eDoc. This function is designed to assist in encoding health records through scanning and uploading them individually into the system.

2. Online Patient Registration. In this feature, the complete information regarding patients and their intake can be uploaded and accessed online.

3. Scheduling. This includes hassle-free facilitation of patients' visit schedules and appointments. The feature is easy to navigate since it was designed with drag and drop menu functions.

4. Catch Missed Notes. In instances when patient volumes are too high and there is barely enough time to finish documenting patients' notes, this feature allows the practitioner to complete these notes at a later time.

5. Appointment Reminders. This feature helps practitioners keep set appointments with their patients through email and phone or text messaging reminders. However, text-messaging reminders are limited to only 100 per month, but there is an option to increase the limit by paying extra for added number of reminders per month. $25 would yield an additional 100 appointment reminders, $100 would be for 500, and $350 would add 2,000 appointment reminders per month.

6. Home Exercise Program (HEP). The home exercise program is a feature that charges $49 per month for the first clinic and an additional $29 for each extension or annex clinics. The inclusions of this program are:

   a. Using a wide array of multimedia programs to ensure improved patient compliance to treatment regimen.

   b. Allows the therapist to spend more time actually treating patients than retraining them to perform the same exercises again.

   c. Allows the physical therapist to send patients exercise plans through email so those who are busy can review and perform them at their own convenience.

   d. Enables physical therapists to view exercise profiles that are peer-reviewed and integrate them to the treatment flow sheet of a patient.

   e. Gives practitioners the liberty to implement customization into the exercise programs set for patients and their associated instructions.

Kareo Integrated Billing

This service provider charges physical therapists an average $199 for the initial set-up of the EHR program into the office. Kareo also operates using partner modules. The most common product package that therapists use with Kareo is the unlimited claims and eligibility checks. This feature charges $99.50 per month and includes the following features:

   a. Review and Submit Claims. With the use of Kareo PM, providers can carry out reviewing of claims prior to submission and have them approved for accuracy before they are electronically sent to healthcare insurance payers.

   b. Get paid for services rendered. One of the reasons why physical therapists and other health care providers use Kareo is its feature that allows them to access funds online and contact insurance payers.

c. Billing of patients. Kareo PM allow practitioners to set-up an online bills payment system, which can be accessed 24/7. Furthermore, this also allows for sending of digital statements of accounts (or print hard copies of such statements for patients with copay programs), other deductibles, shared insurance provider set-ups and assistance with self-pay scenarios.

Apart from the most basic services that Kareo offers, there are also other options from which practitioners can choose from. These are:

a. PQRS Registry Based Reporting. This service bills for $399 annually for the first facility to be registered with an additional $99 for other clinics that would use the same system for its PQRS reporting.

b. PQRS Claims-Based Reporting. This feature starts to bill $99 annually for use by providers in each clinic location.

Clinics and practitioners who wish to register their EHR under the services of Kareo may choose a combination of several programs they offer. However, these will be billed independently from each other and may incur different charges depending on the registration if the user is a health care provider or a staff member.

Clinicient

This program allows the provider to pay one dollar per visit as long as he or she meets the minimum monthly user's fee of $450 per month. This fee includes use of their features such as registration of patients, scheduling their visits and appointments, and allowing electronic documentation of their clinical records. Practitioners and providers who wish to avail of the all-inclusive billing services of the Clinicient program need to pay at least $3,024 per month as expressed in their revenue cycle service agreement; and training and implementation service fees of $995.

OptimisPT

This EHR program provider offers practitioners and physical therapists the option to choose from 2 different service packages: the Core package and the Complete Package. The Core package includes the basic electronic health records such as patient appointments scheduling, health record documentation and reporting practice management. These services are offered at a rate of $0.85 per patient visit, but the rates are lowering considerably as the volume of patient visits are increasing. In some instances when the practitioner does not have too many patient visits, OptimisPT charges a minimum rate of $200 per month for patient visits below 235. If the practitioner wishes to avail of the complete package, however, the price is $1.25 per patient visit. The rate also goes lower as the number of patient visits increase, but similar to the Core, there is also a minimum usage fee of $300 per month. This applies to patient visits of 240 or less.

Providers who avail of programs from OptimisPT get 3 weeks of unlimited training with the program, ongoing technical support through voice calls, and online support via the Support Tab within the program. Furthermore, updates made into the system are continuously being relayed to the users to ensure the system runs effectively and smooth. In using the OptimisPT program, therapists and practitioners should bear in mind that the charging is based on the time the patient visit is decked into the system. This actually allows the practitioner to enter into the system what is being done on the patient in real-time. If there are concerns about the patient being billed too much, the system also has a solution for that since it does not make any charges on the patient's record once the patient makes changes with the appointment, cancels it or if the visit is not performed. Furthermore, the system allows the practitioner to create as many documents needed based on the date when visits are done so that the patients' care is documented chronologically and as concisely as possible. One thing that makes OptimisPT one of the services of choice for most providers is that the program does not charge an upfront service or installation fees, allows for more flexible contracts and does not charge different rates if the user belongs in another clinic location.

As a checks-and-balance system, there are five different clearinghouses with which OptimisPT works. These clearinghouses are distinct entities from each other and are separate from OptimisPT itself. This makes the system in place reliable since there is an external check-and-balance apart from the internal quality assurance that OptimisPT does. Providers who wishes to use the Complete OptimisPT package should understand these clearinghouses are integral to the package, and there may be a need to contact concerned clearinghouses every once in a while.

In an effort for OptimisPT to show practitioners its product and how to use it efficiently, it offers practitioners a free billing demonstration every Monday until Thursday, from 8am to 2pm PDT. The following are the website addresses and contact details of the clearinghouses for those who wish to avail of the Complete OptimisPT package.

a. Office Ally.

    a. Web address: www.officeally.com

    b. Phone number: (866) 575-4120

c. Gateway EDI

    a. Web address: www.gatewayedi.com

    b. Phone number: (888) 697 1011

c. MD Online

    a. Web address: www.mdon-line.com

    b. Phone number: (973) 734-9900

c. Claim Remedi

      a. Web address: www.claimremedi.com

      b. Phone number: (800) 763-8484

    c. ZirMed

      a. Physical address: 888 W. Market St., Suite 400, Louisville, KY 40202

      b. Web address: www.zirmed.com

Theraoffice

Theraoffice provides practitioners numerous features along with its EHR programs. Developed by a company known as Hands On Technology, Inc., the program is designed to assist practitioners with coding, billing, and payment claims through electronically storing, managing and retrieving patients' medical records. Practitioners who want to avail of the product usually get a proposal from the company listing the services they offer as well as the associated cost of each service.

The most common features of TheraOffice that make it one of the EHR program developers being availed by practitioners are its phone and live technical support, real time email support system, and automatic system. It also offers an easier system for training users as it makes the training module available through internet, thereby not requiring future users to skip long hours off work just to train. However, there is also a need for the physical therapist and other users to undergo an hour of personal training with the system that allows them to ask their questions and have them answered.

Also with TheraOffice, there is an integration of the system with Zirmed due to the use of the same clearinghouse setup. The program is offered to future users with the IT standard proposal and price matrix. Subscription to the program is normally offered together with technical support or assistance and regular program updates. Compared with other programs, setup fees with TheraOffice can be waived depending on the service agreement between Hands On Technology and the practitioner.

Installation of the software including the associated technical support is charged a one-time payment of $725. The training cost is $150. These fees are fixed regardless of the number of participants in the training. Monthly fees vary depending on who uses the system. Clinicians who engage in the work and use TheraOffice on a full time basis are charged $125 per month, while a part time licensed clinician only pays $100 per month. Staffs of the facility such as office staff, administrative staff and billers are charged $25 for every month of use.

TheraOffice also allows its users to avail of added products and services even after signing up. Different pricing and payment options are available to practitioners depending on their need and the nature of their practice. Normally, when a new database needs to be set up, especially if there is a new tax ID involved, therapists and practitioners are charged $500. Those who consider using TheraOffice may contact the program developer Hands On Technology via their website www.rehabsoftware.com or their phone numbers (630) 455-2863 ext 112.

Therabill

Therabill is another EHR program provider that practitioners can avail. Under Therabill, different payment schemes are available depending on how many practitioners are using the system. Below is a summary of its charges as compared with the number of practitioners using Therabill.

a. Solo Practice. This option is most recommended for a single physical therapy practice and is charged $80 per month. This is optimized for those who are just starting out in their respective practices and have a very meager amount of clients being treated (usually below 7). The company offers these therapists with a small client volume a 3 month-starter package to better take advantage of the system and integrate it to their practice. Those who have below 7 clients are charged only $50, but this can only last for 3 months from the day they started using the system.

b. Group Practice. This is best recommended for those facilities with fewer than 4 therapists on deck and bills facilities $150 monthly. If there are more than three therapists using the system, the company would need to pay an additional $25 for each additional therapist. However, since there is a considerable amount of therapists using the system, accounts used by office staff are free. When Group Practice is availed by the facility, the program includes an unlimited number of user accounts for the office staff, capacity to be used in different office locations at no extra cost, email support and phone support (unlimited for the first 3 months of subscription) and the privilege of having unlimited documentation, patient appointment scheduling and claim options.

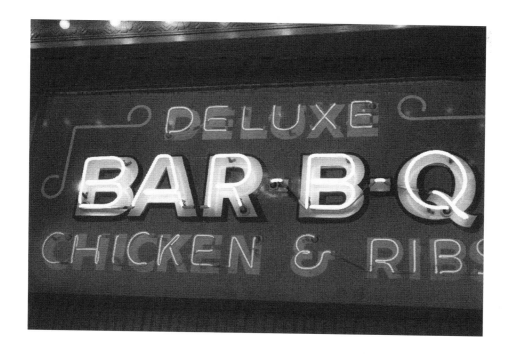

The Group Practice option also provides its users 2 gigabytes of storage space for attachments associated with medical records. However, if the facility goes beyond this capacity, it is to be billed with $20.00 for each gigabyte in excess of the allotment per month. There is also a single time training schedule via remote site that can be availed by the facility upon their request.

Therabill claims they do not charge hidden fees, do not use the services of clearinghouses to make their services faster and more efficient, and they do not require their users to pay upfront set-up fees.

Free PT

This EHR program provider offers a premium edition for its program and charges users an average of $149 per month. **Moreover**, it also affords its users online support and assistance via its website.

	Features	FREE EDITION	PLUS EDITION	PREMIUM EDITION
	Price	Free	$69/Mo. Per Provider	$149/Mo. Per Provider
A	Cloud Based, HIPAA Secure, State-of-the-art Features			
1.	No Contract, Month-to-Month, Just Sign Up and Get Started	✓	✓	✓
2	Unified, End-to-End Cloud Based System: Scheduling, Billing, HER, Web Portal and KIOSK	Choose EHR w/ Scheduler or Billing w/ Scheduler	✓	✓
3	ICD10 Operational: 5010, HIPAA, HITECH & OMNIBUS Compliant	✓	✓	✓
4	Choose Complete Medical Billing Software, or **PT, OT**, or **SLP** Soap Note HER	Choose EHR or Billing Free	Need Both? Add $49/Mo.	EHR, Billing & EDI w/ Full Practice Mgmt.
5	Powerful, Flexible Patient Appointment Scheduler!	✓	✓	✓
6	No Setup Fee, No Monthly - Truly 100% FREE Software	✓	$69 Setup, Config. EDI, Text, eFax	$149 Setup, Config. EDI, Text, eFax
7	No Intrusive Ads. No Potential Patient Privacy Violations	✓	✓	✓

(Continued)

	Features	FREE EDITION	PLUS EDITION	PREMIUM EDITION
8	You Own and Maintain Complete Control of Your Data. Export Upon Request	✓	✓	✓
9	Number of Users	One User	2 Users	Unlimited
10	Unlimited Electronic Commercial Claims	25 Claims Mo.	✓	Unlimited
11	Unlimited Electronic Commercial ERA and Auto Posting	✗	✓	Unlimited
12	Unlimited Electronic Non Commercial ERA and Auto Posting	✗	100 Claims and ERAs	Unlimited
13	Unlimited Real-time Eligibility Verification	✗	$0.24ea	✓
14	File Electronic Secondary Claims	✗	100 per Mo.	✓
15	Unlimited Print Paper Claims	25 Claims Mo.	✓	✓
16	Unlimited Print Patient Statements	25 Per Mo.	✓	✓
17	Unlimited Text Message Appointment Reminders	✗	75 Messages	Unlimited
18	Non-Commercial Claims Clearinghouse Enrollment - Emdeon/ RelayHealth (e.g. Medicare, BC/BS, Tri-Care & Railroad	✗	$95 OT	$95 OT
B	Access, Security, Backup and Storage			
1	Works on Tablet, **iPad,** Desktop and Laptop	✓	✓	✓
2	Works on Windows, Android, **Mac** and Linux	✓	✓	✓
3	Works on IE, Chrome, **Safari,** Firefox and others	✓	✓	✓
4	Secure Data Backup: Incremental (Every 5 Minutes), Full (Daily)	✓	✓	✓
5	Enterprise Class Systems: LINUX, APACHE, ORACLE, JAVA and Web 3.0	✓	✓	✓

(Continued)

	Features	FREE EDITION	PLUS EDITION	PREMIUM EDITION
C	Maintenance, Release, Updates and Support			
1	All Maintenance, Releases and Updates	✓	✓	✓
2	Step-by Step **Free Video Instruction** (Over 100 Training Videos!)	✓	✓	✓
3	**Free Training** via Weekly Live Webinars	✓	✓	✓
4	Comprehensive User Guide	✓	✓	✓
5	Unlimited Email & Instant Chat Support	✓	✓	✓
6	Unlimited Telephone Support	✓	✓	✓
D	Front Office - Appointment Scheduler - Key Features			
1	Double, Triple Book, User Definable Time Slots	✓	✓	✓
2	Instantly Search for Patients or Appointment Times	✓	✓	✓
3	360 Degree Patient Financial View	✗	✓	✓
4	Patient Kiosk - Self Check-in. (Hardwar not included) Setup $195 OT	✗	✗	$39/Mo.
5	Enter Payments and Co-pays from Appointment Calendar	✓	✓	✓
6	Set Recurring Appointments	✗	✓	✓
7	Customize Appointment Color by Type and Length	✗	✓	✓
8	View Scheduler by Day, Week, Month	✓	✓	✓
9	Comprehensive Patient Ledger and Demographics	✓	✓	✓
10	Scan and Upload Documents: Insurance Cards, Driver's License	✗	✓	✓
11	Print Patient's Future Appointments	✓	✓	✓

(Continued)

	Features	FREE EDITION	PLUS EDITION	PREMIUM EDITION
12	Upload Patient's Picture	✗	✓	✓
13	View Appointment Hx	✓	✓	✓
E	ICD10 Features			
1	ICD9, ICD10 Dual Mode Billing Software	✓	✓	✓
2	Print New ICD10 Dual Mode CMS 1500 Claim Form	✓	✓	✓
3	ICD10: Code up to 12 Diagnoses	✓	✓	✓
4	Instant ICD10 Lookup for ICD9 Codes (GEM Crossover)	✗	✗	✓
5	ICD10 Claim Validator⊠	✗	✗	✓
6	ICD10 Super-Bill Convertor⊠	✗	✓	✓
F	Claim Management & Financial Reporting			
1	Pre-Billing Charges Report (Review Charges Before Transmitting)	✓	✓	✓
2	Automatically Push Charges to Billing from HER!	✗	$29/Mo.	✓
3	Encounter Activities Report (All Charges in Detail)	✓	✓	✓
4	Deposit Report - End of Day Reconciliation	✓	✓	✓
5	Payment & Adjustment Activity Report	✓	✓	✓
6	Summary A/R by Payer	✓	✓	✓
7	Detailed A/R by Payer	✓	✓	✓
8	Summary A/R by Patient/Guarantor	✓	✓	✓
9	Practice Financial Summary (Charges, Payments, Adjustments)	✓	✓	✓
10	Patient Financial Summary by Referring Physician	✓	✓	✓
11	Cash Practice Analytical Reporting	✓	✓	✓

(Continued)

	Features	FREE EDITION	PLUS EDITION	PREMIUM EDITION
G	Clinical Office: Key Features			
1	Soap Note EMR Specifically Designed for **PT, OT,** and **SLP**	✓	✓	✓
2	Therapist Friendly Charting - Resembles Paper Charting	25 Encounters Mo.	✓	✓
3	**Copy Last Note, Modify and Save!**	✗	✓	✓
4	Comprehensive Encounter Sheets: Initial, Daily and Final Eval.	✗	✓	✓
5	Health Information Exchange, Gateway Connection	✓	✓	✓
6	Outstanding Documents - Dictate, Type, Point and Click	✓	✓	✓
7	Continuity of Care Reporting and Documentation	✓	✓	✓
8	Easily Export Superbills for Remote Biller	✗	✓	✓
H	Clinical Reporting			
1	Incomplete Notes Reporting	✓	✓	✓
2	Pending Notes Reporting	✓	✓	✓
3	PQRS Meaningful Use Dashboard	✓	✓	✓
4	Real-time Meaningful Use **Alerts**	✗	✓	✓
I	Billing Office: Key Features	✓	✓	✓
1	Manage Multiple Cases: Self-Pay, PI, WC and MVA	✓	✓	✓
2	Connectivity to National Payer Base of Over 1600 Payers	✓	✓	✓
3	**Instant Repeat Billing**	✗	✓	✓
4	Unlimited Insurance Contracts / Fee Schedules	✗	✓	✓
5	Charges on Hold (Charges Queued that Require Attention)	✗	✓	✓

(Continued)

	Features	FREE EDITION	PLUS EDITION	PREMIUM EDITION
6	Aging Claim Sorted by Insurance	✓	✓	✓
7	Aging Receivables by Patient	✓	✓	✓
8	Payment & Adjustment Posting	✓	✓	✓
J	Premium Front Office Features			
1	Multiple Offices, Multiple Tax IDs and Multiple NPIs	✘	✘	✓
2	Single Sign-on Across Multiple Offices and Multiple Legal Entities	✘	✘	✓
3	Inter Office Communication - Unifies Entire Practice	✘	✘	✓
4	Generate Custom Mail-Merge Letters & Forms	✘	✘	✓
5	Employee Time-card and Payroll Report	✘	✘	✓
6	Resources and Equipment Scheduling	✘	✘	✓
7	Scan and Upload Assignment Forms, Intake Forms, Registration Forms	✘	✘	✓
8	Fraud Prevention: Front Office Payments & Superbill Reconciliation Reporting	✘	✘	✓
9	Text Message / Email Notification for Missed, Cancelled Appts.	✘	✘	✓
10	Scheduling Alerts, Patient Balance Alerts, Authorization Alerts	✘	✘	✓
11	Track Visits Used and Visits Remaining	✘	✘	✓
12	Track Patient Referral Source	✘	✘	✓
13	Auto Generate Recall Letters	✘	✘	✓
14	Create and Print Custom Labels	✘	✘	✓
15	User Level Productivity Monitoring	✘	✘	✓
K	Premium Billing Office Features	✘	✘	✓

(Continued)

	Features	FREE EDITION	PLUS EDITION	PREMIUM EDITION
1	Flexible Month-end Financial Close (4 Types of Closes to Choose From)	✗	✗	✓
2	Powerful Collections and Denials Workbench	✗	✗	✓
3	Low Reimbursements Alerts and Reporting	✗	✗	✓
4	Unbilled Visits Report (Reconcile Visits to Superbills = Unbilled Charges)	✗	✗	✓
5	Month End Reconciliation Report by User	✗	✗	✓
6	Drill Down Revenue and Financial Dashboard Reporting	✗	✗	✓
7	Cash Flow Blocker Indicators	✗	✗	✓
8	View Financial Health of Entire Practice At-a-Glance	✗	✗	✓
9	Patient Payment Plan and Installment Billing	✗	✗	✓
10	Pre-Collection Management	✗	✗	✓
11	Send PI, WC and MVA Claims Electronically	û	û	Opt-in

Intouch EMR

This program provider for EHR charges its clients $49 per month of use of their basic program and $149 per month for their Biller Pro program. The main difference between the two programs is that the Biller Pro offers its users increased access to the program, assistance with scheduling patient appointments and visits, verifying eligibility of health care insurance plans of the patient, billing and coding support, ERAs and utilization of clearinghouses. The Biller Pro service is available to clients on a 12-month contract, while the basic Intouch is used on a monthly term.

Collection

Collecting payment from your clients, regardless if they have chosen to pay cash or via credit card or check, needs practical management and systematized procedures. Before all else, you must have a presentable bill, and be sure that the person that you hire to handle the front office is a trustworthy individual since he or she will be collecting the payment.

At the time of service, have the receptionist ask the patient for his or her Social Security Number (which is required for collection), a copy of his or her driver's license, and the name of an emergency contact (Halley, 2008).

Make sure that the patient receives a brochure containing the list of offered services and corresponding fees, a financial policies notice, and a privacy practice notice. After treatment, provide a service fee slip. For patients with delinquent accounts who need to be reminded, you can call them at home, get payment by credit card, send a collection letter, or have a collection agency help you out.

2
CHAPTER

BASICS OF MEDICARE

In 1965, the government implemented a healthcare insurance program called Medicare. The main goal of this program was to give ample health insurance coverage to the elderly population or those who have already retired from their jobs or professions (Centers for Medicare & Medicaid Services, 2012).

Medicare and Medicaid are administered by Centers for Medicare and Medicaid Services. On the other hand, the Social Security Administration (SSA) determines an individual's Medicare eligibility and also processes the premium payments for the Medicare program. To carry out Medicare's mission, Centers for Medicare and Medicaid Services have contracted private companies to act as intermediaries for the government and healthcare providers. Contracted private companies are usually in the insurance or healthcare fields. These mediators manage claims and payment, call center services (for customer service and support), clinician enrollment, and investigations of fraud. Medicare is divided into four parts: Part A—Hospital Insurance, Part B—Medical Insurance, Part C—Medicare Advantage, and Part D—Prescription Drugs. For the benefit of this book, just Medicare Part B will be discussed (Centers for Medicare & Medicaid Services, 2012).

Medicare Part B

The coverage of Part B comprises medically necessary physician services, outpatient care, and services that Part A does not cover. Part B also includes preventive services. Payments are established in the physician fee schedule for each unit of service, regardless of where the services are provided. As with most services covered under Part B, Medicare pays 80% of the payment amount, and the beneficiary is responsible for a 20% coinsurance. In 2006, Medicare payments for outpatient therapy totaled $4.07 billion (Ciolek & Hwang, 2008). Physical therapy services make up about 75% of this spending, with occupational and speech therapies making up the remaining 25%. Two services (therapeutic exercise and therapeutic activities) accounted for almost half of all therapy spending.

Of the 45.5 million Medicare Part B beneficiaries in 2006, 9.7% received therapy, 8.5% of which received physical therapy. The majority of those Medicare Part B participants (22.1%) were age 65-69. Those who utilized therapy services tended to be in an older age range. The peak age of physical therapy users was 70-74; however, the peak age for occupational and speech therapy users was 80-84 (Ciolek&Hwang 2008).

Medicare Part B covers the following:

- Bone mass measurement (biannually).

- Cardiovascular screenings (triglyceride, lipid, and cholesterol levels every five years).

- Colorectal cancer screening: (a) annual fecal occult blood test, (b) flexible sigmoidoscopy (every four years), (c) screening colonoscopy (every ten years), or (d) barium enema (every four years).

- Diabetic screenings, in case of having high blood pressure, dyslipidemia, obesity, or high blood sugar.

- Diabetic self-management training (must be prescribed by physician).

- Diabetic supplies (monitors, test strips, lancet devices, and therapeutic shoes).

- Dialysis.

- Flu shots (annually, during flu season).

- Glaucoma tests (should be performed annually by a licensed eye examiner).

- Hearing and balance exams.

- Hepatitis B shots.

- Hospital services.

- Lab services (blood tests, urinalysis).

- Limited prescription drugs.

- Mammograms.

- Medical nutrition therapy.

- Mental health care.

- Occupational therapy.

- Outpatient surgery service and supplies.

- Pap tests or pelvic exams.

- Physical therapy.

- Practitioner services.

- Preventive shots.

- Prosthetic devices.

- Transplant services.

Medicare Part B covers limited, reasonable, and medically necessary part-time care and services. This includes skilled nursing care, physical therapy, occupational therapy, speech-language pathology, and medical social services. Home use medical equipment and chiropractic services are also covered. An ambulance would be provided if any other form of transportation would not be appropriate for the condition of the patient. Since Part A only covers blood transfusion during hospital stay, Part B covers outpatient blood transfusions. If used for preventive reasons, clinical trials are also covered. Ambulatory surgery fees will be covered on the grounds that the service is approved. Emergency room services are covered. Eyeglasses are also covered, but are only limited to a pair after a cataract surgery (Centers for Medicare & Medicaid Services, 2012).

Underpayment usually happens in outpatient physical therapy claims in Medicare because guidelines on top of the ICD-10 CM codes are not properly followed. Medicare, in the most ideal sense, is bound to reimburse for their patients' payments made for outpatient physical therapy services, but certain considerations need to be made. The following points are worth considering when claiming for Medicare reimbursement, most especially for outpatient physical therapy:

a. Physical therapy availed on outpatient basis is generally reimbursed and covered by Medicare Part B.

b. Outpatient physical therapy includes settings such as the patients' homes, facilities where assisted living is offered; home-care settings and others that do not fall within the definition of institutional care.

c. There is a limit for reimbursement of services rendered by a physical therapist. Currently, this cap is $1940 (APTA, 2015).

d. There is involvement of the physician in furnishing the needed documents when making payment claims. This involvement is normally on certifying documents and evaluating patient progress during therapy.

e. Although the physical therapists may use the assistance of aides in providing care, the involvement of aides are not billable under Medicare.

Therapy Students

Only the services of the therapist can be billed and paid under Medicare Part B. The services performed by a student are not reimbursed even if provided under "line of sight" supervision of the therapist. However, the presence of the student "in the room" does not make the service unbillable. Medicare Part B will pay for the direct (one to one) patient contact services of the physician or therapist provided to Medicare B patients. Group therapy services performed by a therapist or physician may be billed when a student is also present "in the room".

Aides

Services provided by aides, even if under the supervision of a therapist, are not therapy services in the outpatient setting and are not covered by Medicare. Although an aide may help the therapist by providing unskilled services, those services that are unskilled are not covered by Medicare and shall be denied as not reasonable and necessary if they are billed as therapy services. The supporting personnel must be employees of the therapist.

Supplies

The cost of supplies (e.g., theraband, hand putty, electrodes, looms, ceramic tiles or leather) used in furnishing covered therapy care is included in the payment for the HCPCS codes billed by the physical therapist and are, therefore, not separately billable. The restriction on separate coverage and billing does not apply to items meeting the definition of a brace.

Private Insurances

Apart from Medicare and Medicaid, there are numerous private health insurance providers that patients use for paying for their health care bills. In the situation of having physical therapy done on an outpatient basis, several aspects become a concern for therapists and billers when the time comes for them to charge for their health care services. In an article posted in the American Physical Therapy Association (2014) site, it was mentioned that when patients avail of physical therapy outside confinement or as an outpatient care, one of the things that private insurance providers determine is the presence of a medical need for the services availed by the insured party (in this case, the patient). It then becomes a responsibility for the individual physical therapists to ensure that they have valid documents supporting their bills when claiming payments.

Most of these private health insurance providers increase their focus on controlling the costs of care they have to shoulder in behalf of the policy owners. Different insurance providers may have different definitions for what is a medical necessity for justifying physical therapy when claiming payments, and this is where some of the problems occur. This issue prompted the board of directors of the American Physical Therapy Association to take some action and made a position on the most basic yet important definition of terms. On August of 2011, the board adopted a guideline entitled *Defining Medically Necessary Physical Therapy Services.*

In the said published document, it is emphasized that physical therapists are indeed licensed and therefore have the authority to make responsible decisions regarding the care of their patients. This means that when services are provided to patients, they are to be seen as medically necessary and so payment claims need to be processed if this is part of the coverage availed by an insured patient. Physical therapists are also to express the need or purpose of their services to their patients, apart from the medical reason behind it. In a simpler sense, expressing whether physical therapy is done to improve mobility and independence on the part of the patients or to minimize impairments due to disease states would give more substance to justifying its need. Physical therapists are also required to list down any restrictions imposed upon their patients, whether these are enforced during or after therapy sessions (APTA, 2014; CMS, 2014).

Claiming payments from private insurance providers for outpatient physical therapy also requires the practitioners and the billers to provide documents that prove that the care given to patients follows the standards of care for physical therapy. These documents can be in the form of an evaluation tool, an intervention checklist or a guideline that is recognized by an authority. And lastly, to make certain that physical therapy claims are not underpaid, it is important for the billers to make sure when filing documents for claims, apart from following the coding guidelines, the amount of the services rendered and for how long they were performed should be part of the claims form. As long as these are followed and provided in the manner that insurance companies are requiring, claiming payments for outpatient physical therapy needs not to be as complicated as it seems (Wojciechowski, 2009).

Claiming for payments from private insurance providers is a complicated matter, but filing for claims from Medicare may be more complicated. Apart from the documentation requirements, physical therapists and billers should familiarize themselves with the different aspects of payment claims submission (APTA, 2014).

Medicare Skilled Guidelines

A written plan of treatment must be furnished for the therapy. It should have measurable goals and time periods indicated by the physician or therapist taking care of the patient. It should also be approved and signed by the physician. The service to be rendered must be complex and sophisticated, and the sole performer of the service is a qualified therapist under the supervision of the physician.

Medical Necessity

A service or treatment complies with medical necessity if the following conditions are met:

- It follows the accepted standards of medical practice with a specific and effective treatment for the patient's condition.

- The amount of improvement anticipated should be reasonable when compared to amount of therapy required to achieve goals.

- The exacerbation of chronic illness or significant change of condition should have significant potential for improvement in response to therapy.

- It requires unique skills of a therapist in order to make functional improvements.

- Impaired functions should be restored with realistic functional outcomes.

- It allows for sufficient improvement for the patient to live at home independently or with family assist rather than in an institution.

- The goal is not to return to labor market, leisure, or play.

Expressing Medical Necessity and Skilled Care

Without the evidence of medical necessity, the claim can be denied. Third-party payers say that a patient's visit must be medically necessary and must also require skilled intervention. Medical necessity and skilled care are expected to be supported by evidence in a patient's record. Here are some suggestions of how to support these in a clinical documentation:

- A brief evaluation/assessment of the patient's reaction or response to the interventions must be indicated during each visit or instance.

- The provider's clinical decision-making process must be documented. A provider (such as a speech-language pathologist) should explain why there is a change in the patient's treatment.

- Once a payer gives a request for the documentation of a certain date of service, the provider must take the time to review the note. The provider might need to provide supporting documentations.

Advance Beneficiary Notice

If a provider believes that a Medicare service claim can be denied, the patient must be informed and then must decide if the test or service will still be performed. If the patient agrees to carry on the test or service, an Advance Beneficiary Notice (ABN) should be provided with the signature of the patient. Without an ABN, the test or service cannot be billed. An ABN must meet the following requirements:

- It should be given to the patient before the test or service is administered.

- It must contain the name of the patient, date, and description of test or procedure.

- The reasons for the assumption that the test/procedure may not be medically necessary or reasonable must also be stated.

- The patient must sign the ABN (with date) and a waiver that states that he or she is willing to pay for the test/services in the event that Medicare denies the claim.

In order to comply with the new guidelines for medical necessity, physicians are advised to order tests that are needed for the diagnosis and treatment of their patients, and to be sure of the appropriate and accurate entry of ICD-9 codes in patient files and test request forms (these two should completely match each other). In case of doubt, an ABN should be signed and dated by the patient. Also, to guarantee that services comply with medical necessity, coverage policies are made in order to define certain clinical requirements, and the required ICD and CPT codes. The coverage criteria must be met by the services.

The ABN notice is given to beneficiaries in Original Medicare to communicate that Medicare most likely will deny coverage in a particular case. "Notifiers" include any physicians, healthcare providers, practitioners and suppliers paid under Part B. The ABN must be completed and delivered to affected beneficiaries or their representative prior to implementing services that may not be covered. (Note: skilled nursing facilities (SNFs) have to use the revised ABN for Part B items and services.) As of March 1, 2009, the ABN-G and ABN-L became invalid, and now notifiers must use the revised Advance Beneficiary Notice of Non-coverage (CMS-R-131).

The ABN must be discussed verbally with the beneficiary or his/her representative, and all questions need to be answered before the document is signed. In order for the beneficiary to make an informed choice and have time to consider all options, the ABN must be delivered in advance. The ABN may be delivered by the notifier or employees or subcontractors of the notifier as well. In emergency situations, an ABN is never required. After the document is completed and signed, the beneficiary receives a copy and the notifier must keep the original ABN on file.

The ABN is a collection of formal information subject to approval by the Executive Office of Management and Budget (OMB) under the Paperwork Reduction Act of 1995 (PRA). Every three years, the ABN is made available for public comments and subject to re-approval. This revised ABN takes into consideration input from notifiers, changes necessary based on consumer testing and other means, and any relevant Medicare policy changes and clarifications that have been implemented in the previous three year period.

Prior to this revision, the ABN was only required for denials recognized under section 1879 of the Paperwork Reduction Act. The revised version may also be used to give voluntary notification of financial liability, which should eliminate the need for the Notice of Exclusion from Medicare Benefits (NEMB) in voluntary notification situations.

Instructions for completion of the ABN form included below can be found on the CMS website. Regarding the ABN, relevant policy on billing and coding of claims and coverage determinations are also found in the CMS manual system or website (www.cms.hhs.gov).

Notice to Beneficiaries

Contractors will advise providers/suppliers to notify beneficiaries of the therapy financial limitations at their first therapy encounter. Providers/suppliers should inform beneficiaries that beneficiaries are responsible for 100% of the costs of therapy services above each respective therapy limit, unless this outpatient care is furnished directly or under arrangements by a hospital when outpatient hospital therapy services are excluded from the limitation.

Providers are now encouraged to use either a form of their own design, or the Advanced Beneficiary Notice of Non-coverage (ABN, Form CMS-R131) as a voluntary notice. When using the ABN form as a voluntary notice, the form requirements specified for its mandatory use do not apply. The provider should, however, include the beneficiary's name on the form and the reason that Medicare may not pay in the space provided within the form's table.

After the cap is exceeded, voluntary notice via a provider's own form or the ABN is appropriate, even when services are exempt from the cap. The ABN is also used BEFORE the cap is exceeded when notice about non-covered services is mandatory. For example, whenever the clinician determines that the services being provided are no longer expected to be covered because they do not satisfy Medicare's medical necessity requirements, an ABN must be issued before the beneficiary receives that service. At the time the clinician determines that skilled services are not medically necessary, the clinical goals have been met, or there is no longer potential for the rehabilitation of health and/or function in a reasonable time, the beneficiary should be informed. If the beneficiary requests further services, beneficiaries should be informed that Medicare most likely will not provide additional coverage, and the ABN should be issued prior to delivering any services. The ABN informs the beneficiary of his/her potential financial obligation to the provider and provides guidance regarding appeal rights.

If a Part B patient or designated representative requests further services but staff feels that services won't be covered by Medicare, provide ABN (CMS-R-131). See below for an example of an ABN form:

Maintenance Programs

During the last visits for rehabilitative treatment, the qualified professional may develop a maintenance program. The goals of a maintenance program would be, for example, to maintain functional status or to prevent decline in function.

The specialized skill, knowledge and judgment of a therapist may be required, and their services covered, to design or establish the maintenance program, assure patient safety, train the patient, family members, caregiver, and/or unskilled personnel and make infrequent but periodic re-evaluations of the program.

The services of a qualified professional are not necessary to carry out a maintenance program, and are not covered under ordinary circumstances. The patient may perform such a program independently or with the assistance of unskilled personnel or family members. Where a maintenance program is not established until after the rehabilitative physical therapy program has been completed (and the skills of a therapist are not necessary), development of a maintenance program would not be considered reasonable and necessary for the treatment of the patient's condition unless the patient's safety was at risk.

Evaluation and Maintenance Plan without Rehabilitative Treatment

After the initial evaluation of the extent of the disorder, illness, or injury, if the treating qualified professional determines that the potential for rehabilitation is insignificant, an appropriate maintenance program may be established prior to discharge. Since the skills of a therapist are required for the development of the maintenance program and training the patient or caregivers, this service is covered.

Skilled Maintenance Therapy for Safety

If the services required to maintain function involve the use of complex and sophisticated therapy procedures, the judgment and skill of a therapist may be necessary for the safe and effective delivery of such services. When the patient's safety is at risk, those reasonable and necessary services shall be covered, even if the skills of a therapist are not ordinarily needed to carry out the activities performed as part of the maintenance program.

For example, where there is an unhealed, unstable fracture that requires regular exercise to maintain function until the fracture heals, the skills of a therapist would be needed to ensure that the fractured extremity is maintained in proper position and alignment during maintenance range of motion exercises.

Individual Activities Concurrent with Rehabilitative Treatment

An individualized plan of exercise and activity for patients and their caregiver(s) may be developed by clinicians to maintain and enhance a patient's progress during the course of skilled therapy, as well as after discharge from therapy services. Such programs are an integral part of therapy from the start of care and should be updated and modified as the patient progresses. Therapist skills are required to develop and revise the program and to train the patient and/or caregiver to follow it. As the patient or caregiver masters an activity or exercise, transition to a maintenance program for completion of the activity or exercise is expected.

A. Notifier:

B. Patient Name: **C. Identification Number:**

Advance Beneficiary Notice of Noncoverage (ABN)

<u>NOTE:</u> If Medicare doesn't pay for **D.** _____ below, you may have to pay.
Medicare does not pay for everything, even some care that you or your health care provider have good reason to think you need. We expect Medicare may not pay for the **D.** _____ below.

D.	E. Reason Medicare May Not Pay:	F. Estimated Cost

WHAT YOU NEED TO DO NOW:
- Read this notice, so you can make an informed decision about your care.
- Ask us any questions that you may have after you finish reading.
- Choose an option below about whether to receive the **D.** _____ listed above.
  Note: If you choose Option 1 or 2, we may help you to use any other insurance that you might have, but Medicare cannot require us to do this.

G. OPTIONS: **Check only one box. We cannot choose a box for you.**
☐ **OPTION 1.** I want the **D.** _____ listed above. You may ask to be paid now, but I also want Medicare billed for an official decision on payment, which is sent to me on a Medicare Summary Notice (MSN). I understand that if Medicare doesn't pay, I am responsible for payment, but **I can appeal to Medicare** by following the directions on the MSN. If Medicare does pay, you will refund any payments I made to you, less co-pays or deductibles.
☐ **OPTION 2.** I want the **D.** _____ listed above, but do not bill Medicare. You may ask to be paid now as I am responsible for payment. **I cannot appeal if Medicare is not billed**.
☐ **OPTION 3.** I don't want the **D.** _____ listed above I understand with this choice I am **not** responsible for payment, and **I cannot appeal to see if Medicare would pay.**

H. Additional Information:

This notice gives our opinion, not an official Medicare decision. If you have other questions on this notice or Medicare billing, call **1-800-MEDICARE** (1-800-633-4227/**TTY:** 1-877-486-2048).
Signing below means that you have received and understand this notice. You also receive a copy.

I. Signature:	J. Date:

According to the Paperwork Reduction Act of 1995, no persons are required to respond to a collection of information unless it displays a valid OMB control number. The valid OMB control number for this information collection is 0938-0566. The time required to complete this information collection is estimated to average 7 minutes per response, including the time to review instructions, search existing data resources, gather the data needed, and complete and review the information collection. If you have comments concerning the accuracy of the time estimate or suggestions for improving this form, please write to: CMS, 7500 Security Boulevard, Attn: PRA Reports Clearance Officer, Baltimore, Maryland 21244-1850.

Form CMS-R-131 (03/11)   Form Approved OMB No. 0938-0566

Evaluation and Maintenance Program without Rehabilitation Therapy

When there is no expectation of significant functional improvement, therapy may be covered for the establishment of a safe and effective maintenance program to maintain or prevent decline in function. Maintenance program development and periodic monitoring are covered if the specialized knowledge and judgment of a therapist is required to design or establish the plan, assure patient safety, train the patient, family members and/or unskilled personnel, and make infrequent but periodic re-evaluations of the plan.

When patients with chronic progressive conditions experience a deterioration of function, rehabilitative therapy may be appropriate and reasonable to assist the patient in restoring lost function. Other times, the intent of therapy is not necessarily rehabilitative, but to develop a maintenance program to delay or minimize functional deterioration. Instructing patients and/or caregivers in a maintenance program required to delay or minimize functional deterioration in patients suffering from a chronic disease is not expected to require more than 2 to 4 visits. Supporting documentation is required to justify more than 4 visits. In addition, therapy may be intermittently necessary to determine the need for assistive equipment and/or establish/revise a program to maximize function.

Non-covered indications for maintenance programs include the following services:

- Non-individualized services.

- Services considered being routine or non-skilled (e.g., supportive nursing services).

- Exercises or activities that could have been transitioned to an independent or caregiver assisted program (e.g., consistently repetitive exercises/activities).

- Continuation of treatment solely for the purpose of staff training and education, or development of a formal maintenance program after rehabilitative therapy has been completed.

Maintenance Therapy Lawsuit

On January 24th, 2013, the U.S. District Court of Vermont approved the settlement agreement for the class action lawsuit of Jimmo vs. Sebelius specific to Medicare Part A and Part B coverage of "maintenance" therapy. The Center for Medicare Advocacy alleged that Medicare claims involving skilled care were being inappropriately denied due to a lack of a beneficiary's restorative potential, even though skilled care was required. Medicare beneficiaries were denied coverage for conditions that were chronic, stable or did not present improvement.

The settlement clarified that coverage cannot be denied based on the potential for improvement. Skilled services cannot be denied when they prevent further deterioration of the patient. These settlements DOES NOT imply that Medicare automatically covers maintenance therapy.

Medicare Appeal Deadlines

Medicare Audit Recovery

The Medicare Modernization Act of 2003 established the Medicare Recovery Audit Contractor to identify and recover assumed overpayments to healthcare providers. The Tax Relief and Health Care Act of 2006 made this program permanent. The Centers for Medicare and Medicaid Services launched the program all over the United States in 2010. Recovery Audit Contractors identify improper payments caused by incorrect billing, non-covered services (including services that are not reasonable and necessary), incorrectly coded services (including DRG miscoding), and duplicate services.

The objective of audits by the Recovery Audit Contractor is different than other Medicare audits. The conventional Medicare audit process was designed to target providers with limited budget and technology. On the other hand, Recovery Audit Contractor audits are accomplished outside this traditional framework, done by modern medical collection agencies. The objective of Centers for Medicare and Medicaid Services is to make sure that providers will adopt Medicare's evidence-based criteria of payment and required elements of documentation with a high level of commitment.

The Centers for Medicare and Medicaid Services pay permanent Recovery Audit Contractors with roughly 10% of every dollar identified and recovered in assumed overpayments. Quality Improvement Organizations are not paid any more for similar services.

It is a common misconception that Recovery Audit Contractor auditors are bounty hunters. Recovery Audit Contractor auditors are collection companies or recovery firms hired by Centers for Medicare and Medicaid Services. Recovery Audit Contractor auditors are contracted to impose the evidence-based coverage policies and payment criteria for billing and submission of claims set by Medicare (Centers for Medicare & Medicaid Services, 2012).

Another misconception is that Recovery Audit Contractor audits were designed to thwart Medicare fraud. Actually, Recovery Audit Contractors are designed to identify overpayments and cut down any "abuse" providers are assumed to be doing. The Recovery Audit Contractor Statement of Work nevertheless requires reports on potential fraud to Centers for Medicare and Medicaid Services or the Office of Inspector General (Centers for Medicare & Medicaid Services, 2012).

The following table outlines the appeals process for Medicare (CMS 2015):

Level	Stage	Reviewing Entity	Filing Deadline
1st	Redetermination	Medicare Administrative Contractor (Medicare Administrative Contractor)	120 days of receiving notice of initial determination
2nd	Reconsideration	Qualified Independent Contract (QIC)	180 days of receiving notice of redetermination decision

(Continued)

Level	Stage	Reviewing Entity	Filing Deadline
3rd	Hearing	Administrative Law Judge (ALJ)	60 days of receipt of the QIC's decision
4th	Administrative Review (HHS)	Medicare Appeals Council (Medicare Administrative Contractor)	60 days of receipt of the ALJ's decision
5th	Judicial Review	Federal District Court	60 days of receipt of the Medicare Administrative Contractor's decision

The schedule above is strictly followed.

Appealing Recoupment

A provider has a choice to refute any potential recoupment action. This can be done within 15 days upon notice of any possible recoupment. A statement to the claims processing contractor with evidence to prove that overpayment has not occurred can be written by a provider.

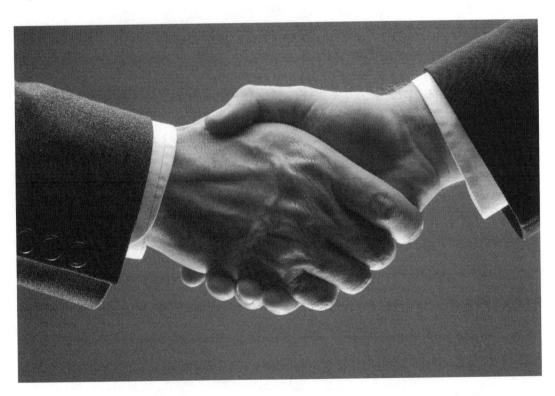

Sample Letters of Appeal

To Whom It May Concern:

Please review the following information for the reconsideration of [therapy service provided] for services for the month of _____.

Mr./Mrs. _____ is a _____ year old male/female who was referred for [therapy services] because of [state problems]. He/She has a medical history of:

His/Her prior level of function was [be specific as related to the functional areas treated].

He had/had not received prior OT/PT/ST therapy. [Dates and outcome]

Upon evaluation, Mr./Mrs. ____ presented with [details]

His/Her goals are: ____

Therapy consisted of: ____

Education was provided to ____ related to ____

He/she progressed to ____

Skilled therapy was required to ____

Therapy meets Medicare's reasonable and necessary requirements because ____

Thank you for reconsidering this claim.

EFFECTIVE DOCUMENTATION

Basics of Documentation

For the past 50 years, physical therapists have been required to provide documentation of services. The Social Security Act of 1965 declared practitioners must document patient care. This is necessary to prove the necessity of the care (Shamus & Stern, 2004).

Vital information about the patient must be included in the documentation for the purpose of identification. This consists of the patient's full name and identification number (also included on all official documents).

All entries should have a date and should be authenticated along with the full name of the provider and the appropriate designation. If required by state laws, the license number and printed name of the provider must be indicated. The provider of the service must be specific and clear in the documentation. For example, indicate if the provider was a physical therapist or a physical therapist assistant. Referral mechanisms must be included in documentation. It may include one of the following: (a) direct access, (b) request for consultation from another practitioner, or (c) referral from practitioner authorized to refer per state practice act.

The documentation in a patient's medical record should be sufficient to justify plan of care and to identify potential changes in patient's medical condition. Skilled services, particularly therapy services, should be properly tailored to the individualized goals of the patient.

A malpractice judgment can seriously harm a provider's professional life. Your documentation may be the only thing between your word and that of a patient. Your proper documentation may be the sole item of evidence in a case and therefore is essential for avoiding adverse legal action.

Remember that your documentation may be subject to a subpoena. You must be comfortable in the knowledge that someone could be reading your notes. View your patient as a unique individual with a distinct set of cultural values, beliefs, and attitudes. Never alter a patient's records. Altering records is a criminal act. It can be especially devastating if any alteration is done after a civil action is filed.

Record your patient's responses to what you do and say. Document what is spoken or avoided, tone of voice, and any changes to the initial mood, attitude, actions, gestures, and body language. This is particularly important with patients who are at risk of harming themselves or others, have cognitive distortions or begin a cycle of devaluation.

Indicate what you plan to do about the patient's response to therapy. Establish any follow-up measures necessary to support the successful implementation of the plan of action.

Documentation is crucial, and mistakes in documentation may lead to insurance denials. Mistakes to avoid when doing a medical documentation include:

- Wrong use of the form (i.e., form for physical therapy was used in place of occupational therapy form).

- Insufficient information.

- Erroneous billing information.

- Inappropriate treatment goal.

- Undocumented results.

- Unnecessary, repetitive, and non-skilled exercises.

- Undocumented visits or treatment. (American Physical Therapy Association, 2010).

One of the standard operational procedures of any medical clinic is the provision of client intake forms, which are to be duly completed and then submitted by every client. Such forms provide practitioners in the fields of physical therapy, occupational therapy, and chiropractic care with all the necessary information regarding the personal background, referral information, payment method, etc. Returning patients also benefit from these forms since it makes it easier for them and their healthcare provider to trace their past medical history and monitor any progress or diagnose any new ailment.

Other necessary items related to this standard operational procedure include patient charts, clipboards, alphabetizing stickers, sign-in sheets, and paper clips to keep related papers together. On the clipboard, you must include a brochure containing the list of the clinic's offered services and corresponding fees, your clinic's financial and company policies, as well as a notice of privacy practice. As you may well guess, these additional forms provide the client with convenient information about your clinic's policies. This prevents clients from claiming that they were not informed about some policy of your clinic if they ever file certain kinds of lawsuits. Attached to the patient chart is the fee slip for the provider to mark. An Assignment of Benefits Form may or may not be added, depending upon your discretion (Halley, 2008).

It is worth mentioning that poor quality paper deteriorates much faster especially in hot and humid environments. When producing intake forms and other related documents, try having them done using the most affordable first-rate paper. You do not want your important patient files to simply just tear, easily crumple, or develop molds quickly. Patient intake forms must be well organized for easy retrieval and stored in file cabinets for convenience and safekeeping. Alphabetize the forms by your clients' surnames with the help of alphabetizing stickers. It is best that you regularly go through these documents to check if there are any missing forms or if the papers are dirty or damaged (i.e., by mildew, accumulated dust). Intake forms will have to include company policies. They are there to facilitate smooth service transactions between you and your client.

Some examples of important company policies are given below:

Late Policy "10 Minutes"

Clients who are late over ten minutes will have to reschedule for another appointment or wait for another available slot or cancellation. Overlapping appointments is prohibited since this compromises the service of another client.

24-Hour Advance Notice Fee

Changing or cancellation of an appointment requires a minimum of 24-hour advance notice and failing to do so will result in a __ dollar penalty fee.

Penalty for No-show clients

Patients that do not show up without any warning will have all their future appointments cancelled.

Evaluation

Place Logo Here

PATIENT INFORMATION & MEDICAL HISTORY

In order to provide you with the most appropriate treatment, please complete the following questionnaire.

All information is strictly confidential.

Name _____

DOB ____/____/____ Age _____ Sex _____

Address _____ City _____ State _____ Zip Code _____

Cell Phone _____ Home Phone _____

E-Mail Address _____ How did you hear about us? _____

Medical Information   Do you have any of the following medical conditions? (Please circle all that apply).

Cancer	Vitiligo	Diabetes	High Blood Pressure	Herpes Simplex	Frequent Cold Sores
Depression	Psoriasis	Eczema Thyroid Imbalance		Muscle Weakness	Seizure Disorder
Paralysis	Arthritis	Neurological Disorder		Auto- Immune Disorder	Keloid Skin Lesions
Hepatitis	HIV/AIDS	Hormone Imbalance		Pacemaker/Defibrillator	Blood Clotting Disorder

Are you currently under the care of a Physician? Y or N (Please specify.)_____

Do you have any other current or past health problems or medical conditions? Y or N (Please specify.)_____

Please list any known allergies, and/ or past allergic reactions_____

Current Medications Please list all oral and topical medications you are presently taking: (including antibiotics, hormone therapy, blood thinners, mood altering medications OTC medications) _____

Please list all vitamins and/or herbal supplements you are presently taking: _____

Lifestyle   Do you (Please circle all that apply).

smoke	drink	have sun exposure that changed your skin color
exercise use tanning beds		recently used any self-tanning lotions of spray tans/treatments

For our female patients only: Are you (Please circle all that apply).

currently on birth control pregnant	lactating	trying to become pregnant
get hyperpigmentation during your pregnancy		menopausal
When was the last day of your last menstrual period?		

Occupation: _____

Employer Name:_____

Employer Phone Number:(_____)_____

My condition is related to: Work   Auto Accident (State_____)   Other_____

Work Status: Currently Employed   Retired   Disabled (__Total or ___Temporary)   Student

II. REFERRAL INFO (ALL INFO REQUIRED)

How did you hear about us? _____

If by a friend or family member, please give their phone number and address below that we may send a thank you note and a small gift.

_____

_____

_____

Primary or Referring Physician Name:_____

Street Address: _____

Phone No._____ Fax_____ E-mail Address_____

Do you have a follow up appointment with this physician? _____ If yes, when?_____

PAYMENT INFO (Circle One)

I am paying by CASH, CHECK, CREDIT and would like a . . .

- 20% discount by paying at the time of service.
- Payment plan. Fees may apply.

I have INSURANCE and would like to. . .

- Have you directly deal with them. I will assign my benefits to you by completing the "Assignment of Benefits Form." Fees may apply. The following information is required prior to first visit. My coinsurance /copay is $_____My deductible is $_____
- Get a 20% discount by paying the entire bill at the time of service. I will get reimbursement on my own. (Ask the front desk person for details)

I have an ATTORNEY and would like to. . .

- Get a 20% discount by paying up front. I will get reimbursed after my case settles.
- Wait until my case settles before paying. I will complete the "Attorney Lien" form. Fees may apply.

CREDIT CARD ON FILE (SAFE AND SECURE. I understand I will be notified of any and all charges prior to processing.)

VISA   Master Card   American Express Discover Card

Credit Card No._____ Name on Card_____

Exp Date_____ CVV Code_____

I have read and agree to all the policies on this form.

(Continued)

Clinic Policies

- No children under 12 allowed in the lobby without adult supervision. (Your Clinic) is not responsible for childcare during your treatment.
- Only the person receiving treatment is allowed in the room, unless the person being treated is a minor.
- Pre- paid packages require full payment at the time of first treatment to receive discounted price, a separate service agreement will be given.
- Specials, promotional pricing, series or package pricing cannot be refunded, combined, transferred, exchanged, or given to someone else. Any specials circumstances will be subject to review by management.
- All prices are base prices only and are subjected to a consultation.
- Prices are subject to change without notice.
- (Your Clinic) does hold the right to refuse service.

In consideration of the services rendered to me by (Your Clinic), I am obligated to pay said office in accordance with the credit terms and policies. I understand that payment is due in full at each appointment at the time of service, unless the service has been pre- paid. We kindly ask for a 24-hour notice for all appointment changes or cancellations.

I understand that (Your Clinic) will use/ and or disclose my personal health information for the sole purpose of carrying out treatment, obtaining payment, evaluating the quality of services provided and any administrative operations. I understand that I have the right to restrict how my information is used for treatment, payment, or administrative operations if I notify the practice of my wishes. I understand that (Your Clinic) does not allow the use of my information for marketing, fundraising, solicitation, or research studies. I hereby consent to the use and disclosure of my personal health information for the provision of treatment, facilitation of payment, evaluation of service quality, or administrative operations. I hereby release (Your Clinic), its medical staff and technicians from any liability arising out of the services associated with the above treatment. I certify that the preceding medical, personal, and skin histories are true and correct. I am aware of the above stated spa policies and will abide by them. I am aware that it is my responsibility to inform the technician, esthetician, or nurse of any medical changes, health changes, skincare regimen, new or changed medications, or recent sun exposure as this will alter the results of my treatment. A current medical history is essential for the caregiver to execute the appropriate treatment procedures.

Print Patient Name: _____   Date: _____

Patient Signature: _____

(Parent or Guardian if patient is under 18)

Tech Signature: _____   Date: _____

MD Signature: _____

After the intake forms have been completed, the patient must then undergo an evaluation procedure to be conducted by the attending health professional. The aim of the evaluation is for the health professional to assess the patient's overall physical condition through several attributes before moving on to any other procedures (Halley, 2008). This is extremely necessary in order for the health professional to better understand the patient's complaint and reach a well-informed decision about appropriate treatment.

The evaluation procedure should start off with the health professional taking a brief medical history of the patient by asking the client several questions. This is then to be followed by an analysis of the patient's flexibility, muscle strength, gait, mobility, balance, coordination, and function through certain tests. These tests include movement analysis, postural screening, flexibility tests, muscle strength tests, sensory and neurological tests, coordination tests, joint motion tests, and observation, palpation, and balance tests. The health professional must then ask the patient to perform a variety of specific movements as well as assume different positions for the duration of the evaluation.

Aside from the evaluation procedure tools (which include the goniometer, reflex hammer, pin wheel, hand dynamometer, step stool, X-ray, manual muscle tester, etc.), there are several necessary forms that the therapist must provide. These include the following:

- Pre-exam form, to be filled out by the patient

- Travel card, evaluation form

- Patient role sheet: precautions, home exercise program

- Prescription note pad: teacher, employer

- MD request form for a script: home TENS, extend script, request for orthosis

- Disabilities recommendation form

An example of an evaluation form to be completed by the health professional is provided. It is just a sample and there are actually various kinds of evaluations depending on your specific medical field as well as your personal judgment. Some may even be downloaded from the Internet for a certain fee.

Evaluation procedures should be handled with care and accuracy. Administer the various assessment measures to the best of your ability in order to have precise measurements and relevant comments. Then, record your findings accordingly (Halley, 2008). Give the client your best and you will see that they will remember to come back to you for further services or treatments.

Physical Therapy

PT Evaluation and Plan of Treatment

| | Provider: |
| | NPI: |

Identification Information

	Patient:		Start of Care:	
	Payer:		Hospitalization:	
	MRN:
	Diagnoses
	DOB:

Type	Code	Description	Onset
Tx	719.7	DIFFICULTY IN WALKING	
Tx	728.87	MUSCLE WEAKNESS (GENERALIZED)	
Med	V57.89	REHABILITATION PROCEDURE NEC	

Plan of Treatment

Short-Term Goals   Assistance   Target Date:

#1.0	Patient will safely perform bed mobility tasks with
#2.0	Patient will safely perform functional transfers with
#3.0	Patient will safely ambulate on level surfaces
#4.0	Patient will safely

Long-Term Goals

#1.0	Patient will safely perform bed mobility tasks with
#2.0	Patient will safely perform functional transfers with
#3.0	Patient will safely ambulate on level surfaces
#4.0	Patient will safely

Treatment Approaches May Include

| PT evaluation (97001) | Therapeutic exercises (97110) | Gait training therapy (97116)
| PT re-evaluation (97002) | Neuromuscular reeducation (97112) | Therapeutic activities (97530)

Frequency: _____ time(s)/week

Duration: _____ week(s)

Intensity: _____ minutes

Patient Goals: _____

Potential for Achieving Goals: Patient demonstrates excellent rehab potential as evidenced by high PLOF, ability to follow multi-step directions, recognizes familiar situations/routines, recognition of familiar people, active participation w/POT, motivation to return to PLOF, ability to learn new information, supportive staff and decreased anxiety.

Participation: Patient/Caregiver participated in establishing POT

Original Signature: _____ Date

I certify the need for these medically necessary services furnished under this plan of treatment while under my care.

Physician Signature: _____ Date

Initial Assessment / Current Level of Function & Underlying Impairments

Factors Supporting Medical Necessity

Referral Source: Physician

Clinical Program: General Functional Decline, Ortho, Balance

Reason for Referral: Patient referred to PT due to decline of strength, functional mobility, ambulation, balance, neuromotor control, functional activity tolerance, postural alignment, coordination, static and dynamic balance, increased need for assistance from others and ADL participation and patient is now unable to ambulate without assistance, maintain balance, transfer without assistance, position self in bed without assistance, perform car transfers, maintain skin integrity and negotiate environmental barriers secondary to lack of spontaneous recovery.

Current Medical Hx: _____

Past Medical History: _____

Prior Living: _____

Anticipated D/C Plan: _____

Measure #130: Documentation of Current Medications: _____

PLOF: _____

Background Assessment

Precautions _____

Previous Tx _____

Joint ROM/Goniometric Measurements

LE ROM (B) LE ROM: WFL

Strength / Manual Muscle Testing

LE Strength at least 3/5

RLE _____

LLE _____

Balance

Sitting Balance | **Standing Balance**

Static Sitting _____ | Static Standing _____

Dynamic Sitting _____ | Dynamic Standing _____

Additional Abilities/Underlying Impairments

Measure #131: Pain Assessment and Follow-Up | **Coordination** | Gross Motor Coordination = Intact

Patient reports no recent or exacerbation of musculoskeletal pain

Other Pain | **Tone** | LE Muscle Tone = Normal

Chronic/Musculoskeletal/Other Pain = Patient reports no other pain | **Posture** | Kyphotic posture

Measure #182: Functional Outcome Assessment

Bed Mobility	Current	PLOF
rolling		
supine <-> sit		

Underlying impairments	Body awareness deficits, Decreased safety awareness, Fine motor coordination, Fine motor control, Static and dynamic balance, Strength, Static balance and Functional activity tolerance.

Transfers	Current	PLOF
sit <-> stand		
bed <-> chair		

Underlying impairments	Body awareness deficits, Decreased safety awareness, Fine motor coordination, Fine motor control, Static and dynamic balance, Strength, Static balance and Functional activity tolerance.

Gait	Current	PLOF
Status/ Assistance		
Distance		
Assistive device		

Gait Analysis	Patient exhibits forward lean of trunk which are associated with the underlying causes of lack of/impaired coordination, impaired proprioception, improper adjustment of assistive device and reduced functional activity tolerance.
Gait Pattern:	The patient exhibits the following characteristics during gait: uneven step length and abnormalities in posture.

Measure 154: Falls: Risk Assessment/ Fall predictors	Asymmetrical stance.

	Current	PLOF
W/C Mobility		
Stairs		
Other Areas		

Assessment Summary

Summary of Findings:	Resident presents with decrease in strength, balance and coordination. Resident requires extensive (A) in bed mobility, transfers and ambulation.
Skilled Justification:	Patient requires skilled PT services to evaluate need for assistive device, facilitate (I) with gait, facilitate (I) with all functional mobility, increase (I) with transfers, promote safety awareness, improve dynamic balance, facilitate coordination and facilitate discharge planning in order to enhance patient's quality of life by improving ability to safely return to private residence.
Risk Factors:	Due to the documented physical impairments and associated functional deficits, the patient is at risk for: compromised general health, decreased circulatory function, decrease in level of mobility, decreased leisure task participation, decreased skin integrity, depression, dehydration, DVT, falls, further decline in function, limited out-of-bed activity and social isolation.
Focus of POT	Restoration
Is Supervision of Plan of Tx being transferred?	No

Procedures

PQRS

Measure #131: Pain Assessment and Follow-Up	G8730: Pain assessment documented as positive utilizing a standardized tool AND a follow-up plan is documented		
	G8731: Pain assessment documented as negative, no follow-up plan required		
Measure #182: Functional Outcome Assessment	G8942: Documented functional outcomes assessment and care plan within the previous 30 days		
	G8540: Documentation that the patient is not eligible for a functional outcome assessment using a standardized tool		

	attests to documenting the patient's current medications to the best of his/her knowledge and ability		
Measure #130: Documentation of Current Medications:	G8430: Eligible professional attests the patient is not eligible for medication documentation		
Measure #128 (NQF 0421): Preventive Care and Screening: Body Mass Index (BMI) Screening and Follow-Up	G8420: Calculated BMI within normal parameters and documented		
	G8417: Calculated BMI above normal parameters and a follow-up plan was documented		
	G8418: Calculated BMI below normal parameters and a follow-up plan was documented		

Primary Functional Limitation

		Modifier Impairment Limitation Restriction
G8978 Mobility: walking and moving around functional limitation, current status		
G8979 Mobility: walking and moving around functional limitation, projected goal status		CH 0 percent impaired, limited or restricted
G8980 Mobility: walking and moving around functional limitation, discharge status		CI At least 1 percent but less than 20 percent impaired, limited or restricted
		CJ 40 percent impaired, limited or
		CK 60 percent impaired, limited or
		CL 80 percent impaired, limited or
		CM 100 percent impaired, limited or
		CN restricted

Treatment

After you have evaluated your patient's problem or difficulty through taking the client's problem history and by performing particular tests and measures, you must now move on to the treatment phase. You'll need to formulate a treatment plan that has specific goals directly based on the findings of the earlier evaluation, including the patient's past medical history (Halley, 2008). Once a suitable treatment plan has been finalized, you must then administer the said treatment to the patient. Monitor the patient's progress and make the proper adjustments with the treatment plan and goals as you see fit. Your general goal here is to facilitate a faster recovery of a problem or physical dysfunction, so always be watchful just in case changes need to be made in the treatment plan due to a new development in the client's health.

Part of being a responsible physical, occupational therapist, or chiropractor is consulting with other health professionals about your treatment system to facilitate the better recovery of your patients. Within your treatment system, you must also include patient education that will teach your patients how to deal with their current problems as well as prevent future problems. Use equipment and aids that facilitate postural reeducation and movement awareness among your patients undergoing treatment (Halley, 2008). These, along with therapeutic exercise instructions from you, will help your clients restore their strength, movement, balance, or coordination, serving as guides toward complete functional recovery.

Modalities serve to decrease pain and increase bodily movement and function, making use of properties of heat, cold, air, light, water, electricity, ultrasound, and traction. Myofascial release, TENS (Transcutaneous Electrical Nerve Stimulation), electrical stimulation, whirlpools, ultrasound, traction, cold packs, hot packs, and intermittent compression pumps are some of the most commonly applied techniques. Integrate these into your treatment system when the need calls for it, especially when the patient complains of pain.

Your health facility must also engage in functional training as treatment for particular patients who have issues that are related to work, home activities, recreational and sports pursuits. Exercise, therefore, must be among the elements of your treatment system. Determine the most suitable kind of exercise for a certain patient's case and use an exercise log to monitor his or her progress. An example of an exercise log you can use in your clients' treatment is provided.

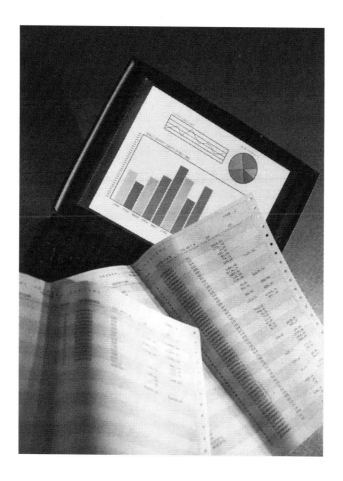

Sample of an Exercise Log:

EXERCISE LOG

Patient Name: _____

           Last Name   **First Name**   **Middle Name**

DATE: _____ **Male**   **Female**   **Age:**_____

DAY: M   Tu   W   Th   Fr   Sa   Su

Contraindications/Precautions: Yes   No

If Yes, specify: _____

_____

_____

_____

WEIGHT:_____ **lbs**

Name of Exercise	SETS	REPS	REST	TIME	DIST	NOTES

(Continued)

Name of Exercise	SETS	REPS	REST	TIME	DIST	NOTES

You must remember that in developing and pursuing your treatment system, you have to be patient, observant, and considerate of the needs and feelings of your patient. Having a good relationship with your patient is almost as important as your treatment methods, so be as supportive as you can, especially if you see that the patient is feeling down or discouraged. Be the best therapist or chiropractor you can with your treatment system. Your clients will remember you for it and may even refer you to others in the future.

Late Entries and Supplemental Notes

If you need to add late entries and supplemental notes in the medical record, and when some vital omissions are discovered, you must write "Late Entry" at note's preface. Refer to the original entry or the date that is being addressed (i.e., late entry for October 30, 2010). Put the date when the late entry was written, and sign. For supplemental notes, write "Supplemental Note" at the note's beginning. This will ensure that you are not suspected of falsifying the records after the fact.

The late entry or supplemental note must be written by the therapist that rendered the care. The clinician must be knowledgeable of the care being delivered. When some parts of the evaluation form are not filled out and the physician has noticed this before signing the evaluation, a late entry should be made. If the incomplete data is discovered after the physician has signed the evaluation, the addition should be noted as "Supplemental Note."

Documentation Requirements

A patient's medical record documentation should contain the following: evaluation and plan of care, certification and recertification, progress reports, treatment notes, and discharge notes (Centers for Medicare and Medicaid Services, 2012).

Therapy services shall be payable when the medical record and the information on the claim form consistently and accurately report covered therapy services. Documentation must be legible, relevant and sufficient to justify the services billed. In general, services must be covered therapy services provided according to the requirements in Medicare manuals. Documentation must comply with all legal/regulatory requirements applicable to Medicare claims. Please review Local Coverage determination (LCD) for Outpatient Physical and Occupational Therapy Services (L29833).

The documentation guidelines identify the minimal expectations of documentation by providers or suppliers or beneficiaries submitting claims for payment of therapy services to the Medicare program. State or local laws and policies, or the policies of the profession, the practice, or the facility may be more stringent. Additional documentation not required by Medicare is encouraged when it conforms to state or local law or to professional guidelines of the American Physical Therapy Association. It is encouraged but not required that narratives that specifically justify the medical necessity of services be included in order to support approval when those services are reviewed. Services are medically necessary if the documentation indicates they meet the requirements for medical necessity including that they are skilled rehabilitative services provided by clinicians (or qualified professionals when appropriate) with the approval of a physician/non-physician practitioner, safe, and effective (i.e., progress indicates that the care is effective in rehabilitation of function).

Documentation Required upon Request

The following types of documentation of therapy services are expected to be submitted in response to any requests for documentation, unless the contractor requests otherwise. The timelines are minimum requirements for Medicare payment. Document as often as the clinician's judgment dictates but no less than the frequency required in Medicare policy:

- Evaluation and Plan of Care (may be one or two documents). Include the initial evaluation and any re-evaluations relevant to the episode being reviewed.

- Certification (physician/non-physician practitioner approval of the plan) and recertification when records are requested after the certification/recertification is due. Certification (and recertification of the plan when applicable) is required for payment and must be submitted when records are requested after the certification or recertification is due.

- Progress Reports (including Discharge Notes, if applicable) when records are requested after the reports are due.

- Treatment Notes for each treatment day (may also serve as Progress Reports when required information is included in the notes).

Limits on Requirements

Only a clinician may perform an initial examination, evaluation, re-evaluation and assessment and establish a diagnosis or a plan of care. As part of the evaluation or re-evaluation, the clinician may include objective measurements or observations made by a PTA within their scope of practice, but the clinician must actively and personally participate in the evaluation or re-evaluation rather than just summarize the work of others.

The initial evaluation, which must be performed by a clinician, should document the medical necessity of a course of therapy through objective findings and subjective patient self-reporting, as well as the conditions being treated and any complexities in the case. Where it is not obvious, describe the impact of the conditions and complexities so that it is clear to the medical reviewer that the services planned are appropriate for the individual.

The initial evaluation establishes the baseline data necessary for assessing expected rehabilitation potential, setting realistic goals and measuring progress. Initial evaluations need to provide objective, measurable documentation of the patient's impairments and how any noted deficits affect ADLs/IADLs and result in functional limitations. Functional limitations refer to the inability to perform actions, tasks and activities that constitute the "usual activities" for the patient. Functional limitations must be meaningful to the patient and caregiver, and must have potential for improvement. In addition, the remediation of such limitations must be recognized as medically necessary.

To support medical necessity, the evaluation should include the following items.

- Presenting condition or complaint.

- A significant change from the patient's "usual" physical or functional ability to warrant an evaluation.

- An objective and detailed description of the changes in function that now necessitate skilled therapy.

- Diagnosis and description of specific problem(s) to be evaluated.

- Area of the body that is affected as well as the conditions and complexities that could impact treatment.

- Subjective complaints and date of onset.

- Applicable medical history, medications, comorbidities (factors that make therapy more complicated or require extra precautions).

- Prior level of function and prior diagnostic imaging/testing results.

- Prior therapy history for the same diagnosis, illness or injury.

- Patient's living environment, mobility status, self-care dependence and access to care/support.

- The level of independence required for the patient to be safe in the home environment.

- Functional testing.

- Meaningful ADLs/IADLs.

- Pain and how it limits function.

If recent therapy was provided, documentation must clearly establish that additional therapy is reasonable and necessary.

Use concise, objective measurements. Avoid minimal/moderate/severe types of descriptions when more specific definitions or measurements are available.

Certifications and Recertifications

Medicare beneficiaries receiving outpatient therapy services must be under the care of a physician/non-physician practitioner. Orders (sometimes called referrals) and certifications are common means of demonstrating such evidence of physician involvement.

Certification, which is a coverage condition for therapy payment, requires a dated physician/non-physician practitioner signature on the therapy plan of care or some other document that indicates approval of the plan of care. A certification often differs from an order or referral in that it must contain all required elements of a plan of care. To assist medical review in determining that the certification requirements are met, certifications/recertifications should include the following elements:

- The date from which the plan of care being sent for certification becomes effective (for initial certifications, the initial evaluation date will be assumed to be the start date of the certified plan of care).

- Diagnoses.

- Long-term treatment goals.

- Type, amount, duration and frequency of therapy services.

- Signature, date and professional identity of the therapist who established the plan.

- Dated physician/non-physician practitioner signature indicating that the therapy service is or was in progress and the physician/non-physician practitioner makes no record of disagreement with the plan. (Note: The CORF benefit does not recognize a non-physician practitioner for certification.)

As was effective from January 1, 2008, the interval length shall be determined by the patient's needs, not to exceed 90 days. Certifications that include all the required plan of care elements will be considered valid for the longest duration in the plan (such as three times per week for six weeks which will be considered as a total of 18 treatments). If treatment continues past the longest duration specified, a recertification will be required.

Dictated Documentation

For Medicare purposes, dictated therapy documentation is considered completed on the day it was dictated. The qualified professional may edit and electronically sign the documentation at a later date.

Dates for Documentation

The date the documentation was made is important only to establish the date of the initial plan of care because therapy cannot begin until the plan is established, unless treatment is performed or supervised by the same clinician who establishes the plan. However, contractors may require that treatment notes and progress reports be entered into the record within one week of the last date to which the Progress Report or Treatment Note refers.

Evaluation/Re-Evaluation and Plan of Care

The initial evaluation, or the plan of care including an evaluation, should document the necessity for a course of therapy through objective findings and subjective patient self-reporting. As stated above, only a clinician may perform an initial examination, evaluation, re-evaluation and assessment or establish a diagnosis or a plan of care.

Evaluation shall include a diagnosis (where allowed by state and local law) and description of the specific problem(s) to be evaluated and/or treated. In many cases, both a medical diagnosis (obtained from a physician/non-physician practitioner) and an impairment-based treatment diagnosis related to treatment are relevant. Where a diagnosis is not allowed, use a condition description similar to the appropriate ICD-9-CM or ICD-10-CM code. For example, the medical diagnosis made by the physician is CVA; however, the treatment diagnosis or condition description for physical therapy may be abnormality of gait. Physical therapists should be sure to include the body part evaluated. Include all conditions and complexities that may impact the treatment. A description might include, for example, the premorbid function, date of onset, and current function.

Documentation supporting illness severity or complexity includes:

- Identification of other health services concurrently being provided for this condition (e.g., physician, PT, OT, SLP, chiropractic, nurse, respiratory therapy, social services, psychology, nutritional/dietetic services, radiation therapy, chemotherapy, etc.).

- Identification of durable medical equipment needed for this condition.

- Identification of the number of medications the beneficiary is taking (and type if known).

- Complexity and its effect on the beneficiary.

- Generalized or multiple conditions and cognitive or mental disorders. The beneficiary has, in addition to the primary condition being treated, another disease, condition or disorder being treated, or generalized musculoskeletal conditions, or conditions affecting multiple sites and these conditions will directly and significantly impact the rate of recovery.

- Identification of factors that impact severity including age, time since onset, cause of the condition, stability of symptoms, how typical/atypical are the symptoms of the diagnosed condition, availability of an intervention/treatment known to be effective, predictability of progress.

Documentation supporting medical care prior to the current episode, if any, (or document none) includes:

- Record of discharge from a Part A qualifying inpatient, SNF, or home health episode within 30 days of the onset of this outpatient therapy episode.

- Identification of whether beneficiary was treated for this same condition previously by the same therapy discipline (regardless of where prior services were furnished).

- Documentation required to indicate beneficiary health related to quality of life, specifically.

- The beneficiary's response to the following question of self-related health: "At the present time, would you say that your health is excellent, very good, fair, or poor?" If the beneficiary is unable to respond, indicate why

Documentation that indicates beneficiary social support includes:

- Beneficiary's living arrangements for the duration and conclusion of the outpatient therapy episode.

- Beneficiary's immediate support/care network and access to in-home care.

Documentation to indicate beneficiary's objective, measurable, physical function includes:

- Functional assessment individual item and summary scores (and comparisons to prior assessment scores) from commercially available therapy outcomes instruments other than those listed above.

- Functional assessment scores (and comparisons to prior assessment scores) from tests and measurements validated in the professional literature that are appropriate for the condition/function being measured.

- Clinician's clinical judgments or subjective impressions that describe the current functional status of the condition being evaluated, when they provide further information to supplement measurement tools; and

- A determination that treatment is not needed, or, if treatment is needed a prognosis for return to premorbid condition or maximum expected condition with expected time frame and a plan of care.

Additional Components of Evaluation/Reevaluation

REASON FOR REFERRAL (state the condition of the patient):

Example: This [age] year old [gender] underwent a [condition] due to [reason] on [date]. The patient shows impaired function in [functional activities] and difficulty in [functional activities]. Skilled therapy is necessary to improve [function]; without therapy, patient is at risk for [list complications].

MEDICATIONS (List of side effects and how they affect therapy):

Angina medication: at risk for dizziness, headache or tachycardia

Anti-anxiety medication: at risk for decreased ability to sustain attention for speech sessions, decreased endurance, decreased exercise tolerance, loss of appetite impacts dysphagia treatment.

Anti-arrhythmic agents: at risk for arrhythmias, confusion, EKG changes, hallucinations, hepatotoxicity, increased blood pressure, increased heart rate, lethargy or toxicity (increased left ventricular performance and aerobic capacity).

Anti-coagulants: at risk for excessive bruising, hemorrhage (including rectal bleeding and coughing up blood), heparin-induced thrombocytopenia (hit syndrome); dietary restrictions: green leafy vegetables, broccoli, & liver may be restricted; cranberry products & juice are forbidden, risk of bleeding with aggressive therapy, falls.

Anti-depressants: at risk for weight loss, decreased ability to sustain attention for speech sessions, decreased endurance and exercise tolerance, loss of appetite.

Anti-hypertensive: at risk for at risk for chest pain, cough, depression, dizziness, fainting, GI disturbances, headache, lethargy, lightheadedness, nausea, orthostatic, hypotension, pedal edema, possible exercise intolerance or tachycardia

Anti-psychotics: at risk for decreased exercise tolerance, difficulty with mobility & exercise, uncontrollable muscle movement of the articulators.

Bronchodilators: at risk for GI disturbances, nervousness, restlessness, tachycardia, trembling.

Corticosteroids: at risk for decreased exercise/activity tolerance due to weakness, pain.

Dementia/Alzheimer's medications: at risk for anorexia, diarrhea, dizziness, hepatoxicity, lethargy, loss of appetite, muscle cramping, nausea, ulcers, vomiting or weight loss.

Diabetic medications: increased risk of hypoglycemia with excessive exercise.

Diuretics: at risk for electrolyte imbalance, which can cause impaired concentration, attention & overall decreased cognitive-linguistic function, potential for dehydration.

GERD medications: at risk for headache, nausea, stomach pain or vomiting, dehydration.

Goiter medications: at risk for anxiety, GI disturbances, insomnia, lethargy, mood swings and weakness.

Hypothyroid medications: at risk for anxiety which can impact attention and concentration; weight loss; dehydration.

Muscle relaxers: at risk for confusion which can impact treatment; difficulty with activity & exercise, lethargy.

Narcotic pain medications: at risk for addiction potential, GI irritation, liver toxicity, mental clouding, respiratory depression or withdrawal risk.

Non-steroidal anti-inflammatory: at risk for bleeding of stomach and GI tract, irritation or ulceration.

Parkinson's medications: at risk for behavioral issues, dyskinesia or GI disturbances (becomes less effective the longer the patient takes medication).

Zollinger-Ellison syndrome medications: at risk for diarrhea, headache, nausea or stomach pain, vomiting, dehydration.

ANALYSIS OF FUNCTIONAL OUTCOMES & CLINICAL IMPRESSION:

Example: Change in status has resulted in setback in [area] due to [reason], requiring patient to need more assist for [task].

Example: Improvement in [impairment] allows patient to tolerate higher levels of challenges in [specific task].

SKILLED SERVICES PROVIDED SINCE LAST REPORT:

Example: Analysis of [function] resulted in an adjustment to treatment plan of [specifics].

PATIENT & CAREGIVER TRAINING:

Example: Patient & caregiver education initiated with [caregiver] focusing on [focus].

REMAINING FUNCTIONAL DEFICITS:

Example: Patient continues to have deficits in [deficit area] which limit ability to [functional ability].

IMPACT ON DAILY LIFE:

Example: Patient's setbacks in [function or task] due to [cause], have caused in increase in burden of care for [specific tasks]. It is expected, however, that the patient will improve once [reason]. The patient has shown gains in [function or task] which allowed for [improvement].

UPDATES TO TREATMENT APPROACH:

Example: Continued [patient] training required in [area] to improve safety in [functional activity]. Short-term goals related to [goal specifics] have been met and new short-term goals to be added as appropriate for patient.

REASONS FOR MISSED TREATMENT:

Example: Schedule conflict due to [reason].

SUMMARY OF SKILLED SERVICES SINCE START OF CARE (SOC):

Skilled services provided since start of care included [all treatment techniques and skills provided] which improved patient's abilities in [functional activities].

ENVIRONMENTAL FACTORS/SOCIAL SUPPORT:

Example: Environmental home factors include [number] of steps with [equipment] for entry into home. Patient has [caregiver] help at home who will be able to provide [level of assist] assistance upon discharge.

PRIOR RESIDENCE AND LIVING ARRANGEMENT:

Example: Patient lived at home and was [level of independence] in self-care and household activities, but required assistance for [functional activities] and was responsible for own [activity].

DISCHARGE PLANS:

Example: Discharge home with [full time/part time] caregiver assist from [caregiver] with continued [home health or outpatient therapy].

When the Evaluation Serves as the Plan of Care

When an evaluation is the only service provided by a provider/supplier in an episode of treatment, the evaluation serves as the plan of care if it contains a diagnosis, or in states where a therapist may not diagnose, a description of the condition from which a diagnosis may be determined by the referring physician/non-physician practitioner. The goal, frequency, and duration of treatment are implied in the diagnosis and one-time service.

The referral/order of a physician/non-physician practitioner is the certification that the evaluation is needed and the patient is under the care of a physician. Therefore, when evaluation is the only service, a referral/order and evaluation are the only required documentation. If the patient presented for evaluation without a referral or order and does not require treatment, a physician referral/order or certification of the evaluation is required for payment of the evaluation. A referral/order dated after the evaluation shall be interpreted as certification of the plan to evaluate the patient.

The time spent in evaluation shall not also be billed as treatment time.

Re-Evaluations

Re-evaluation documentation must include clear justification for the need for further tests and measurements after the initial evaluation, such as new clinical findings, a significant, unanticipated change in the patient's condition, or failure to respond to the interventions in the plan of care. It is expected that clinicians continually assess the patient's progress as part of the ongoing therapy services. This assessment is not considered a formal re-evaluation; the time of any assessment is included and billed within the appropriate treatment intervention CPT code.

Re-evaluations must be performed by clinicians and contain all applicable components of the initial evaluation. Resolved problems do not need to be re-evaluated; only new or ongoing problems may need to be re-evaluated, especially if there is an anticipated change to the long-term goals. A re-evaluation may be appropriate prior to planned discharge for the purposes of determining whether goals have been met, or for the use of the physician or the treatment setting at which treatment will be continued.

Re-evaluations are distinct from therapy assessments. Assessments are considered a routine aspect of intervention and are not billed separately from the intervention. For example, a patient is being seen in physical therapy for shoulder pain and limited shoulder functional range of motion due to capsular tightness. Prior to performing shoulder joint mobilizations, the therapist assesses the patient's ROM and pain level/pattern to determine the effect of prior treatment and, if further mobilization is warranted, to determine the appropriate mobilizations. After the mobilizations are completed, the ROM is assessed again to determine the effects of the treatment just performed. The time required to assess the patient before and after the intervention is added to the minutes of the treatment intervention (code 97140 in this example). Continuous assessment of the patient's progress is a component of the ongoing therapy services, and is not payable as a re-evaluation.

Do not bill for re-evaluations as unlisted codes (97039, 97139, 97799) or test and measurement, ROM, MMT codes (95831-95834, 95851-95852, 97750, 97755).

Progress Reports

A progress report must be completed at least once every 10 treatment days or 30 calendar days (whichever is less). Writing progress notes more frequently than the minimum is encouraged to support the medical necessity of treatment. A progress report is not a separately billable service.

Clinician participation in treatment is required during the progress report period. Signature and professional identification of the qualified professional who wrote the report and the date it was written, objective reports of the patient's subjective statements, objective measurements, and extent of progress (or lack thereof) toward each goal should be included. Plans for continuing treatment, treatment plan revisions, and changes to long- or short-term goals, discharge, or an updated plan of care should be sent to the physician/non-physician practitioner for certification.

In CMS Publication 100-02, Medicare Benefit Policy Manual, chapter 15, sections 220-230, Medicare defines the minimum REQUIRED elements of a progress report. It is essential that clinicians include all required elements in their documentation (either in a progress report or treatment note).

Progress note elements include:

- Date of the beginning and end of the reporting period that this report refers to.

- Date that the report was written by the clinician, or, if dictated, the date on which it was dictated.

- Objective reports of the patient's subjective statements, if they are relevant.

- Objective measurements (impairment/function testing) to quantify progress and support justification for continued treatment.

- Description of changes in status relative to each goal currently being addressed in treatment.

- Assessment of improvement, extent of progress (or lack thereof) toward each goal.

- Plans for continuing treatment, including documentation of treatment plan revisions as appropriate.

- Changes to long or short-term goals, discharge or an updated plan of care that are sent to the physician/non-physician practitioner for certification of the next interval of treatment.

- Signature with credentials of the clinician who wrote the report.

No specific format is required to demonstrate patient progress as long as all information noted in the bullets above is included at least once in the medical record for each progress report period (10 treatment days or 30 calendar days, whichever is less). During each progress report period, the clinician must personally furnish in its entirety at least one billable service on at least one day of treatment. Verification of the clinician's treatment shall be documented by the clinician's signature on the treatment note and/or progress report.

The progress report provides justification for the medical necessity of treatment. Contractors shall determine the necessity of services based on the delivery of services as directed in the plan and as documented in the treatment notes and progress report. For Medicare payment purposes, information required in progress reports shall be written by a clinician that is, either the physician/non-physician practitioner who provides or supervises the services, or by the therapist who provides the services and supervises an assistant. It is not required that the referring or supervising physician/non-physician practitioner sign the progress reports written by a PT.

The minimum progress report period shall be at least once every 10 treatment days. The first day of the episode of treatment counts as the beginning of the first reporting period, regardless of whether the service provided on that day is an evaluation, re-evaluation or treatment. The next treatment day after the 10th treatment day (or after 30 days from the beginning of the reporting period) begins the next reporting period. The progress report period requirements are complete when both the elements of the progress report and the clinician's active participation in treatment have been documented.

It should be emphasized that the dates for recertification of plans of care do not affect the dates for required progress reports. (Consideration of the case in preparation for a report may lead the therapist to request early recertification. However, each report does not require recertification of the plan, and there may be several reports between recertifications). In many settings, weekly progress reports are voluntarily prepared to review progress, describe the skilled treatment, update goals, and inform physician/non-physician practitioners or other staff. The clinical judgment demonstrated in frequent reports may help justify that the skills of a therapist are being applied, and that services are medically necessary. Particularly where the patient's medical status, or appropriate tapering of frequency due to expected progress towards goals, results in limited frequency e.g., (2-4 times a month), more frequent progress reports can differentiate rehabilitative from maintenance treatment, document progress and justify the continued necessity for skilled care.

Care must be taken to assure that documentation justifies the necessity of the services provided during the reporting period, particularly when reports are written at the minimum frequency. Justification for treatment must include, for example, objective evidence or a clinically supportable statement of expectation that:

- The patient's condition has the potential to improve or is improving in response to therapy.

- Maximum improvement is yet to be attained.

- There is an expectation that the anticipated improvement is attainable in a reasonable and generally predictable period of time.

Objective Evidence

Objective evidence consists of standardized patient assessment instruments, outcome measurement tools or measurable assessments of functional outcome. Use of objective measures at the beginning of treatment, during and/or after treatment is recommended to quantify progress and support justifications for continued treatment. Such tools are not required, but their use will enhance the justification for needed therapy.

Absences

Holidays, sick days or other patient absences may fall within the Progress Report Period. Days on which a patient does not encounter qualified professional or qualified personnel for treatment, evaluation or re-evaluation do not count as treatment days. However, absences do not affect the requirement for a Progress Report at least once during each Progress Report Period. If the patient is absent unexpectedly at the end of the reporting period, when the clinician has not yet provided the required active participation during that reporting period, a Progress Report is still required, but without the clinician's active participation in treatment, the requirements of the Progress Report Period are incomplete.

Delayed Reports

If the clinician has not written a Progress Report before the end of the Progress Reporting Period, it shall be written within 7 calendar days after the end of the reporting period. If the clinician did not participate actively in treatment during the Progress Report Period, documentation of the delayed active participation shall be entered in the Treatment Note as soon as possible. The Treatment Note shall explain the reason for the clinician's missed active participation. Also, the Treatment Note shall document the clinician's guidance to the assistant or qualified personnel to justify that the skills of a therapist were required during the reporting period. It is not necessary to include in this Treatment Note any information already recorded in prior Treatment Notes or Progress Reports.

The contractor shall make a clinical judgment whether continued treatment by assistants or qualified personnel is reasonable and necessary when the clinician has not actively participated in treatment for longer than one reporting period. Judgment shall be based on the individual case and documentation of the application of the clinician's skills to guide the assistant or qualified personnel during and after the reporting period.

Early Reports

Often, Progress Reports are written weekly, or even daily, at the discretion of the clinician. Clinicians are encouraged, but not required, to write Progress Reports more frequently than the minimum required in order to allow anyone who reviews the records to easily determine that the services provided are appropriate, covered and payable.

Elements of Progress Reports may be written in the Treatment Notes if the provider/supplier or clinician prefers. If each element required in a Progress Report is included in the Treatment Notes at least once during the Progress Report Period, then a separate Progress Report is not required. Also, elements of the Progress Report may be incorporated into a revised Plan of Care when one is indicated. Although the Progress Report written by a therapist does not require a physician/non-physician practitioner signature when written as a stand-alone document, the revised Plan of Care accompanied by the Progress Report shall be re-certified by a physician/non-physician practitioner.

Progress Reports for Services Billed Incident to a Physician's Service

The policy for incident to services requires, for example, the physician's initial service, direct supervision of therapy services, and subsequent services of a frequency, which reflects his/her active participation in, and management of the course of treatment. Therefore, supervision and reporting requirements for supervising physician/non-physician practitioners supervising staff are the same as those for PTs supervising PTAs with certain exceptions noted below.

When a therapy service is provided by a therapist, supervised by a physician/non-physician practitioner and billed incident to the services of the physician/non-physician practitioner, the Progress Report shall be written and signed by the therapist who provides the services.

When the services incident to a physician are provided by qualified personnel who are not therapists, the ordering or supervising physician/non-physician practitioner must personally provide at least one treatment session during each Progress Report Period and sign the Progress Report.

Documenting Clinician Participation in Treatment in the Progress Report

Verification of the clinician's required participation in treatment during the Progress Report Period shall be documented by the clinician's signature on the Treatment Note and/or on the progress report. When unexpected discontinuation of treatment occurs, contractors shall not require a clinician's participation in treatment for the incomplete reporting period.

Assistant's Participation in the Progress Report

PTAs may write elements of the Progress Report dated between clinician reports. Reports written by assistants are not complete Progress Reports, but are meant to give supplemental information regarding treatment and progress. The clinician must write a Progress Report during each Progress Report Period regardless of whether the assistant writes other reports. However, reports written by assistants are part of the record and need not be copied into the clinicians report.

Descriptions shall make identifiable reference to the goals in the current plan of care. Since only long-term goals are required in the plan of care, the Progress Report may be used to add, change or delete short-term goals. Assistants may change goals only under the direction of a clinician. When short-term goal changes are dictated to an assistant or to qualified personnel the change, clinician's name and date should be reported. Clinicians verify these changes with co-signatures on the report or in the clinician's Progress Report. The evaluation and plan of care are considered incorporated into the Progress Report, and information in them is not required to be repeated in the report.

Any consistent method of identifying the goals may be used. Preferably, the long-term goals may be numbered (1, 2, 3,) and the short-term goals that relate to the long-term goals may be numbered and lettered 1.A, 1.B, etc. The identifier of a goal on the plan of care may not be changed during the episode of care to which the plan refers. A clinician, an assistant on the order of a therapist or qualified personnel on the order of a physician/non-physician practitioner shall add new goals with new identifiers or letters. Omit reference to a goal after a clinician has reported it to be met, and that clinician's signature verifies the change.

Discharge Notes

Discharge notes are required in progress report format and should be written by the clinician covering the reporting period from the last progress report to the date of discharge. In the case of a discharge anticipated within three treatment days of the progress report, the clinician may provide objective goals that, when met, will authorize the assistant or qualified auxiliary personnel to discharge the patient. In that case, the clinician should verify that the skilled services provided are required prior to discharge. There must be indication that the clinician has reviewed the treatment notes and agrees to the discharge.

In the case of an unanticipated discharge, the clinician may base any judgments required in the report on the treatment notes and verbal reports of the assistant or qualified auxiliary personnel.

A discharge note is required for each episode of treatment and must be written by the clinician. The discharge note may be considered the last opportunity to justify the medical necessity of the entire treatment episode and, as a result, if a discharge summary has been completed, it may be prudent to submit it with any request of records for medical review, even if the claim under review is for a treatment period prior to the date of discharge.

At the discretion of the clinician, the discharge note may include additional information; for example, it may summarize the entire episode of treatment, or justify services that may have extended beyond those usually expected for the patient's condition. Clinicians should consider the discharge note the last opportunity to justify the medical necessity of the entire treatment episode in case the record is reviewed. The record should be reviewed and organized so that the required documentation is ready for presentation to the contractor if requested.

Treatment Notes

The total timed code treatment minutes should reflect actual treatment time. Do not include time for services that are not billable (i.e., calling physician, rest periods, documentation time). Signature and credentials of the treating therapist should be included.

The type of treatment includes the type of therapy discipline operating under this POC (PT) and should describe the types of treatment modalities, procedures or interventions to be provided.

Amount of Treatment: Refers to the number of times in a day the type of treatment will be provided. Where not specified, one treatment session a day is assumed. More than one session per day per discipline will require additional documentation to support this amount of therapy.

Frequency of Treatment: Refers to the number of times in a week that the type of treatment is provided. Treatment more than two or three times a week is expected to be a rare occurrence. Treatment frequency of greater than three times per week requires documentation to support this intensity.

Duration of Treatment: Refers to the number of weeks, or the number of treatment sessions, for this plan of care. Clinicians could also estimate the duration of the entire episode of care in this setting.

Medical record documentation is required for every treatment day and every therapy service to justify the use of codes and units on the claim.

The treatment note must include the following required information:

- Date of treatment.

- Identification of each specific treatment, intervention or activity provided in language that can be compared with the CPT codes to verify correct coding.

- Record of the total time spent in services represented by timed codes under timed code treatment minutes.

- Record of the total treatment time in minutes, which is a sum of the timed and untimed services; signature and credentials of each individual(s) that provided skilled interventions.

In addition, the treatment note may include any information that is relevant in supporting the medical necessity and skilled nature of the treatment, such as:

- Patient comments regarding pain, function, completion of self-management home exercise program (HEP), etc.

- Significant, unusual or unexpected changes in clinical status.

- Parameters of modalities provided and/or specifics regarding exercises such as sets, repetitions, weight, etc.

- Communication/consultation with other providers (e.g., supervising clinician, attending physician, nurse, another therapist).

- Communication with patient, family, caregiver.

If grid or checklist forms are used for daily notes or exercise/activity logs, include the signature and credentials of the qualified professional/auxiliary personnel providing the service each day. Listing of exercise names (e.g., pulleys, UBE, TKE, SLR) does not alone imply that skilled treatment has been provided, especially if the exercises have been performed over multiple sessions. Be sure to occasionally document the skilled components of the exercises so they do not appear repetitive and therefore, unskilled. Documenting functional activities performed (e.g., "ambulated 35 feet with min assist", "upper body dressing with set up and supervision") also does not imply that skilled treatment was provided. The skilled components/techniques of the qualified professional used to improve the functional activity should be occasionally documented to support medical necessity.

When documenting treatment time, consistently use the CMS language of total "Timed Code Treatment Minutes" and "Total Treatment Time." Do not use other language or abbreviations when referring to treatment minutes, as it may be difficult for medical review to determine the type of minutes documented.

Do not record treatment time as "Time in / Time out" for the entire session as this does not accurately reflect the actual treatment time. Do not "round" all treatments to 15-minute increments, but rather record the actual treatment time. Also do not record as "units" of treatment, instead of minutes.

Only "intra-service care" of skilled therapy services should be reflected in the time documentation. Do not include unbillable time, such as time for changing, waiting for treatment to begin, waiting for equipment, resting, toileting, or performing unskilled or independent exercises or activities.

The **Treatment Note** is not required to document the medical necessity or appropriateness of the ongoing therapy services. Descriptions of skilled interventions should be included in the plan or the Progress Reports and are allowed, but not required daily. Non-skilled interventions need not be recorded in the treatment notes as they are not billable. However, notation of non-skilled treatment or report of activities performed by the patient or non-skilled staff may be reported voluntarily as additional information if they are relevant and not billed. Specifics such as number of repetitions of an exercise and other details included in the plan of care need not be repeated in the Treatment Notes unless they are changed from the plan.

Documentation of each **Treatment** shall include the following required elements:

- Date of treatment.

- Identification of each specific intervention/modality provided and billed, for both timed and untimed codes, in language that can be compared with the billing on the claim to verify correct coding. Record each service provided that is represented by a timed code, regardless of whether or not it is billed, because the unbilled timed services may impact the billing.

- Total timed code treatment minutes and total treatment time in minutes. Total treatment time includes the minutes for timed code treatment and untimed code treatment. Total treatment time does not include time for services that are not billable (e.g., rest periods). The billing and the total timed code treatment minutes must be consistent.

- Signature and professional identification of the qualified professional who furnished or supervised the services and a list of each person who contributed to that treatment (i.e., the signature of Kathleen Smith, PTA, with notation of phone consultation with Judy Jones, PT, supervisor, when permitted by state and local law). The signature and identification of the supervisor need not be on each Treatment Note, unless the supervisor actively participated in the treatment. Since a clinician must be identified on the Plan of Care and the Progress Report, the name and professional identification of the supervisor responsible for the treatment is assumed to be the clinician who wrote the plan or report. When the treatment is supervised without active participation by the supervisor, the supervisor is not required to cosign the Treatment Note written by a qualified professional. When the responsible supervisor is absent, the presence of a similarly qualified supervisor on the clinic roster for that day is sufficient documentation and it is not required that the substitute supervisor sign or be identified in the documentation.

If a treatment is added or changed under the direction of a clinician during the treatment days between the Progress Reports, the change must be recorded and justified on the medical record, either in the Treatment Note or the Progress Report, as determined by the policies of the provider/supplier. New exercises added or changes made to the exercise program help justify that the services are skilled. For example: The original plan was for therapeutic activities, gait training and neuromuscular re-education. "On Feb. 1 clinician added electrical stimulation to address shoulder pain."

Documentation of each treatment may also include the following optional elements to be mentioned only if the qualified professional recording the note determines they are appropriate and relevant. If these are not recorded daily, any relevant information should be included in the progress report.

- Patient self-report.

- Adverse reaction to intervention.

- Communication/consultation with other providers (e.g., supervising clinician, attending physician, nurse, another therapist, etc.).

- Significant, unusual or unexpected changes in clinical status.

When indicating precautions, you have to be clear, accurate, and specific. This is to inform other medical practitioners of the risks and things they have to avoid or provide to the patient. If precautions are not clearly stated, or misunderstood by other practitioners, it may cause harm to the patient and damage your facility's reputation as well (Shamus & Stern, 2004). The following are some examples of precautions you have to take and indicate in the patient's medical records:

- Aspiration precautions: honey, nectar liquids, no straws, NPO, mechanical soft diet, pudding, puree diet, swallow precautions.

- Cardiac: Hypertension, orthostatic hypotension.

- Compromised respiratory status: O2 dependent, O2 prn.

- Contact precautions: Methicillin-resistant Staphylococcus aureus (MRSA), Clostridium difficile (C-diff), Vancomycin-resistant Enterococcus (VRE).

- Diabetic precautions.

- Equipment/ Lines: NG tube, PEG (Percutaneous Endoscopic Gastrostomy) tube, Foley catheter, Restraints.

- Fall risk.

- Low vision.

- Risk for dehydration.

- Skin integrity.

- Surgical precautions: Back, Cervical, Cardiac, Total hip, Total knee, Shoulder precautions, Sternal precautions.

- Weight bearing status: None weight bearing, partial weight bearing, Toe Touch weight bearing, and weight bearing as tolerated.

- Wounds.

Describing Pain

Pain has no definite description in coding. A narrative report about the description of pain will be of great help to get a clear picture of what kind of pain afflicts the patient. The following are some descriptive words that are associated with pain: aching, burning, cramping, discomforting, distressing, dull, exhausting, excruciating, gnawing, sharp, shooting, and stabbing.

Justification for Skilled Services

Providing patients with skilled services of a physical therapist needs to be justified for medical necessity. The following are some medically necessary reasons why a patient needs a therapist's service:

- To administer physical agent modalities.

- To instruct in home exercise program.

- To assess functional abilities; to assess need for environmental adaptations.

- To develop rehabilitation nursing program or functional maintenance program.

- To fabricate a splint; to instruct in compensatory strategies.

- To evaluate need for assistive device; facilitate independence with gait.

- To facilitate independence with transfers.

- To facilitate coordination.

- To teach compensatory/adaptation techniques.

- To teach energy conservation techniques.

Risk Factors

Risks serve as a warning for any impending worse situation. Indicate if the patient is at risk of the following:

- Compromised general health, contracture.

- Decreased circulatory function.

- Decrease in level of mobility.

- Decreased participation with functional tasks.

- Decreased skin integrity.

- Depression.

- Dehydration.

- Falls.

- Decline in function.

- Malnutrition.

- Pneumonia.

- Pressure sores.

- Social isolation.

- Weight loss.

Documenting a Patient's Potential for Rehabilitation

Another factor in proving the medical necessity of skilled services is the rehabilitation potential of a patient. There must be a justifiable reason why a patient is provided with skilled services. The reason may include the patient's demonstration of the following:

- Ability to follow multi-step directions.

- Ability to learn new information.

- Active participation in skilled treatment.

- Compliance with skilled training.

- High cognitive functioning.

- High prior level of function.

- Insight regarding functional deficits and recent onset of the condition.

Creating Goals

To make it simple, goals should be measurable, have a specific time frame, and be functional. The appropriateness of goals must always be considered because it can cause denials when the claim for a service is submitted. Goals are always patient-centered and usually begin with "Patient will..." There are two types of goals: the long-term goal and the short-term goal. The long-term goals reflect the functional outcome at the end of therapy treatments. If the goal established is not suitable for the condition of the patient, reimbursements can be denied.

Here are some goals to use for balance and transfers:

Example: Patient will improve standing balance to (grade):

- In order to reduce the risk for falls.

- Facilitate upright posture.

- Safely shift weight to opposite lower extremity.

- Prepare for transfers.

- Participate in edge of bed activities.

- Ambulate without restrictions.

- Increase participation with functional tasks of choice and decrease dependency on caregivers during functional tasks.

Here are some goals you can use for rest periods:

Example: Patient will transfer from bed to wheelchair (assistance) with (number of rest periods):

- For push up from arms of chair.

- For use of energy conservation techniques.

- For use of grab bars.

- For maintain upright sitting.

- For use of compensatory strategies due to proprioception impairments.

- For compensatory strategies due to language impairments and for compensatory tech due to cognitive-communicative impairments.

Here are some bed mobility goals:

Example: Patient will roll to the left (assistance):

- Using side rails in order to decrease risk for skin breakdown.

- To prepare for use of bedpan.

- To increase ability to pull garments up over hips.

- To participate in edge of bed activities.

- To prepare for transfers.

- To get in/out of bed.

- Interaction opportunities in environment.

- Enhance safe functional mobility and reduce risk for falls.

Here some examples to add a skilled component to transfers and ambulation goals:

Example: Patient will ambulate with a rolling walker (assistance):

- Without signs and symptoms of medical complications.

- Without signs and symptoms of physical exertion.

- With stable vital signs.

- While maintaining oxygen saturation > 98%.

- Without falls.

- Without shortness of breath.

- Without loss of balance.

- With implementation of compensatory strategies and in response to environmental modifications.

Here are examples of different conditions to use for ambulation:

- On level surfaces.

- On level and uneven surfaces.

- Outdoors.

- With ad lib conditions within facility.

- Throughout nursing facility.

- Under high attention demand situations.

Here are more examples of goals:

Activity tolerance (includes sitting and standing tolerance):

The patient will increase upright sitting tolerance in the chair to (5) minutes (moderate) assistance while maintaining proper positioning to increase upper body trunk strength, sitting tolerance, and to increase interaction in his/her environment.

Adaptive equipment:

The patient will effectively utilize adaptive equipment to complete (tasks) with (minimal) assistance.

Ambulation (includes stair negotiation; specify deviations and assistive device):

The patient will negotiate (5) steps with (1) handrail (contact guard) assist.

The patient will ambulate (10) feet safely with (rolling walker) (moderate) assistance on (level surfaces) in order to (skilled need).

Balance (includes sitting and standing balance):

The patient will increase sitting balance to (balance grade) and tolerate for (number) minutes to (skilled need).

The patient will increase the Tinetti balance score to (increments 1) /16 and the gait score to (increments 1) /12 for a total balance and gait score of (increments 1), relating to the (Tinetti score risk) fall risk category, due to improvement in (specifics), which will decrease risk for falls and improve functional mobility.

Bed mobility includes rolling and supine <-> sit:

The patient will safely roll (moderate) assistance in order to (skilled need).

Incontinence:

The patient will have a reduction in episodes of urinary incontinence to (increments 1) per day to increase safety and reduce risk of (risk area).

Pain:

The patient will have decreased pain in (location) to in order to perform (functional task). (pain scale) /10 in order to perform (functional task).

Positioning:

The patient will demonstrate optimal positioning of (body areas) in (position and space) in order to achieve (functional activity) or in order to reduce pressure areas and reduce risk for skin breakdown.

ROM:

The patient will (change) (rom) of (extremities) (joint & movement) to (degrees) to (degrees) to achieve functional range of motion for daily living.

Strength:

The patient will improve muscle strength to (grade) of (joint and movement) in order to (functional need).

The patient will increase (extremities) (which finger) pinch strength to (increments 1) pounds(s) in order to (UE targets).

Toileting:

The patient will achieve balance on toilet/commode to complete toilet hygiene and clothing management utilizing (ADL device) increasing to (level of assistance) (initiation cue) (percent) (verbal cueing).

Transfer: includes bathing prep, bathing, bed<>wheelchair, sit <> stand, toilet

The patient will perform (transfers) transfers increasing to (level of assistance) (initiation cue) (percent) (verbal cueing) in order to (functional task).

Wheelchair mobility (include distance, surfaces):

The patient will efficiently propel wheelchair (feet) (locations) using (extremities) increasing to (level of assistance) (initiation cue) (percent) (verbal cueing) to increase independence in environment.

Wound care (include stage of pressure ulcer and location):

The patient will show increased healing of (location) (wound type) measuring (cm) cm(s) length by (cm) cm(s) width with an area of (area cm) cm(s) 2 by (cm) cm(s) depth by (wound treatment) in order to decrease pain and increase (tasks). Wound site characteristics include (wound bed description), (wound color), (wound drainage), and (wound tissue type).

The patient will demonstrate healing of (location) wound to (wound stage) in order to allow for improved skin integrity and reduce risk of (risk).

Plan of Care

The evaluation and plan may be reported in two separate documents or a single combined document.

The services must relate directly and specifically to a written treatment plan. The plan (also known as a plan of care or plan of treatment) must be established before treatment is begun. The plan is established when it is developed (e.g., written or dictated).

The signature and professional identity of the person who established the plan, and the date it was established must be recorded with the plan. Establishing the plan, which is described below, is not the same as certifying the plan.

Outpatient therapy services shall be furnished under a plan established by:

- A physician/non-physician practitioner (consultation with the treating physical therapist is recommended.

- The physical therapist that will provide the physical therapy services.

The plan may be entered into the patient's therapy record either by the person who established the plan or by the provider's or supplier's staff when they make a written record of that person's oral orders before treatment is begun.

Treatment under a Plan

The evaluation and treatment may occur and are both billable either on the same day or at subsequent visits. It is appropriate that treatment begins when a plan is established. Therapy may be initiated by qualified professionals or qualified personnel based on a dictated plan. Treatment may begin before the plan is committed to writing only if the treatment is performed or supervised by the same qualified clinician who establishes the plan. Payment for services provided before a plan is established may be denied.

Two Plans

It is acceptable to treat with two separate plans of care when different physicians/non-physician practitioners refer a patient for different conditions. It is also acceptable to combine the plans of care into one plan covering both conditions if one or the other referring physician/non-physician practitioner is willing to certify the plan for both conditions. The Treatment Notes continue to require timed code treatment minutes and total treatment time and need not be separated by plan. Progress Reports should be combined if it is possible to make clear that the goals for each plan are addressed. Separate Progress Reports referencing each plan of care may also be written, at the discretion of the treating clinician, or at the request of the certifying physician/non-physician practitioner, but shall not be required by contractors.

Contents of Plan

The plan of care shall contain, at minimum, the following information as required:

- Diagnoses.
- Long-term treatment goals.
- Type, amount, duration and frequency of therapy services.

The plan of care shall be consistent with the related evaluation, which may be attached and is considered incorporated into the plan. The plan should strive to provide treatment in the most efficient and effective manner, balancing the best achievable outcome with the appropriate resources.

Long-term treatment goals should be developed for the entire episode of care in the current setting. When the episode is anticipated to be long enough to require more than one certification, the long-term goals may be specific to the part of the episode that is being certified. Goals should be measurable and pertain to identified functional impairments. When episodes in the setting are short, measurable goals may not be achievable; documentation should state the clinical reasons progress couldn't be shown.

The type of treatment is physical therapy, or, where appropriate, the type may be a description of a specific treatment or intervention. For example, when there is a single evaluation service, but the type is not specified, the type is assumed to be consistent with the therapy discipline (physical therapy) ordered, or of the therapist who provided the evaluation. When a physician/non-physician practitioner establishes a plan, the plan must specify the type (physical therapy) of therapy planned.

There shall be different plans of care for each type of therapy discipline. When more than one discipline is treating a patient, each must establish a diagnosis, goals, etc., independently. However, the form of the plan and the number of plans incorporated into one document are not limited as long as the required information is present and related to each discipline separately. For example, a physical therapist may not provide services under an occupational therapist plan of care. However, both may be treating the patient for the same condition at different times in the same day for goals consistent with their own scope of practice.

The frequency refers to the number of times in a week the type of treatment is provided. When frequency is not specified, one treatment is assumed. If a scheduled holiday occurs on a treatment day that is part of the plan, it is appropriate to omit that treatment day unless the clinician who is responsible for writing progress reports determines that a brief, temporary pause in the delivery of therapy services would adversely affect the patient's condition.

The duration is the number of weeks, or the number of treatment sessions, for this plan of care. If the episode of care is anticipated to extend beyond the 90-calendar day limit for certification of a plan, it is desirable, although not required, that the clinician also estimate the duration of the entire episode of care in this setting.

It may be appropriate for therapists to taper the frequency of visits as the patient progresses toward an independent or caregiver-assisted self-management program with the intent of improving outcomes and limiting treatment time. For example, treatment may be provided three times a week for two weeks, then two times a week for the next two weeks, then once a week for the last two weeks. Depending on the individual's condition, such treatment may result in better outcomes, or may result in earlier discharge than routine treatment three times a week for four weeks.

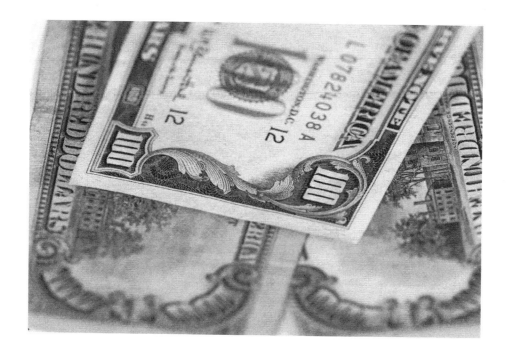

Starting your Own Practice from Scratch

When tapered frequency is planned, the exact number of treatments per frequency level is not required to be projected in the plan, because the changes should be made based on assessment of daily progress. Instead, the beginning and end frequencies shall be planned. For example, amount, frequency and duration may be documented as "once daily, three times a week, tapered to once a week over six weeks". Changes to the frequency may be made based on the clinicians clinical judgment and do not require recertification of the plan unless requested by the physician/non-physician practitioner. The clinician should consider any comorbidity, tissue healing, the ability of the patient and/or caregiver to do more independent self-management as treatment progresses, and any other factors related to frequency and duration of treatment.

Changes to the Therapy Plan

Changes are made in writing in the patient's record and signed by one of the following professionals responsible for the patient's care:

- The physician/non-physician practitioner.

- The qualified physical therapist (in the case of physical therapy).

- The registered professional nurse or physician/non-physician practitioner on the staff of the facility pursuant to the oral orders of the physician/non-physician practitioner or therapist.

While the physician/non-physician practitioner may change a plan of treatment established by the therapist providing such services, the therapist may not significantly alter a plan of treatment established or certified by a physician/non-physician practitioner without their documented written or verbal approval. A change in long-term goals (for example, if a new condition was to be treated) would be a significant change. Physician/non-physician practitioner certification of the significantly modified plan of care shall be obtained within 30 days of the initial therapy treatment under the revised plan.

A treatment plan or plan of care must contain session notes, frequency, duration, diagnosis, long-term treatment goals, and date of treatment. Identify each specific intervention in language that can be compared with current procedural terminology (CPT) codes. Record each service provided that is represented by a timed code, regardless of whether or not it is billed.

4
CHAPTER

ICD-9-CM/ICD-10-CM AND CPT CODES

An attempt to classify diseases dates back to as early as 1785 and was originally implemented to categorize causes of death. Over the years, revisions and updates to the original list of diseases and causes of death evolved. In 1948, during the sixth revision, the World Health Organization (WHO) incorporated an International Classification into the *Manual of the International Statistical Classification of Diseases, Injuries, and Causes of Death*. In 1975, the ninth revision of the ICD was established for worldwide use. http://www.who.int/classifications/icd/en/HistoryOfICD.pdf

In 1979, the United States developed the International Classification of Diseases Clinical Modification (ICD-9-CM) for surgical, diagnostic, and therapeutic procedures. ICD-9-CM assigns codes to diagnoses and procedures in the United States associated with hospital utilization. As of 1999, the ICD-10 replaced the ICD-9 to code mortality data from death certificates, but ICD-9-CM is still in place, for now. The Centers for Medicare and Medicaid Services and the National Center for Health Statistics (NCHS) oversee any changes to the ICD-9-CM. ICD - ICD-9-CM - International Classification of Diseases, Ninth Revision, Clinical Modification

When a patient comes to physical therapy with a prescription from the doctor, the diagnosis given by the doctor is accompanied by a code that represents that diagnosis. The code is currently the ICD-9-CM, but as of October 1, 2015, it will need to be the ICD-10-CM. According to the Centers for Disease Control and Prevention, the ICD-10-CM will provide the following benefits:

- addition of information regarding ambulatory and managed care encounters

- expansion of injury codes

- creation of combination diagnosis/symptom codes to reduce the number of codes needed to accurately describe a condition

- addition of sixth and seventh characters

- incorporation of common 4th and 5th digit sub-classifications

- laterality

- increased specificity in code assignment ICD - ICD-10-CM - International Classification of Diseases, Tenth Revision, Clinical Modification

A presentation from the APTA Learning Center from March 27, 2014, discusses the integration of the ICD-10-CM codes. A summary of the chart from this presentation for understanding the difference between the ICD-9 codes and the updated ICD-10 codes follows:

- The ICD-9 codes have 3 to 5 digits; ICD-10 have 3 to 7 digits

- The ICD-9 codes have Alpha "E" and "V" on first character; ICD-10 have alpha or numeric character for any

- The ICD-9 codes have no place holder characters; ICD-10 have place holder characters

- The ICD-9 codes have limited severity parameters; ICD-10 have extensive severity parameters

- The ICD-9 codes have 14,000 codes; ICD-10 have 69,000 codes

- The ICD-9 codes have limited combination codes; ICD-10 combination codes are common

- The format of the code sets is similar for ICD-9 and ICD-10

The www.CMS.gov/ICD10 website has a wealth of up-to-date information on ICD-10 as the newest implementation date approaches. Providers, payers, and all groups under the Health Insurance Portability and Accountability Act (HIPAA) will be affected by the change. The advice given for medical practice regarding ICD-10 is summarized as follows:

- Identify where ICD-9 is currently used in your practice (documentation, superbills, practice management system, electronic medical record system, etc.), because ICD-10 codes will be replacing them.

- Discuss with your practice management system vendor how they plan to implement the ICD-10 codes. Make sure your system is upgraded to 5010 standards. Find out what updates are to be made to your practice management system and when they will be installed (and ask if upgrades are included in your contract agreement). Make sure any new system you may soon purchase is prepared for ICD-10.

- Know the plan for ICD-10 implementation plans regarding your clearinghouses, billing services, and payers for a seamless transition.

- Find out if your payers will be changing contracts, payment schedules, or reimbursement because of the implementation of the more specific ICD-10 codes. Identify what may have to change regarding business processes and clinical documentation.

- Know which members of your staff need to undergo training to learn the nuances of ICD-10 codes. Identify the resources around for training, possibly from other local healthcare providers. Training is recommended 6 months before the ICD-10 compliance deadline.

- Set a new budget for time and costs to implement ICD-10, including expenses for staff training and resource materials, any system changes, and costs of any software updates or fabrication of new superbills.

- Perform test transactions with ICD-10 codes with your payers and clearinghouses to make sure they are actually being transmitted and received by your payers and billing service or clearinghouse.

The suggestions listed above also apply to those physical therapists working in small and rural practices. An essential step in the transition to using ICD-10-CM is identifying where ICD-9-CM codes are currently used in practice, whether on paper or in electronic medical records. Forms need to be changed and systems need to be updated appropriately and in a timely matter in order to support the submission of documentation and billing claims. Training staff members on the ICD-10-CM coding before transition is a worthwhile effort in the long run.

ICD codes (International Statistical Classification of Diseases and Related Health Problems) classify and categorize diseases, injuries, or conditions along with its signs, symptoms, implications, and external causes of injury and disease. This system enables every health condition to be assigned with a unique code under a unique category. The World Health Organization published the International Classification of Diseases, which is specially used for reimbursements systems for its high level of specificity. These codes are also used for the uniform collection, processing, classification, and presentation of statistics (Centers for Medicare and Medicaid, 2012).

Codes are being updated from time to time, and a coder must be informed immediately of these significant changes. The diagnosis information on therapy claims is poor. Thus, for example, the most common therapy code used for PT services is HCPCS code V57.1, which stands for encounter for physical therapy. Other top diagnoses are often vague or describe the location of pain, such as pain in shoulder (HCPCS code 719.41) and pain in limb (HCPCS code 729.5), as opposed to the patient's diagnosis. The poor state of diagnoses coding limits the development of a classification system and a risk adjustment methodology needed to establish a prospective payment system for these services.

Another problem with the diagnosis coding is that although a single claim may include more than one type of therapy furnished during the visit, providers are not required to list separate diagnoses for each service rendered. As a result, the diagnoses associated with OT and SLP are more likely to describe the condition motivating PT service use, the more frequently provided service. For example, "abnormality of gait" is a common diagnosis for beneficiaries receiving SLP services (American Physical Therapy Association, 2003).

With these limitations in mind, six of the top ten diagnoses for patients receiving PT services were musculoskeletal-related. Among OT users, stroke was the most frequent diagnosis, though it accounted for only 4% of OT claims. In contrast, SLP diagnoses were more concentrated—28% of claims were for patients with swallowing disorders (Ciolek & Hwang, 2004).

The sequential order when coding ICD-9 codes is most important. ICD-9 codes don't differentiate between medical diagnosis and treatment diagnosis. The highest level of specificity is needed in coding to avoid denials. ICD-9 codes all begin with three digits, usually an alphanumeric combination, or just numeric. Behind a decimal point, there will be a fourth or fifth digit, whenever necessary.

Basic Guidelines in Using ICD-9 codes

Appropriate codes should be indicated on the claim form based on the ICD-9-CM code range 001.0 through V82.9 for the identification of conditions, diagnoses, symptoms, and any other reason for providing the procedure or service. Codes 001.0–999.9 are used to classify diseases and injuries. Codes describing symptoms must be supported by a physician's documentation with the highest level of diagnostic certainty. V-codes 01.0 to 82.9 are for circumstances other than disease or injury.

The "first listed diagnosis" is the primary diagnosis. The "highest level of specificity" is needed to list ICD-9 codes. If there is no five-digit sub-classification for a category, three or four digits can be used. Codes with insufficient digits can cause a claim's denial.

V codes are used when there are circumstances that have to be identified caused by any reason other than illness or injury (i.e., immunization). V codes are also utilized to cite problems and factors that may affect the patient care. For example, an individual diagnosed with a disease, condition or injury, regardless of its status (current or resolving) receives chemotherapy for a malignant tumor from a healthcare facility. Another example is when an individual has an allergy—this problem is not an illness or injury.

V codes can be categorized as: Problems, Services, or Factual, based on the circumstances mentioned earlier. V codes can also be classified as History Codes, Status Codes, Aftercare Visit Codes and Follow up Codes. V codes can be used as a principal code and a secondary code. If coding a complication, instead of using V codes, codes under categories 001–799 must be used.

E codes describe and classify environmental factors and circumstances that caused an injury, poisoning and other negative side effects. ICD codes under 001–999 classification can be assigned with an appropriate E code that specifies any external cause of an injury or a condition. E codes cannot stand alone; therefore, they should not be used as principal diagnostic codes. Since details of an accident are signified by E codes, insurance companies can issue faster reimbursements.

Other terms that maybe encountered when using ICD-9 codes are:

Not Otherwise Specified (NOS). There is a lack of detail in the diagnosis statement, and cannot be assigned with a more specific subdivision.

Not Elsewhere Classified (NEC). This term is used to alarm the coder that a specific form of a condition was classified differently.

Coding Guidelines

A medical diagnosis is one of the most important factors looked for when billing a patient for physical therapy services. When a valid medical diagnosis is made and attached to the billing documents, payment processing becomes much easier. Accomplishing forms such as billing, especially those that pertains to services rendered by physical therapists, needs to follow the Guide to Physical Therapist Practice Patient/Client Management Model (American Physical Therapy Association, 2014).

The ICD-10-CM code for billing, which is used in most health care institutions, has proven to be a challenging tool to use. When using this guideline, the biller should know the most accurate definition of the medical condition that the patient comes seeking treatment for based on the signs and symptoms they present with upon entering a facility. This means that there is a possibility that when a patient presents with more than one health problem, there is a need to accurately list the symptoms related to each one and the appropriate treatment for each listed diagnosis (CMS, 2014).

Physical therapy services have been using billing codes for payments, but more importantly, this is also done for easier data management as well. When services rendered by physical therapists are billed, observance of the ICD-10-CM requires practitioners to include the exact medical diagnosis that required physical therapy interventions (Centers for Medicare and Medicaid Service, 2010). This would entail the physical therapist to identify the diagnosis as either a primary problem, an acquired impairment or a complication of the condition (Guide to Physical Therapy Practice, 2014).

In the goal of conforming to the guidelines of the ICD-10-CM, several practitioners have been lodging their queries with the APTA (American Physical Therapy Association). Most of these queries include asking for reasons why their claims for payments are being rejected by the HMOs. According to the CMS (2014), one of the primary reasons for underpayment or non-payment for physical therapy bills is the use of an invalid coding pursuant to the ICD-10-CM. Although not a major issue at the moment, it will be worth noting that the use of codes would have to be mastered by billers and practitioners. Starting October of 2015, billing that does not conform to the ICD-10-CM guidelines may have a hard time collecting for payments, or worse, may not be paid their dues (CMS, 2014; APTA, 2014). The implication of this would be to enforce among physical therapists the need to know which specific codes to use in billing for services in line with a valid medical diagnosis.

Transitioning to the ICD-10 Codes

The ICD-9 code sets used to report medical diagnoses and inpatient procedures will be replaced by ICD-10 code sets by October 1, 2015.

ICD-10 ICD-10-CM/PCS (International Classification of Diseases, 10th Edition, Clinical Modification /Procedure Coding System) consists of two parts:

1. ICD 10 CM for diagnosis coding

2. ICD-10-PCS for inpatient procedure coding ICD-10-CM is for use in all U.S. health care settings.

Diagnosis coding under ICD-10-CM uses three to seven digits instead of the three to five digits used with ICD-9-CM, but the format of the code sets is similar. ICD-10-PCS is for use in U.S. inpatient hospital settings only. ICD-10 PCS uses seven alphanumeric digits instead of the three or four numeric digits used under ICD-9-CM procedure coding. Coding under ICD-10-PCS is much more specific and substantially different from ICD-9-CM procedure coding. The transition to ICD-10 is occurring because ICD-9 produces limited data about patients' medical conditions and hospital inpatient procedures. ICD-9 is 30 years old, has outdated terms, and is inconsistent with current medical practice. Also, the structure of ICD-9 limits the number of new codes that can be created, and many ICD-9 categories are full. ICD-10 will affect diagnosis and inpatient procedure coding for everyone covered by Health Insurance Portability Accountability Act (HIPAA), not just those who submit Medicare or Medicaid claims. The change to ICD-10 does not affect CPT coding for outpatient procedures. Health care providers, payers, clearinghouses, and billing services must be prepared to comply with the transition to ICD-10, which means: All electronic transactions must use Version 5010 standards, which have been required since January 1, 2012. Unlike the older Version 4010/4010A standards, Version 5010 accommodates ICD-10 codes. ICD-10 diagnosis codes must be used for all health care services provided in the U.S., and ICD-10 procedure codes must be used for all hospital inpatient procedures. Claims with ICD-9 codes for services provided on or after the compliance deadline cannot be paid.

It is important to prepare now for the ICD-10 transition. The following are steps you can take to get started: Providers: Develop an implementation strategy that includes an assessment of the impact on your organization, a detailed timeline, and budget. Check with your billing service, clearinghouse, or practice management software vendor about their compliance plans. Providers who handle billing and software development internally should plan for medical records/coding, clinical, IT, and finance staff to coordinate on ICD-10 transition efforts. Review payment policies since the transition to ICD-10 will involve new coding rules.

Sample Documentation Requirements for Fractures of the Radius	Documentation Requirements
Fracture Type	Open Closed Pathologic Physeal (Growth Plate) Fractures Neoplastic Disease Torus (Buckle) Fractures Green Stick Fractures Stress Fractures Orthopedic Implant (fractures associated with) Bent Bone
Healing	Routine Delayed Nonunion Malunion
Localization	Shaft Lower End Upper End Head Neck Styloid Process
Encounter	Initial Subsequent Sequelae
Displacement	Displaced Non-displaced
Classification	Salter Harris I Salter Harris II Salter Harris III Salter Harris IV Gustilo Type I or II Gustilo Type IIIA, IIIB, or IIIC
Laterality	Right Left Unspecified Side Unilateral Bilateral
Joint Involvement	Intra-articular Extra-articular
Fracture Pattern	Transverse Oblique Spiral Comminuted (many pieces) Segmental
Named Fractures	Colles' Galleazzi's Barton's Smith's

The Centers for Medicare and Medicaid Services (CMS) and the National Center for Health Statistics (NCHS) provide the following guidelines for coding and reporting using the International Classification of Diseases, 10th Revision, Clinical Modification (ICD-10-CM). These guidelines should be used as a companion document to the official version of the ICD-10-CM as published on the NCHS website.

Adherence to these guidelines when assigning ICD-10-CM diagnosis codes is required under the Health Insurance Portability and Accountability Act (HIPAA). The diagnosis codes (Tabular List and Alphabetic Index) have been adopted under HIPAA for all healthcare settings. A joint effort between the healthcare provider and the coder is essential to achieve complete and accurate documentation, code assignment, and reporting of diagnoses and procedures. These guidelines have been developed to assist both the healthcare provider and the coder in identifying those diagnoses and procedures that are to be reported. The importance of consistent, complete documentation in the medical record cannot be overemphasized. Without such documentation accurate coding cannot be achieved. The entire record should be reviewed to determine the specific reason for the encounter and the conditions treated.

These guidelines are not intended to replace any guidelines in the main body of the ICD-10-CM Official Guidelines for Coding and Reporting.

All claims involving inpatient admissions to general acute care hospitals or other facilities are subject to a law or regulation mandating collection of present on admission information.

1. The Alphabetic Index and Tabular List

   The ICD-10-CM is divided into the Alphabetic Index, an alphabetical list of terms and their corresponding code, and the Tabular List, a chronological list of codes divided into chapters based on body system or condition. The Alphabetic Index consists of the following parts: the Index of Diseases and Injury, the Index of External Causes of Injury, the Table of Neoplasms and the Table of Drugs and Chemicals.

2. Format and Structure:

   The ICD-10-CM Tabular List contains categories, subcategories and codes. Characters for categories, subcategories and codes may be either a letter or a number. All categories are three characters. A three-character category that has no further subdivision is equivalent to a code. Subcategories are either four or five characters. Codes may be three, four, five, six or seven characters. That is, each level of subdivision after a category is a subcategory. The final level of subdivision is a code. Codes that have applicable seventh characters are still referred to as codes, not subcategories. A code that has an applicable seventh character is considered invalid without the seventh character.

3. Use of codes for reporting purposes

   For reporting purposes only codes are permissible, not categories or subcategories, and any applicable seventh character is required.

4. Placeholder character

   The ICD-10-CM utilizes a placeholder character "X". The "X" is used as a placeholder at certain codes to allow for future expansion.

5. Seventh Characters

   Certain ICD-10-CM categories have applicable seventh characters. The applicable seventh character is required for all codes within the category, or as the notes in the Tabular List instruct. The seventh character must always be the seventh character in the data field. If a code that requires a seventh character is not six characters, a placeholder X must be used to fill in the empty characters.

6. Abbreviations

    a. Alphabetic Index abbreviations

    NEC "Not elsewhere classifiable"

    This abbreviation in the Alphabetic Index represents "other specified". When a specific code is not available for a condition, the Alphabetic Index directs the coder to the "other specified" code in the Tabular List.

    NOS "Not otherwise specified"

    This abbreviation is the equivalent of unspecified.

    b. Tabular List abbreviations

    NEC "Not elsewhere classifiable"

    This abbreviation in the Tabular List represents "other specified". When a specific code is not available for a condition the Tabular List includes an NEC entry under a code to identify the code as the "other specified" code.

    NOS "Not otherwise specified"

    This abbreviation is the equivalent of unspecified.

7. Punctuation

    [ ] Brackets are used in the Tabular List to enclose synonyms, alternative wording or explanatory phrases. Brackets are used in the Alphabetic Index to identify manifestation codes.

    () Parentheses are used in both the Alphabetic Index and Tabular List to enclose supplementary words that may be present or absent in the statement of a disease or procedure without affecting the code number to which it is assigned. The terms within the parentheses are referred to as nonessential modifiers.

    : Colons are used in the Tabular List after an incomplete term which needs one or more of the modifiers following the colon to make it assignable to a given category.

8. Use of "and"

    When the term "and" is used in a narrative statement it represents and/or.

9. Other and Unspecified codes

   a. "Other" codes

   Codes titled "other" or "other specified" are for use when the information in the medical record provides detail for which a specific code does not exist. Alphabetic Index entries with NEC in the line designate "other" codes in the Tabular List. These Alphabetic Index entries represent specific disease entities for which no specific code exists so the term is included within an "other" code.

   b. "Unspecified" codes

   Codes titled "unspecified" are for use when the information in the medical record is insufficient to assign a more specific code. For those categories for which an unspecified code is not provided, the "other specified" code may represent both other and unspecified.

10. Etiology/manifestation convention ("code first", "use additional code" and "in diseases classified elsewhere" notes)

    Certain conditions have both an underlying etiology and multiple body system manifestations due to the underlying etiology. For such conditions, the ICD-10-CM has a coding convention that requires the underlying condition be sequenced first followed by the manifestation. Wherever such a combination exists, there is a "use additional code" note at the etiology code, and a "code first" note at the manifestation code.

    In most cases the manifestation codes will have in the code title, "in diseases classified elsewhere." "In diseases classified elsewhere" codes are never permitted to be used as first-listed or principal diagnosis codes. They must be used in conjunction with an underlying condition code and they must be listed following the underlying condition. Dementia in other diseases classified elsewhere, is an example of this convention.

There are manifestation codes that do not have "in diseases classified elsewhere" in the title. For such codes a "use additional code" note will still be present and the rules for sequencing apply.

In the Alphabetic Index both conditions are listed together with the etiology code first followed by the manifestation codes in brackets. The code in brackets is always to be sequenced second.

An example of the etiology/manifestation convention is dementia in Parkinson's disease. In the Alphabetic Index, code G20 is listed first, followed by code F02.80 or F02.81 in brackets. Code G20 represents the underlying etiology, Parkinson's disease, and must be sequenced first, whereas codes F02.80 and F02.81 represent the manifestation of dementia in diseases classified elsewhere, with or without behavioral disturbance.

"Code first" and "Use additional code" notes are also used as sequencing rules in the classification for certain codes that are not part of an etiology/ manifestation combination.

General Coding Guidelines

1. Locating a code in the ICD-10-CM

   The Alphabetic Index does not always provide the full code. Selection of the full code, including laterality and any applicable seventh character can only be done in the Tabular List. A dash (-) at the end of an Alphabetic Index entry indicates that additional characters are required.

2. Level of Detail in Coding

   Diagnosis codes are to be used and reported at their highest number of characters available. ICD-10-CM diagnosis codes are composed of codes with three, four, five, six or seven characters. Codes with three characters are included in ICD-10-CM as the heading of a category of codes that may be further subdivided by the use of fourth and/or fifth characters and/or sixth characters, which provide greater detail.

   A three-character code is to be used only if it is not further subdivided. A code is invalid if it has not been coded to the full number of characters required for that code, including the seventh character, if applicable.

3. Code or codes from A00.0 through T88.9, Z00-Z99.8

   The appropriate code or codes from A00.0 through T88.9, Z00-Z99.8 must be used to identify diagnoses, symptoms, conditions, problems, complaints or other reason(s) for the encounter/visit.

4. Signs and symptoms

   Codes that describe symptoms and signs, as opposed to diagnoses, are acceptable for reporting purposes when a related definitive diagnosis has not been established (confirmed) by the provider.

5. Conditions that are an integral part of a disease process

   Signs and symptoms that are associated routinely with a disease process should not be assigned as additional codes, unless otherwise instructed by the classification.

6. Conditions that are not an integral part of a disease process

   Additional signs and symptoms that may not be associated routinely with a disease process should be coded when present.

7. Multiple coding for a single condition.

   In addition to the etiology/manifestation convention that requires two codes to fully describe a single condition that affects multiple body systems, there are other single conditions that also require more than one code. "Use additional code" when a secondary code is useful to fully describe a condition. The sequencing rule is the same as the etiology/manifestation pair.

"Code first" notes are also under certain codes that are not specifically manifestation codes but may be due to an underlying cause. When there is a "code first" note and an underlying condition is present, the underlying condition should be sequenced first.

"Code, if applicable, any causal condition first", notes indicate that this code may be assigned as a principal diagnosis when the causal condition is unknown or not applicable. If a causal condition is known, then the code for that condition should be sequenced as the principal or first-listed diagnosis.

Multiple codes may be needed for late effects, complication codes and obstetric codes to more fully describe a condition. See the specific guidelines for these conditions for further instruction.

8. Acute and Chronic Conditions

If the same condition is described as both acute (subacute) and chronic, and separate subentries exist in the Alphabetic Index at the same indentation level, code both and sequence the acute (subacute) code first.

9. Combination Code

A combination code is a single code used to classify:

Two diagnoses, or

A diagnosis with an associated secondary process (manifestation)

A diagnosis with an associated complication

Assign only the combination code when that code fully identifies the diagnostic conditions involved or when the Alphabetic Index so directs. Multiple coding should not be used when the classification provides a combination code that clearly identifies all of the elements documented in the diagnosis. When the combination code lacks necessary specificity in describing the manifestation or complication, an additional code should be used as a secondary code.

10. Late Effects (Sequela)

A late effect is the residual effect (condition produced) after the acute phase of an illness or injury has terminated. There is no time limit on when a late effect code can be used. The residual may be apparent early, such as in cerebral infarction, or it may occur months or years later, such as that due to a previous injury. Coding of late effects generally requires two codes sequenced in the following order: The condition or nature of the late effect is sequenced first. The late effect code is sequenced second.

An exception to the above guidelines are those instances where the code for late effect is followed by a manifestation code identified in the Tabular List and title, or the late effect code has been expanded (at the fourth, fifth or sixth character levels) to include the manifestation(s). The code for the acute phase of an illness or injury that led to the late effect is never used with a code for the late effect.

11. Reporting Same Diagnosis Code More than Once

Each unique ICD-10-CM diagnosis code may be reported only once for an encounter. This applies to bilateral conditions when there are no distinct codes identifying laterality or two different conditions classified to the same ICD-10-CM diagnosis code.

12. Laterality

For bilateral sites, the final character of the codes in the ICD-10-CM indicates laterality. An unspecified side code is also provided should the side not be identified in the medical record. If no bilateral code is provided and the condition is bilateral, assign separate codes for both the left and right side.

All official authorized addenda through October 1, 2013, have been included in this revision. The complete official authorized addenda to ICD-10-CM, including the "ICD-10-CM Official Guidelines for Coding and Reporting," can be accessed at the following website:

www.cdc.gov/nchs/icd/icd10cm.htm

A description of the ICD-10-CM updating and maintenance process can be found at the following website:

http://www.cdc.gov/nchs/icd/icd9cm_maintenance.htm

Steps in Coding

The ICD-9-CM V-code coding guidelines included in this article preview coding practices in ICD-10-CM for factors influencing health status and contact with health services. The coding guidelines between the two coding classification systems are the same unless otherwise specified.

A significant change between the two coding classifications is that ICD-9-CM's supplementary codes are incorporated into the main classification in ICD-10-CM. The ICD-10-CM Tabular List categorizes codes to represent reasons for encounters as Z codes instead of V codes. ICD-10-CM codes have three to seven characters, but Z-code categories Z00–Z99 consist of three to six characters. Additional ICD-10-CM information is available on the National Center for Health Statistics Web site at www.cdc.gov/nchs/icd/icd10cm.htm.

Aftercare codes identify specific types of continuing care after the initial treatment of an injury or disease. V-code subcategories for orthopedic aftercare (V54.1 and V54.2) specify encounters following initial treatment of fractures. Coding guidelines state that a fracture code from the main classification can be used only for an initial encounter. Subsequent encounters that usually occur in an outpatient, home health, or long-term care facility now have the ability to report the type and site of fractures within the new subcategory sections.

Orthopedic aftercare visit coding guidelines differ in ICD-10-CM in that Z codes should not be used if treatment is directed at the current injury. If treatment is directed at the current injury, the injury code should be reported with a seventh-character extension to identify the subsequent encounter. The purpose of assigning the extension is to be able to track the continuity of care while identifying the type of injury.

While aftercare codes are used for a resolving or long-term condition, follow-up codes are used for conditions that require continuing surveillance following completed treatment of a disease, condition, or injury. ICD-9-CM coding guidelines state that follow-up codes are listed first unless a condition has recurred on the follow-up visit, then the diagnosis code should be listed first in place of the follow-up code.

Below is a complete listing of the most commonly used ICD-10 codes in table format:

TRAUMA & INJURY

AMPUTATION, TRAUMATIC

	Thumb	Index	Middle	Ring	Little	Other	Unspecified
Finger, metacarpophalangeal							
Complete	S68.01xx	S68.11xx	S68.11xx	S68.11xx	S68.11xx	S68.118x	S68.119x
Partial	S68.02xx	S68.12xx	S68.12xx	S68.12xx	S68.12xx	S68.128x	S68.129x
Transphalangeal							
Complete	S68.51xx	S68.61xx	S68.61xx	S68.61xx	S68.61xx	S68.618x	S68.619x
Partial	S68.52xx	S68.62xx	S68.62xx	S68.62xx	S68.62xx	S68.628x	S68.629x

6th character "x": C, 2, 4, 6 right 1, 3, 5, 7 left; For categories S68.0 and S68.5: 1 right 2 left 9 unspecified

	Foot/ankle	Midfoot	Foot, level unsp	Great toe	1 Lesser toe	≥2 Lesser toes	
Foot, complete	S98.01xx	S98.31xx	S98.91xx	S98.11xx	S98.13xx	S98.21xx	
Partial	S98.02xx	S98.32xx	S98.62xx	S98.12xx	S98.14xx	S98.22xx	

	Shoulder/upr arm	Elbow/forearm	Hip/thigh	Knee/lower Leg	Foot	Hand	
Limb							
Complete							
At/through joint (proximal) (upper)	S48.01xx	S58.01xx	S78.01xx	S88.01xx	S98.01xx	S68.41xx	
Mid (limb) (tarsal) (carpal) level	S48.11xx	S58.11xx	S78.11xx	S88.11xx	S98.31xx	S68.71xx	
Unspecified level	S48.91xx	S58.91xx	S78.91xx	S88.91xx	S98.91xx	S98.91xx	
Partial							
At/through joint (proximal)	S48.02xx	S58.02xx	S78.02xx	S88.02xx	S98.02xx	S68.42xx	

Mid (limb) (tarsal) (carpal) level	S48.12xx	S58.12xx	S78.12xx	S88.12xx	S98.32xx	S68.72xx
Unspecified level	S48.92xx	S58.92xx	S78.92xx	S88.92xx	S98.92xx	

6th character "x": 1 right 2 left 9 unspecified

7th character "x": D subsequent encounter S sequela

CONTUSION

Extremity, lower

Foot (except toes)	Ankle	Knee	Lower leg	Thigh	Hip
S90.3xxx	S90.0xxx	S80.0xxx	S80.1xxx	S70.1xxx	S70.0xx

Toe(s)

Great	Great w/ nail damage	Lesser	Lesser w/ nail damage
S90.11xx	S90.21xx	S90.12xx	S90.22xx

Extremity, upper

Elbow	Forearm	Hand (except fingers)	Shoulder	Wrist
S50.0xxx	S50.1xxx	S60.22xx	S40.01xx	S60.21xx

Finger

Thumb	Thumb w/ nail damage	Index	Index w/ nail damage	Middle	Middle w/ nail damage
S60.01xx	S60.11xx	S60.05xx	S60.15xx	S60.03xx	S60.13xx
Little	Little w/ nail damage	Ring	Ring w/ nail damage	Unspecified	Unsp w/ nail damage
S60.05xx	S60.15xx	S60.04xx	S30.14xx	S60.00xx	S60.10xx

5th or 6th character "x": 1 right 2 left 0 or 9 unspecified

7th character "x": D subsequent encounter S sequela

DISCLOCATION & SUBLUXATION OF JOINT, TRAUMATIC

Ankle — Subluxation S93.0Xxx | Dislocation S93.0Xxx

Elbow

	Anterior	Lateral	Medial	Posterior	Other	Unspecified
Nursemaid's	—	—	—	—	—	S53.03xx
Radial head, Dislocation	S53.01xx	—	—	S53.02xx	S53.09xx	S53.00xx
Subluxation	S53.01xx	—	—	S53.02xx	S53.09xx	S53.00xx
Ulnohumeral, Dislocation	S53.11xx	S53.14xx	S53.13xx	S53.12xx	S53.19xx	S53.10xx
Subluxation	S53.11xx	S53.14xx	S53.13xx	S53.12xx	S53.19xx	S53.10xx

Foot

	Tarsal	Tarsometatarsal	Other	Unspecified
Foot, dislocation	S93.31xx	S93.32xx	S93.33xx	S93.30xx
Subluxation	S93.31xx	S93.32xx	S93.33xx	S93.30xx

Hip

	Central	Posterior	Obturator	Anterior	Unspecified
Hip, dislocation	S73.04xx	S73.01xx	S73.02xx	S73.03xx	S73.00xx
Subluxation	S73.04xx	S73.01xx	S73.02xx	S73.03xx	S73.00xx

Knee

	Anterior	Lateral	Medial	Posterior	Other
Knee, dislocation	S83.11xx	S83.14xx	S83.13xx	S83.12xx	S83.19xx
Subluxation	S83.11xx	S83.14xx	S83.13xx	S83.12xx	S83.19xx

Patella

	Lateral	Other
Patella, dislocation	S83.01xx	S83.09xx
Subluxation	S83.01xx	S83.09xx

Shoulder

	w/100–200% Displac	w/>200% Displac	Inferior	Posterior	Unspecified
Acromioclavicular, Dislocation	S43.12xx	S43.13xx	S43.14xx	S43.15xx	S43.10xx
Subluxation	S43.11xx	—	—	—	—

Humerus, Dislocation	S43.01xx	S43.03xx	S43.02xx	S43.08xx	S43.00xx
Subluxation	S43.01xx	S43.03xx	S43.02xx	S43.08xx	S43.00xx
Scapula, Dislocation	S43.31xx	—	—	—	—
Subluxation	S43.31xx	—	—	—	—
Sternoclavicular, Dislocation	S43.21xx	—	S43.22xx	—	S43.20xx
Subluxation	S43.21xx	—	S43.22xx	—	S43.20xx

5th or 6th character "x": 1 or 4 right 2 or 5 left 3, 6 or 9 unspecified

Vertebra	C0-C1	C1-C2	C2-C3	C3-C4	C4-C5	C5-C6	C6-C7	Unspecified
Cervical, Dislocation	S13.111x	S12.121x	S13.131x	S13.141x	S13.151x	S13.161x	S13.171x	S13.100x
Subluxation	S13.110x	S13.120x	S13.130x	S13.140x	S13.150x	S13.160x	S13.170x	S13.101x
(level)	T12-L1	L1-L2	L2-L3	L3-L4	L4-L5	Unspecified		
Lumbar, Dislocation	S33.170x	S33.110x	S33.120x	S33.130x	S33.140x	S33.100x		
Subluxation	S33.171x	S33.111x	S33.121x	S33.131x	S33.141x	S33.101x		
(level)	C7-T1	T1-T2	T2-T3	T3-T4	T4-T5	T5-T6	T6-T7	Unspecified
Thoracic, Dislocation	S13.180x	S23.110x	S23.120x	S23.122x	S23.130x	S23.132x	S23.140x	S23.100x
Subluxation	S13.181x	S23.111x	S23.121x	S23.123x	S23.131x	S23.133x	S23.141x	S23.101x
(level)	T7-T8	T8-T9	T9-T10	T10-T11	T11-T12	Unspecified		
Thoracic, Dislocation	S23.142x	S23.150	S23.152x	S23.160x	S23.162x	S23.100x		
Subluxation	S23.143x	S23.151x	S23.153x	S23.161x	S23.163x	S23.101x		

7th character "x": D subsequent encounter S sequela

FRACTURES

	Lat condylar	Medial condylar	Unsp condylar	Lower epiphyseal	Supracond, simple	Supracond, complex
Limb, lower						
Femur						
Lower end, Displaced	S72.42xx	S72.43xx	S72.41xx	S72.44xx	S72.45xx	S72.46xx
Nondisplaced	S72.42xx	S72.43xx	S72.41xx	S72.44xx	S72.45xx	S72.46xx
	Comminuted	Oblique	Segmental	Spiral	Transverse	Other
Shaft, Displaced	S72.35xx	S72.33xx	S72.36xx	S72.34xx	S72.32xx	S72.39xx
Nondisplaced	S72.35xx	S72.33xx	S72.36xx	S72.34xx	S72.32xx	S72.32xx
	Other	Unspecified				
Upper end						
Neck NOS	S72.09xx	S72.00xx				
Base, Displaced	S72.04xx					
Nondisplaced	S72.04xx					
Head NOS	S72.09xx	S72.05xx				

	Apophyseal	Articular	Epiphyseal	Gr. trochanter	Intratrochanter	Less. trochanter
Upper end, Displaced	S72.13xx	S72.06xx	S72.02xx	S72.11xx	S72.14xx	S72.12xx
Nondisplaced	S72.13xx	S72.06xx	S72.02xx	S72.11xx	S72.14xx	S72.12xx
	Bimalleolar	Lateral malleolar	Maisonneuve's	Medial malleolar	Pilon	Trimalleolar

5th or 6th character "x": 1 or 4 right 2 or 5 left 3, 6 or 9 unspecified
7th character "x": D subseq encounter closed fx routine heal E subseq encounter open fx type I/II routine
heal F subseq encounter open fx type III A/B/C routine heal S sequela

Limb, lower (Continued)

Fibula

	Comminuted	Oblique	Segmental	Spiral	Transverse	Unspecified
Lower end, Displaced	S82.84xx	S82.6xXx	S82.86xx	S82.5-Xx	S82.87xx	S82.85xx
Nondisplaced	S82.84xx	S82.6xXx	S82.86xx	S82.5-Xx	S82.87xx	S82.85xx
Shaft, Displaced	S82.45xx	S82.43xx	S82.46xx	S82.44xx	S82.42xx	S82.40xx
Nondisplaced	S82.45xx	S82.43xx	S82.46xx	S82.44xx	S82.42xx	—

Foot

	Anterior process	Avulsion, tuber	Body	Extraarticular	Intraarticular	Unspecified
Calcaneus, Displaced	S92.02xx	S92.03xx	S92.01xx	S92.C5xx	S92.06xx	S92.00xx
Nondisplaced	S92.02xx	S92.03xx	S92.01xx	S92.C5xx	S92.06xx	—

	First	Second	Third	Fourth	Fifth	Unspecified
Metatarsal, Displaced	S92.31xx	S92.32xx	S92.33xx	S92.34xx	S92.35xx	S92.30xx
Nondisplaced	S92.31xx	S92.32xx	S92.33xx	S92.34xx	S92.35xx	S92.30xx

	Avulsion (chip) fx	Body	Dome	Neck	Post Process	Unspecified
Talus, Displaced	S92.15xx	S92.12xx	S92.14xx	S92.11xx	S92.13xx	S92.10xx
Nondisplaced	S92.15xx	S92.12xx	S92.14xx	S92.11xx	S92.13xx	—

	Intermed cuneiform	Lateral cuneiform	Medial cuneiform	Navicular	Unspecified
Tarsal, Other, Displaced	S92.23xx	S92.22xx	S92.24xx	S92.25xx	S92.20xx
Nondisplaced	S92.23xx	S92.22xx	S92.24xx	S92.25xx	—

	Comminuted	Longitudinal	Osteochondral	Transverse	Unspecified
Patella, Displaced	S82.04xx	S82.02xx	S82.01xx	S82.03xx	S82.09xx

Tibia

	Comminuted	Oblique	Segmental	Spiral	Transverse	Unspecified
Nondisplaced	S82.04xx	S82.02xx	S82.01xx	S82.03xx	—	
Shaft, Displaced	S82.25xx	S82.22xx	S82.26xx	S82.24xx	S82.22xx	S82.20xx
Nondisplaced	S82.25xx	S82.22xx	S82.26xx	S82.24xx	S82.22xx	—

	Biocondylar	Lateral condyle	Medial condyle	Tibial spine	Tibial tuberosity
Upper end, Displaced	S82.14xx	S82.12xx	S82.13xx	S82.11xx	S82.15xx
Nondisplaced	S82.14xx	S82.12xx	S82.13xx	S82.11xx	S82.15xx

Limb, upper
Hand & wrist

	Capitate	Hamate body	Hamate hook	Lunate	Pisiform	Trapezium	Trapezoid	Triquetrium
Carpal, Displaced	S62.13xx	S62.14xx	S62.15xx	S62.12xx	S62.16xx	S62.17xx	S62.18xx	S62.11xx
Nondisplaced	S62.13xx	S62.14xx	S62.15xx	S62.12xx	S62.16xx	S62.17xx	S62.18xx	S62.11xx

Humerus

	Lat condyle	Med condyle	Lat epicondyle	Med epicondyle	Other	Comminuted supracon	Simple supracon
Lower end, Displaced	S42.45xx	S42.46xx	S42.43xx	S42.44xx	S42.49xx	S42.42xx	S42.41xx
Nondisplaced	S42.45xx	S42.46xx	S42.43xx	S42.44xx	S42.49xx	S42.42xx	S42.41xx

	Comminuted	Greenstick	Oblique	Segmental	Spiral	Transverse	Unspecified
Shaft, Displaced	S42.35xx	—	S42.33xx	S42.36xx	S42.34xx	S42.32xx	S42.39xx
Nondisplaced	S42.35xx	S42.31xx	S42.33xx	S42.36xx	S42.34xx	S42.32xx	S42.30xx

	Less tuberosity	Gr tuberosity	Surg neck uns	Surg neck 2-pt	Surg neck 3-pt	Surg neck 4-pt	Other
Upper end, Displaced	S42.26xx	S42.25xx	S42.21xx	S42.22xx	S42.23xx	S42.24xx	S42.29xx
Nondisplaced	S42.26xx	S42.25xx	S42.21xx	S42.22xx	S42.23xx	S42.24xx	S42.29xx

	Bennett's	Rolando's	Base	Shaft	Neck	Other	Unspecified
Metacarp, first, Displaced	S62.22xx	S62.22xx	S62.23xx	S62.24xx	S62.25xx	S62.29xx	S62.20xx
Nondisplaced		S62.22xx	S62.23xx	S62.24xx	S62.25xx	—	—

Metacarpal, other

	Second right	Second left	Third right	Third left	Fourth right	Fourth left	Fifth right	Fifth left
Base, Displaced	S62.310x	S62.311x	S62.312x	S62.313x	S62.314x	S62.315x	S62.316x	S62.317x
Nondisplaced	S62.340x	S62.341x	S62.342x	S62.343x	S62.344x	S62.345x	S62.346x	S62.347x

5th or 6th character "x": 1 or 4 right 2 or 5 left 3, 6 or 9 unspecified

7th char "x": D subseq encounter closed fx routine heal E subseq encounter open fx type I / II routine heal

F subseq encounter open fx type III A/B/C routine heal S sequela

Limb, upper, Metacarpal, other (Continued)

	Second right	Second left	Third right	Third left	Fourth right	Fourth left	Fifth right	Fifth left
Neck, Displaced	S62.330x	S62.331x	S62.332x	S62.333x	S62.334x	S62.335x	S62.336x	S62.337x
Nondisplaced	S62.360x	S62.361x	S62.362x	S62.363x	S62.364x	S62.365x	S62.366x	S62.367x
Shaft, Displaced	S62.320x	S62.321x	S62.322x	S62.323x	S62.324x	S62.325x	S62.326x	S62.327x
Nondisplaced	S62.350x	S62.351x	S62.352x	S62.353x	S62.354x	S62.355x	S62.356x	S62.357x

Navicular

	Distal pole	Middle third	Proximal third	Unspecified
Navicular, Displaced	S62.01xx	S62.02xx	S62.03xx	S62.00xx
Nondisplaced	S62.01xx	S62.02xx	S62.03xx	—

Radius

	Barton's	Colles'	Intraarticular, oth	Exraarticular, oth	Smith's
Lower end	S52.56xxx	S52.53xx	S52.57xx	S52.55xx	S52.54xx
Styloid proc, Displaced	S52.51xx	—	—	—	—
Nondisplaced	S52.51xx	—	—	—	—

	Comminuted	Oblique	Segmental	Spiral	Transverse
Shaft, Displaced	S52.35xx	S52.33xx	S52.36xx	S52.34xx	S52.32xx
Nondisplaced	S52.35xx	S52.33xx	S52.36xx	S52.34xx	S52.32xx

	Galeazzi's	Greenstick	Other
Other	S52.37xx	S52.31xx	S52.39xx

	Head	Neck	Other
Upper end, Displaced	S52.12xx	S52.13xx	S52.18xx
Nondisplaced	S52.12xx	S52.13xx	—
Styloid process			Other

Ulna

	Greenstick	Monteggia's	Other
Lower end, Displaced	S52.61xx	S52.69xx	
Nondisplaced	S52.61xx	—	

	Comminuted	Oblique	Segmental	Spiral	Transverse
Shaft, Displaced	S52.25xx	S52.23xx	S52.26xx	S52.24xx	S52.22xx
Nondisplaced	S52.25xx	S52.23xx	S52.26xx	S52.24xx	S52.22xx

Other

	Coronoid process	Olecranon process compl w/ extension	Olecranon process simple/no extension	Other
	S52.21xx	S52.27xx	S52.29xx	
Upper end, Displaced	S52.04xx	S52.03xx	S52.02xx	S52.09xx
Nondisplaced	S52.04xx	S52.03xx	S52.02xx	—

6th character "x": 1 or 4 right 2 or 5 left 3, 6 or 9 unspecified

Phalanges

	Index x	Little x	Middle x	Ring x	Other	Unspecified
Finger, displaced, proximal	S62.61xx	S62.61xx	S62.61xx	S62.61xx	S62.618x	S62.619x
Medial	S62.62xx	S62.62xx	S62.62xx	S62.62xx	S62.628x	S62.629x
Distal	S62.63xx	S62.63xx	S62.63xx	S52.63xx	S62.638x	S62.639x
Finger, nondisplaced, proximal	S62.64xx	S62.64xx	S62.64xx	S62.64xx	S62.648x	S62.649x
Medial	S62.65xx	S62.65xx	S62.65xx	S62.65xx	S62.658x	S62.659x
Distal	S62.66xx	S62.66xx	S62.66xx	S62.66xx	S62.668x	S62.669x

6th character "x" for category S62.6: 0, 2, 4 or 6 right 1, 3, 5 or 7 left

	Distal	Medial	Proximal
Thumb, Displaced	S62.52xx	—	S62.51xx
Nondisplaced	S62.52xx	—	S62.51xx

6th character "x" for category S62.5: 1 or 4 right 2 or 5 left 3 or 6 unspecified

Toes, great, Displaced	S92.41xx	—
Nondisplaced	S92.42xx	—
Toes, lesser, Displaced	S92.52xx	S92.53xx
Nondisplaced	S92.53xx, S92.52xx, S92.51xx	
	6th character "x" for categories S92.4 and S92.5: 1 or 4 right 2 or 5 left 3 or 6 unspecified	

Shoulder	Lateral end	Shaft	Sternal end ant	Sternal end post	Sternal end unsp	Unspecified
Clavicle, Displaced	S42.03xx	S42.02xx	S42.01xx	S42.01xx	—	S42.00xx
Nondisplaced	S42.03xx	S42.02xx		S42.01xx		S42.9xXx

6th character meaning as indicated for S42.0: 1, 4 or 7 right 2, 5 or 8 left 3, 6, or 9 unspecified

7th char "x": D subseq encounter closed fx routine heal E subseq encounter open fx type III A/B/C routine heal S sequela

routine heal F subseq encounter open fx type I/II

FRACTURES (Continued)

	Acrom. process	Body	Coracoid	Glenoid cavity	Neck	Other
Scapula, Displaced	S42.12xx	S42.11xx	S42.13xx	S42.14xx	S42.15xx	S42.19xx
Nondisplaced	S42.12xx	S42.11xx	S42.13xx	S42.14xx	S42.15xx	

6th character "x": 1 or 4 right 2 or 5 left 3, 6 or 9 unspecified

7th char "x": D subseq encounter closed fx routine heal E subseq encounter open fx type I/II

routine heal F subseq encounter open fx type III A/B/C routine heal S sequela

FRACTURE, PHYSEAL

	Salter-Harris I	Salter-Harris II	Salter-Harris III	Salter-Harris IV	Other	Unspecified
Fibula, Lower end	S89.31xx	S89.32xx	—	—	S89.39xx	S89.30xx
Upper end	S89.21xx	S89.22xx	—	—	S89.29xx	S89.20xx
Tibia, Lower end	S89.11xx	S89.12xx	S89.13xx	S89.14xx	S89.19xx	S89.10xx
Upper end	S89.01xx	S89.02xx	S89.03xx	S89.04xx	S89.09xx	S89.00xx
Ulna, Lower & Upper	S59.01xx	S59.02xx	S59.03xx	S59.04xx	S59.09xx	S59.00xx
Humerus, Lower	S49.11xx	S49.12xx	S49.13xx	S49.14xx	S49.19xx	S49.10xx
Upper end	S49.01xx	S49.02xx	S49.03xx	S49.04xx	S49.09xx	S49.00xx

6th character "x": 1 right 2 left 9 unspecified

7th character "x": D subsequent encounter fracture routine healing S sequela

FRACTURE, TORUS

	Femur	Fibula, upper end	Fibula, lower end	Tibia lower end	Tibia, upper end	
Limb, lower	S72.47xx	S82.82xx	S82.81xx	S82.31xx	S82.16xx	
	Humerus, lower end	Humerus, upper end	Radius, lower end	Radius, shaft	Ulna, lower end	Ulna, upper end
Limb, upper	S42.48xx	S42.27xx	S52.52xx	S52.30xx	S52.60xx	S52.01xx

6th character "x": 1 right 2 left 9 unspecified

7th character "x": D subsequent encounter fracture routine healing S sequela

INJURY, CRUSH

	Ankle	Foot	Knee	Leg	Thigh	Hip	Thigh & hip
Extremity, lower	S97.0xXx	S97.8xXx	S87.0xXx	S87.8xXx	S77.1xXx	S77.0xXx	S77.2xXx
Toe(s)	Great — S97.11xx	Lesser — S97.12xx	Unspecified — S97.10xx				
Extremity, upper (Arm, upr/shoulder, Elbow, Forearm, Hand, Wrist, Wrist/hand)	S47.xXXx	S57.0xXx	S57.8xXx	S67.2xXx	S67.3xXx	S67.4xXx	
Finger	Thumb — S67.0xXx	Index — S67.19xx	Middle — S67.19xx	Ring — S67.19xx	Little — S67.19xx	Unspecified — S67.10Xx	

5th or 6th character "x": 1 right 2 left 0 or 9 unspecified

6th character meanings for category S67.1: 0, 2, 4 or 6 right 1, 3, 5 or 7 left

7th character "x": D subsequent encounter fracture routine healing S sequela

SPRAIN

	Calcaneofibular	Deltoid	Other	Tibulofibular	Unspecified	Spine & pelvis	Thoracic
Limb, lower							
Ankle	S93.41xx	S93.42xx	S93.49xx	S93.43xx	S93.40xx		
	Cervical	Neck (other)	Neck (unspecified)	Lumbar	Sacroiliac joint		Thoracic

Region							
Back (spine)	S13.4XXx	S13.8XXx	S13.9XXx	S33.5XXx	S33.6XXx	S33.8XXx	S23.3XXx
Elbow	Radial collateral — S53.43xx	Radiohumeral — S53.41xx	Ulnar collateral — S53.44xx	Ulnohumeral — S53.42xx	Other — S53.49xx	Unspecified — S53.40xx	
Foot	Tarsal ligament — S93.61xx	Tarsometatarsal — S93.62xx	Other — S93.69xx	Unspecified — S93.60xx			
Hip	Iliofemoral — S73.11xx	Ischicapsular — S73.12xx	Other — S73.19xx	Unspecified — S73.10xx			

Knee

Collateral lgmt	Anterior	Lateral	Medial	Posterior	Unspecified
Collateral lgmt		S83.42xx	S83.41xx		S83.40xx
Cruciate lgmt	S83.51xx			S83.52xx	S83.50x
Superior tibio-fibular	S83.6xXx				
Other	S83.8Xxx				

5th or 6th character "x": 1 right 2 left 0 or 9 unspecified

7th character "x": A initial encounter D subsequent encounter S sequela

Meniscus

Meniscus	Bucket handle	Complex	Peripheral	Other	Unspecified
Lateral	S83.25xx	S83.27xx	S83.26xx	S83.28xx	
Medial	S83.21xx	S83.23xx	S83.22xx	S83.24xx	S83.20xx
Unspecified	S83.20xx			S83.20xx	S83.20xx

Limb, upper — Shoulder

	Acromioclaviculr	Coracohumeral	Shoulder girdle	Sternoclavic	SLAP	Unspecified
Shoulder	S43.5xXx	S43.41xx	S43.8xXx	S43.6xXx	S43.42xx	S43.9xXx

		Note: For nontraumatic—see LESION, Shoulder.					
Rotator cuff, traum	S43.01xx						

	Carpal	Thumb, intrphal	Thumb meta-carph	Thumb other	Other	Radiocarpal	Unspecified
Wrist / hand	S63.51xx	S63.62xx	S63.64xx	S63.68xx	S63.8Xxx	S63.52xx	S63.9xXx

STRAIN

Finger	Index finger (rt, lt)	Little finger (rt, lt)	Middle finger (rt, lt)	Ring finger (rt, lt)	Other finger	Unsp finger	Thumb
Flexor (long)	S66.11xx	S66.11xx	S66.11xx	S66.11xx	S66.118x	S66.119x	S66.01xx
Extensor	S66.31xx	S66.31xx	S66.31xx	S66.31xx	S66.318x	S66.319x	S66.21xx
Intrinsic	S66.59xx	S66.59xx	S66.59xx	S66.59xx	S66.598x	S66.519x	S66.41xx

6th character "x": 0, 2, 4 or 6 right 1, 3,5 or 7 left; For category S66.0: 1 right 2 left 9 unspecified

7th character "x": A initial encounter D subsequent encounter S sequela

MUSCULOSKELETAL DISORDERS

ARTHROPATHY

	Ankle/foot	Elbow	Hand	Hip	Knee	Multi/poly	Shoulder	Vertebra	Wrist	Unspecified
Other/unspecified Villonodular synov	M12.27x	M12.22x	M12.24x	M12.25x	M12.26x	M12.29	M12.21x	M12.28	M12.23x	M12.20

6th character "x": 1 right 2 left 9 unspecified

ARTHROPATHY (Continued)

	Ankle/foot	Elbow	Hand	Hip	Knee	Mult/poly	Shoulder	Vertebra	Wrist	Unspecified
Pyogenic arthritis										M00.09
Staphylococcal	M00.07x	M00.02x	M00.04x	M00.05x	M00.06x	M00.09	M00.01x	M00.08	M00.03x	M00.00
	M00.17x M00.12x M00.14x M00.15x M00.16x M00.19 M00.11x M00.18 M00.13x M00.10									
Pneumococcal										
Streptococcus, other	M00.27x	M00.22x	M00.24x	M00.25x	M00.26x	M00.29	M00.21x	M00.28	M00.23x	M00.20
Bacteria, other	M00.87x	M00.82x	M00.84x	M00.85x	M00.86x	M00.89	M00.81x	M00.88	M00.83x	M00.80
Rheumatoid arthritis										M06.9
w/ Rheum factor, oth	M05.87x	M05.82x	M05.84x	M05.85x	M05.86x	M05.89	M05.81x		M05.83x	M05.80
w/ Myopathy	M05.47x	M05.42x	M05.44x	M05.45x	M05.46x	M05.49	M05.41x		M05.43x	M05.40
w/ Polyneuropathy	M05.57x	M05.52x	M05.54x	M05.55x	M05.56x	M05.59	M05.51x		M05.53x	M05.50
w/o Rheum factor	M06.07x	M06.02x	M06.04x	M06.05x	M06.06x	M06.09	M06.01x	M06.08	M06.03x	M06.00
Felty's syndrome	M05.07x	M05.02x	M05.04x	M05.05x	M05.06x	M05.09	M05.01x		M05.03x	M05.00
Traumatic	M12.57x	M12.52x	M12.54x	M12.55x	M12.56x	M12.59	M12.51x	M12.58	M12.53x	M45.50

6th character "x": 1 right 2 left 9 unspecified

BURSITIS

	Ankle/foot	Hand	Olecranon	Elbow	Peripatellar	Knee	Trochanter	Hip	Shoulder	Wrist
Crepitant synovitis	—	M70.04x	—	—	—	—	—	—	—	M70.03x
d/t Overuse	—	M70.1x	M70.2x	M70.3x	M70.4x	M70.5x	M70.6x	M70.7x	M75.5x	—
Other	M71.56x	M71.54x	—	M71.52x	—	M71.56x	—	M71.55x	—	M71.53x

5th or 6th character "x": 1 right 2 left 0 or 9 unspecified

CEREBROVASCULAR DISEASE, LATE EFFECTS (SEQUELAE) OF

	Cerebral infarct	Intracerebral hemorr	Intracranial hemorr	Subarachnoid hemorr	Oth cerebrovascular	Unsp cerebrovascular
(Nontraumatic) (Due To)						
Apraxia	I69.390	I69.190	I69.290	I69.090	I6.890	I69.990
Ataxia	I69.393	I69.193	I69.293	I69.093	I69.893	I69.993

6th character "x" for category I69: 1 rt dom 2 lt dom 3 rt non-dom 4 lt non-dom 5 bilat 9 unspecified

CEREBROVASCULAR DISEASE, LATE EFFECTS (SEQUELAE) OF (Continued)

	Cerebral infarct	Intracerebral hemorr	Intracranial hemorr	Subarachnoid hemorr	Oth cerebrovascular	Unsp cerebrovascular
(Nontraumatic) (Due To)						
Hemiplegia/hemiparesis	I69.35x	I69.15x	I69.25x	I69.05x	I69.85x	I69.95x
Monoplegia, lwr limb	I69.34x	I69.14x	I69.24x	I69.04x	I69.84x	I69.94x

| Monoplegia, upr limb | I69.33x | I69.13x | I69.23x | I69.03x | I69.83x | I69.93x |
| Other paralytic synd | I69.36x | I69.16x | I69.26x | I69.06x | I69.86x | I69.96x |

6th character "x" for category I69: 1 rt dom 2 lt dom 3 rt non-dom 4 lt non-dom 5 bilat 9 unspecified

CONNECTIVE TISSUE DISEASE

	Cervicalgia	Cervi-cobracial syndrome	Cervico-cranial syndrome	Occipital neuralgia	Panniculitis	Radiculop-athy	Radiculop-athy, cervi-cothoracic	Torticollis
Cervical region disorders	M54.2	M53.1	M53.0	M54.81	M54.01	M54.12	M54.13	M43.6

DEFORMITIES (ACQUIRED)

Cavovarus (cavus) of foot	Coxa valga	Cubitus valgus	Cubitus varus	Equinus of foot	Foot drop
M21.6Xx	M21.05x	M21.02x	M21.12x	M21.6Xx	M21.37x
Genu recurvatum	Genu valgum	Genu varum	Wrist drop		
M21.86x	M21.06x	M21.16x	M21.33x		

6th character "x": 1 right 2 left 9 unspecified

DERANGEMENT OF JOINTS

Knee

Instability (knee), chronic	M23.5x					
	Capsular	Lat collateral	Med collateral	Ant cruciate	Post cruciate	Unspecified
Disruption, ligament (old)	M23.67x	M23.64x	M23.63x	M23.61x	M23.62x	M23.60x

6th character "x": 1 or 5 right 2 or 4 left 0 or 9 unspecified

DERANGEMENT OF JOINTS (Continued)

Knee

Meniscus derangement (old)	Lat ant horn	Lat post horn	Lateral Other	Medial ant horn	Medial post horn	Medial other
Knee, specified	M23.34x	M23.35x	M23.36x	M23.31x	M23.32x	M23.33x
	Left	Right	Unspecified			
Knee, unspecified (old)	M23.007	M23.006	M23.009			
Lateral	M23.001	M23.000	M23.002			
Medial	M23.004	M23.003	M23.006			

Other, joint	Ankle	Elbow	Foot	Hand	Hip	Shoulder	Wrist
	M24.87x	M24.82x	M24.87x	M24.84x	M24.85x	M24.81x	M24.83x

6th character "x": 1 or 5 right 2 or 4 left 0 or 9 unspecified

DISORDERS OF JOINTS

	Ankle/foot	Elbow	Hand	Hip	Knee	Shoulder	Wrist	Unspecified
Articular cartilage	M24.17x	M24.12x	M24.14x	M24.15x	M24.16x	M24.11x	M24.13x	M24.10

Chondromalacia	M94.27x	M94.22x	M94.24x	M94.25x	M94.26x	M97.21x	M94.23x	M94.20
Patella	—	—	—	—	M22.4x	—	—	—
Dislocation, recurrent	M24.47x	M24.42x	M24.44x	M24.45x	M24.46x	M24.41x	M24.43x	M24.40
Effusion, joint	M25.47x	M25.42x	M25.44x	M25.45x	M25.46x	M25.41x	M25.43x	M25.40
Hemarthrosis	M25.07x	M25.02x	M25.04x	M25.05x	M25.06x	M25.01x	M25.03x	M25.00
Instability, joint (other)	M25.37x	M25.32x	M25.34x	M25.35x	M25.36x	M25.31x	M25.33x	M25.30
Other specified	M25.87x	M25.82x	—	M24.85x	M24.86x	—	M24.85x	—
Pain	M25.57x	M25.52x	M25.54x	M25.55x	M25.56x	M25.51x	M25.53x	M25.50
Stiffness, joint	M25.67x	M25.62x	M25.64x	M25.65x	M25.66x	M25.61x	M25.63x	M24.60

5th or 6th character "x": 1 right 2 left 0 or 9 unspecified

DISORDERS OF TENDONS

	Ankle/foot	Arm, upper	Forearm	Hand	Leg, lower	Multiple sites	Thigh	Shoulder	Other	Unspecified
Rupture, spontaneous										
Extensor	M66.27x	M66.22x	M66.23x	M66.24x	M66.26x	M66.29	M66.25x	M66.21x	M66.28	M66.20x
Flexor	M66.37x	M66.32x	M66.33x	M66.34x	M66.36x	M66.39	M66.35x	M66.31x	M66.38	M66.30x
Other	M66.87x	M66.82x	M66.83x	M66.84x	M66.86x	M66.89	M66.85x	M66.81x	M66.88	M66.80x
Tenosynovitis	M65.87x	M65.82x	M65.83x	M65.84x	M65.86x	M65.89	M65.85x	M65.81x	M65.88	M65.80x
	Achilles	Patellar	Peroneal	Psoas	Tibial, anterior			Tibial, posterior		

	Ankle/foot	Arm, upper	Forearm	Hand	Hip/thigh	Leg, lower	Shoulder
Tendinitis	M76.6x	M76.5x	M76.7x	M76.1x	M76.81x	M76.82x	M75.3x
Calcific	M65.27x	M65.22x	M65.23x	M65.24x	M65.25x	M65.26x	
	Index	Little	Middle	Ring	Thumb	Unspecified	
Trigger finger	M65.32x	M65.35x	M65.33x	M65.34x	M65.31x	M65.30	

6th character "x": 1 right 2 left 0 or 9 unspecified

DORSOPATHY

	Occipito-atlanto-axial	Mid-cervical	Cervicothoracic	Thoracic	Thoracolumbar	Lumbar	Lumbosacral
Disc (intervertebral) disorder							
Displacement	M50.21	M50.22	M50.23	M51.24	M51.25	M51.26	M51.27
Degeneration	M50.31	M50.32	M50.33	M51.34	M51.35	M51.36	M51.37
w/ Myelopathy	M50.01	M50.02	M50.03	M51.04	M51.05	M51.06	M51.07
w/ Radiculopathy	M50.11	M50.12	M50.13	M51.14	M51.15	M51.16	M51.17

	Cervicalgia	Lumbago w/ sciatica	Lumbago NOS	Occipital neuralgia	Sciatica	Thoracic pain	Unspecified
Dorsalgia (back pain)							
Unspecified	M54.2	M54.4x	M54.5	M54.81	M54.3x	M54.6	M54.9

5th character "x": 1 right 2 left 0 unspecified

DORSOPATHY (Continued)

Dorsalgia (back pain)

	Occip-atla-axial	Mid-cervical	Cervicothoracic	Thoracic	Thoracolumbar	Lumbar	Lumbosacral	Sacral	Multi site
Panniculitis	M54.01	M54.02	M54.03	M54.04	M54.05	M54.06	M54.07	M54.08	M54.09
Radiculopathy	M54.11	M54.12	M54.13	M54.14	M54.15	M54.16	M54.17	M54.18	M54.10

	Occip-atla-axial	Cervical	Cervicothoracic	Thoracic	Thoracolumbar	Lumbar	Lumbosacral	Sacral	Unspecified
Kyphososis									
Flatback synd	—	—	—	—	M40.35	M40.36	M40.37	—	M40.30
Postural	—	—	M40.03	M40.04	M40.05	—	—	—	M40.00
Second, other	—	M40.12	M40.13	M40.14	M40.15	—	—	—	M40.10
Other	—	M40.292	M40.293	M40.294	M40.295	—	—	—	M40.299
Lordosis, postural	—	—	—	—	M40.45	M40.46	M40.47	—	M40.40
Osteochondrosis		—	—			—		—	—
Adult	M42.11	M42.12	M42.13	M42.14	M42.15	M42.16	M42.17	M42.18	M42.10
Juvenile	M42.01	M42.02	M42.03	M42.04	M42.05	M42.06	M42.07	M42.08	M42.00
Scoliosis									
Idiopathic									
Adolescent	—	M41.122	M41.123	M41.124	M41.125	M41.126	M41.127	—	M41.129
Infantile	—	M41.02	M41.03	M41.04	M41.05	M41.06	M41.07	M41.08	M41.00
Juvenile	—	M41.112	M41.113	M41.114	M41.115	M41.116	M41.117	—	M41.119
Other	—	M41.22	M41.23	M41.24	M41.25	M41.26	M41.27	—	M41.20
Neuromuscular	M41.41	M41.42	M41.43	M41.44	M41.45	M41.46	M41.47	—	M41.40
Oth Secondary	—	M41.52	M41.53	M41.54	M41.55	M41.56	M41.57	—	M41.50
Other	—	M41.82	M41.83	M41.84	M41.85	M41.86	M41.87	—	M41.80
Thoracogenic	—	—	—	M41.34	M41.35	—	—	—	M41.30

FASCIITIS

Palmar fascia (Dupuytren's)	Plantar fasciitis	Nodular fasciitis	Other	Unspecified
M72.0	M72.2	M72.4	M72.8	M72.9

LESION

	Carpal tunnel	Ulnar	Radial	Sciatic	Plantar	Tarsal	Femoral
Mononeuropathy	G56.0x	G56.2x	G56.3x	G57.0x	G57.6x	G57.5x	G57.2x
Popliteal	Lateral G57.3x	Medial G57.4x					
Nerve root & plexis	Brachial plexis G54.0	Cervical root G54.2	Lumbosacral plexis G54.1	Lumbosacral root G54.4	Thoracic root G54.3	Phant limb w/ pain G54.6	Phant limb w/o pain G54.7
Nonallopathic	Cervical M99.81	Lower extremity M99.86	Upper extremity M99.87	Lumbar M99.83	Pelvic M99.85	Sacral M99.84	Thoracic M99.82
Shoulder	Adhesive capsulitis M75.0x	Complete —	Derangements M24.81x	Impinge synd M75.4x	Incomplete M75.11x	Other M75.8x	Unspecified M75.10x
Rotator cuff	—	M75.12x	—	—	—	—	—

5th or 6th character "x": 1 right 2 left 0 or 9 unspecified

MUSCLE DISORDERS PRIMARY

Fibromyalgia	Immobility syndrome	Lambert-Eaton	Muscular dystrophy	Myalgia
M79.7	M62.3	G70.80	G71.0	M79.1
Myotonic dystrophy	Poliomyelitis, sequelae	Postpolio syndrome	Rabdomyelitis	Weakness, general
G71.11	B91	G14	M62.82	M62.81
Myasthenia gravis	w/ Acute exacerbation	w/o Acute exacerbation		
	G70.01	G70.00		
Spasm, muscle	Back	Calf	Other	
	M62.830	M62.831	M62.838	

Wasting by site

Ankle & foot	Arm, upper	Forearm	Hand	Lower leg	Multi sites	Other	Shoulder	Thigh
M62.57x	M62.52x	M62.53x	M62.54x	M62.56x	M62.59	M62.58	M62.51x	M62.55

6th character "x": 1 right 2 left 9 unspecified

NEUROPATHIES

Hereditary	Ataxia, hereditary	Charcôt Marie dz	Other	Refsum's dz	Unspecified
	G60.2	G60.0	G60.8	G60.1	G60.9

Mononeuropathy, lwr limb	Causalgia cx pain syn II	Femoral nerve	Mer-algia pares-thetica	Popliteal nerve, lateral	Popliteal nerve, medial	Plantar nerve	Tarsal tunnel	Oth nerve	Unsp nerve
	G57.7x	G57.2x	G57.1x	G57.3x	G57.4x	G57.6x	G57.5x	G57.8x	G57.9x

Upper Limb	Carpal tunnel	Causalgia cx pain syn II	Median nerve oth	Radial nerve	Ulnar nerve	Other nerve	Unsp nerve
	G56.0x	G56.4x	G56.1x	G56.3x	G56.2x	G56.8x	G56.9x

	Critical illness	Guillan-Barre syn.	Inflam, chr demyel	Other	Unspecified
Polyneuropathy	G62.81	G61.0	G61.81	G62.89	G62.9

w/ Motor sensory—see Diabetes Mellitus w/ neurologic complications

5th character "x": 0 unspecified 1 right 2 left

OSTEOARTHRITIS

	Ankle/foot	Elbow	Hand	Hip	Hip d/t dysplasia	Knee	Shoulder	Wrist
Primary, bilateral	—	—	—	M16.0	M16.2	M17.0	—	—
Unilateral	M19.07x	M19.02x	M19.04x	M16.1x	M16.3x	M17.1x	M19.01x	M19.03x
Post-traumatic, bilateral	—	—	—	M16.4	—	M17.2	—	—
Unilateral	M19.17x	M19.12x	M19.14x	M16.5x	—	M17.3x	M19.11x	M19.13x

5th or 6th character "x": 1 right 2 left 0 or 9 unspecified

OSTEOPOROSIS

	Age-related	Other
w/o (Current) path fracture	M81.0	M81.8

OSITIS DEFORMANS

	Ankle & foot	Arm, lower	Arm, upper	Hand	Lower leg
(Paget's disease)	M88.87x	M88.83x	M88.82x	M88.84x	M88.86x
	Multiple sites	Other site(s)	Vertebrae	Unspecified	
	M88.89	M88.88	M88.1	M88.9	

6th character "x": 1 right 2 left 0 or 9 unspecified

PARALYTIC SYNDROMES

	Ataxic	Athetoid	Spastic diplegic	Spastic hemiplegic	Spastic quadraplegic
Cerebral Palsy (infantile)	G80.4	G80.3	G80.1	G80.2	G80.0
	Right dominant	Left dominant	Right nondominant	Left nondominant	Unspecified
Hemiplegia					
Flaccid	G81.01	G81.02	G81.03	G81.04	G81.00
Spastic	G81.11	G81.12	G81.13	G81.14	G81.10
Unspecified	G81.91	G81.92	G81.93	G81.94	G81.90
Monoplegia, lower limb	G83.11	G83.12	G83.13	G83.14	G83.10
Upper limb	G83.21	G83.22	G83.23	G83.24	G83.20
	Diplegia	Paraplegia	Quadriplegia C1-C4	Quadriplegia C5-C7	
Other, complete	G83.0	G82.21	G82.51	G82.53	
Incomplete	—	G82.22	G82.52	G82.54	
Unspecified	—	G82.20	G82.50	G82.50	

POSTPROCEDURAL COMPLICATIONS

Pseudoarthrosis d/t fusion	Postlaminectomy		Postsurgical Lordosis	Postradiation	
	Kyphosis	Syndrome		Kyphosis	Scoliosis
M96.0	M96.3	M96.1	M96.4	M96.2	M96.5

SPONDYLOPATHY

	Occipito-atla-axial	Cervical	Cervicothoracic	Thoracic	Thoracolumbar	Lumbar	Lumbosacral	Sacral
Spondylosis								
Other w/ myelopathy	M47.11	M47.12	M47.13	M47.14	M47.15	M47.16	—	—
Other w/ radiculopathy	M47.21	M47.22	M47.23	M47.24	M47.25	M47.26	M47.27	M47.28
Other w/o myelop or radiculop	M47.811	M47.812	M47.813	M47.814	M47.815	M47.816	M47.817	M47.818
Stenosis, spinal (caudal)	M48.01	M48.02	M48.03	M48.04	M48.05	M48.06	M48.07	M48.08

GENERAL MEDICAL HEALTH STATUS

	Ankle	Elbow	Hip	Knee	Other	Shoulder	Wrist
Status (post), orthopedic implants	Z96.66x	Z96.62x	Z96.64x	Z96.65x	Z63.69x	Z63.61x	Z96.63x

6th character meanings unless otherwise indicated: 1 or 4 right 2 or 5 left 0 or 9 unspecified

PAIN, NEC

Acute	Due to trauma	Postoperative	Other	Post-thoracic			
	G89.11	G89.18	R52	G89.12			
Chronic	Central synd	Due to trauma	Chronic synd	Postoperative	Other	Post-thoracic	
	G89.0	G89.21	G89.4	G89.28	G89.29	G89.22	
Limb	Arm, upr (axilla)	Forearm	Fingers	Hand	Foot	Lower leg	Thigh	Toes
	M79.62x	M79.63x	M79.64x	M79.64x	M79.67x	M79.66x	M79.65x	M79.67x
Myofascial	M79.1	—						
Other pain	Chest, unsp	Jt prosthesis	Generalized	Necplasm-related	Joint x arthralgia		
	R07.9	T84.84Xx	R52	G89.3	M26.62		

6th character meanings unless otherwise indicated: 1 or 4 right 2 or 5 left 0 or 9 unspecified
7th character "x": D subsequent encounter S sequela

OTHER DISEASE / DISORDER

	w/ GI manifestation	w/ Pulmonary manifestation	w/ Other manifestation	Unspecified
Cystic fibrosis	E84.19	E84.0	E84.8	E84.9

Diabetes mellitus w/ complication

Circulatory

	Type I	Type II
Periph angiopath (w/ gangrene)	E10.51	E11.51
w/o Gangrene	E10.52	E11.52
Other	E10.59	E11.59

Neurological

	Type I	Type II
Amyotrophy	E10.44	E11.44
Autonomic (poly) neuropathy	E10.43	E11.43
Mononeuropathy	E10.41	E11.41

Other

	Type I	Type II
Arthropathy, NOS	E10.618	E11.618
Neuropathic	E10.610	E11.610
Dermatitis	E10.620	E11.620

	E10	E11
Other / Polyneuropathy / unspecified	E10.49	E11.49
	E10.42	E11.42
	E10.40	E11.40
Skin / Ulcer / Foot	E10.628	E11.628
	E10.621	E11.621
Other, skin	E10.622	E11.622

SIGNS & SYMPTOMS

Ataxia, NOS R27.0	Coordination, lack of R27.9	Debility R53.81	Develop, lack of normal (child) R62.50	Difficulty walking R26.2	Fatigue, other R53.83	Gait, abn unsp R26.9	Gait, ataxic R26.0
Headache, NOS R51	Incont, urine NOS R32	Invol movmnt, unsp R25.9	Paresthesia, skin R20.2	Wasting, pelvic muscle (female) N81.84	Weakness R53.1	Seizure, post-traumatic R56.1	Tremor, unsp R25.1
Vestibular d/o	Labyrinthitis H83.0x	Labyrinthine dysf H83.2Xx	Labyrinth fistula, unsp H83.1x	Meniere's disease H81.0x	Neuronitis H81.2x	Other H81.8Xx	R25.1
Vertigo	Aural H81.31x	Benign positional H81.1x	Central origin H81.4x	Peripheral H81.39x	Unspecified R42		

5th or 6th character "x": 1 right 2 left 3 bilateral 9 unspecified

General Equivalence Mappings

General Equivalence Mappings (GEMs) attempt to include all valid relationships between the codes in the ICD-9-CM diagnosis classification and the ICD-10-CM diagnosis classification. The tool allows coders to look up an ICD-9 code and be provided with the most appropriate ICD-10 matches and vice versa. GEMs are not a "crosswalk;" they are merely meant to be a guide. Users should exercise clinical judgment when choosing the appropriate code or codes to map between ICD-9 and ICD-10 in either direction. GEMs are a very useful tool, but they are not a substitute for a complete system change over to ICD-10. In some instances, GEMs can be helpful in validating your coding practices to help identify some codes in ICD-10 relative to existing ICD-9 for the purpose of training and validation. The ICD-10 codes will be increasing from approximately 15,000 ICD-9 codes to 150,000 ICD-10 codes, although coders will not need to know every code. Visit the CMS website at www.cms.gov/ICD10 for more information on GEMs.

Step 1:

When choosing the first code to be used (as the principal diagnosis), the first question to be asked is "Is the patient admitted for rehabilitation?" If the patient is admitted for rehabilitation, the number of disciplines that are going to treat the patient should be noted. For multiple therapies, the code to be used is V57.89. If the patient would need to undergo Physical Therapy, the code is V57.1 (Coding, 2010).

V57.1 Encounter for physical therapy

V57.2 Encounter for occupational therapy

V57.3 Encounter for speech therapy

V57.89   Other (multiple therapies) (this code is the best code to use as a Medical Code for Part A patients when more than one discipline is treating and it is the primary reason for admission to the SNF)

Step 2:

For the second step, it must be determined if aftercare code or late effects are appropriate. Aftercare codes are used when initial treatments of a disease or an injury are already provided but patient still needs care because of the long-term effects of the disease or injury are needed to be addressed.

Basically, there are four categories of aftercare codes: (a) Orthopedic, (b) Surgical, (c) Amputation, and (d) acquired absence of an organ. These codes can be used as either the primary codes or principal diagnosis or supporting codes, whichever may apply. Orthopedic after care codes (V54.xx) should be classified as either traumatic fracture or pathologic fracture. Traumatic fractures are caused by accidents or falls. The range of codes that indicate traumatic fractures is from V54.11 to V54.19, based on the location of the fracture and its height of the specificity. For pathologic fractures, which are usually caused by conditions such as osteoporosis and other bone-corrosive diseases, the codes to be used are ranging from V54.21 to V54.29.

After care codes for joint replacements are different. The codes to be used are V54.81, and codes range from V43.61 to V43.66 (the site of the joint replacement).

When using V-codes for aftercare fractures, some exceptions apply, such as a patient or patient of a facility has sustained a fracture and wasn't able to visit a physician and did not receive any treatment outside of the facility. There are multiple codes to choose from, but the location of the fracture and which bone and portion of that bone was broken should be identified.

Coding for surgical after-care is based on the body system, which is involved. The categories are from V58.4 (with a fifth digit) and V58.7 (with a fifth digit).

Amputation codes use two codes. The first code V54.89 is after-care (other, orthopedic) codes. The second code is for the site of the amputation. For the upper limb, the code V49.6 plus the applicable fifth digit is used to specify the site of amputation. For the lower limb, the code V49.7 with the applicable fifth digit is to be used.

Late Effects of Cerebrovascular Disease (438.0–38.9): This category is used to indicate conditions in 430–437 as the cause of the late effects. The "late effects" include conditions specified as such, or as sequelae, which may occur at any time after the onset of the causal condition. Other late effects use the code 438.89 (other late effects). A second code is needed.

Most V-codes are to be utilized as the primary medical diagnoses. An exception to this is the V15.88, history of fall, which should be secondary. If you have more than five diagnoses, then you will need to place additional diagnoses on the medical diagnoses line. In cases of more than five diagnoses, assign diagnoses in order of importance. Complexities and co-morbidities are not the diagnoses therapy is treating and are instead diagnoses that may affect treatment; therefore, these should not be placed as primary diagnoses. Instead, comorbidities and complexities should be assigned as the last diagnoses. For example, if CVA is the cause of the Dysphagia, coding should occur with the Late Effects CVA code first and the type of Dysphagia as the secondary diagnosis. Code 438.82 Late effects CVA/Dyphagia, then code 787.22 Oropharyngeal phase dysphagia.

In coding muscle weakness, the correct code to use is 728.87 (muscle weakness). 728.2 Muscle disuse and atrophy, not elsewhere classified can only be used if the physician documentation supports the true atrophy of the muscle. 780.79 Other malaise and fatigue defined as Asthenia, lethargy postviral syndrome and tiredness, and 780.99 Other general symptoms are not therapy appropriate. The main concept to remember is that ICD-9 codes are the first line of defense against denials. If the codes look correct when billing occurs, it diminishes the chance of a chart being audited.

74-year-old patient fell at home and sustained a subtrochanteric fracture of the left femur and was discharged home. Physician ordered physical therapy for difficulty in walking and exercise three times a week for one month.		
First-Listed Diagnosis	ICD-9-CM	V57.1 Other physical therapy
	ICD-10-CM	S72.22xd Displaced subtrochanteric fracture of left femur, subsequent encounter for closed fracture with routine healing
Additional Diagnosis	ICD-9- ICD-10-CM	719.7 Difficulty in walking V5.13 Aftercare for healing traumatic fracture of hip R26.2 Difficulty in walking, not elsewhere classified

National Center for Health Statistics. "ICD-10-CM Official Guidelines for Coding and Reporting." 2011. www.cdc.gov/nchs/icd/icd10cm.htm#10update.

Step 3:

Determine if there are any pressure ulcers, dysphagia, or musculoskeletal conditions that have been discovered during the evaluation. In case of bilateral ulcers, the site and stage of both ulcers are to be coded. Other musculoskeletal and nervous system types of codes that are appropriate may be discovered in evaluation. For localized osteoarthritis, the code to be used is 715.1 plus the fifth digit representing the joint that is affected.

For ulcer of lower limbs, except pressure ulcer, code any causal condition first: atherosclerosis of the extremities with ulceration (440.23), chronic venous hypertension with ulcer (459.31), chronic venous hypertension with ulcer and inflammation (459.33), diabetes mellitus (249.80–249.81, 250.80–250.83), postphlebitic syndrome with ulcer (459.11), and postphlebitic syndrome with ulcer and inflammation (459.13).

Step 4:

This step is concerned about the issue of complexities that may cause a great impact on the care to be provided. It is recommended to consult the patient's medical record. In the long-term care setting, we frequently see patients due to a decline in function after an illness and no spontaneous recovery. The appropriate-code typically is 799.3 Debility. We should not utilize the urinary tract infection, dehydration, syncope codes as that is not what we are treating. It is very important to use more than one treatment diagnosis if it supports what we are treating. Multiple treatment diagnoses may be appropriate to reflect our interventions.

Acute codes should not be used in the long-term care setting but are reserved for the acute phase of an illness or condition. It is appropriate to use the Aftercare or Late Effects codes in this situation. If a patient is admitted with a diagnosis of acute fracture, the best approach is to get an order for the appropriate V-code that corresponds with the fracture.

Comorbidities and complexities should be assigned as the last diagnoses; therefore, they should only be added last. It is also imperative that the evaluation documentation support the impact of the complexity or co-morbidity.

A medical review will determine if documentation has lack of medical necessity, excessive frequency and duration and insufficient documentation. The goal for a patient is to return to the highest level of function realistically attainable within the context of the disability. The skills of a therapist may not necessarily be required to attain this goal, but may be required initially to ensure safety, select proper modalities for treatment, then transferring the patient to a self-management or caregiver assisted treatment program. Limited services (two to four visits) may be covered to establish and train the patient and/or caregiver in a maintenance program.

History of CPT Codes

The American Medical Association created and now copyrights and maintains the Current Procedural Terminology codes (CPT codes). Medicare began to accept them in 1983; however, CPT codes for outpatient services billing under Medicare Part B did not start until the late 1990s. There are speculations about how it actually started and how it came to affect outpatient service billing practices, as we now know it. The move was initiated in 1992 when a legislation issued by the United States Congress prompted Medicare to implement a new payment system. This was known as RBRVS or the Resource Based Relative Value Scale. The main idea in developing the RBRVS was to have a credible system that would ensure the price paid by Medicare for billed services is based on the actual prevailing cost and that there is no underpayment or overpayment of such. In the system adopted by the RBRVS, there are three categories where costs are divided. These are expense or value of the actual work, the practice expense, and expenses related to malpractice. In making the system easier for practitioners to adopt, work expense was further divided into three different components such as technical expertise, the mental effort and judgment spent on performing a task, and the physical effort needed to accomplish it. However, time was not totally considered as a vital component unless counseling and coordination of care was included and a major part of the meeting with the patient (AMA, 2010; APTA, 2014; CMS, 2014).

Medicare still refused to pay for services billed by physical therapists using E&M codes (Evaluation and Management codes). There was a small number of payers, however, that accepted billing done using E&M codes, but it was later found that therapists using this have the tendency to bill higher than what is accepted since billing is done based on how much time is spent treating the patient instead of the three categories previously described. Unfortunately for physical therapists, they were faced with a myriad of problems related to this, such as having to refund overpayment and court cases related to them (Durham, 2008; AMA, 2011).

There were also problems brought about by this confusion since physical therapists could not perform their jobs effectively trying to figure out the RVUs (relative value units) of treatments being given to their patients to be able to correctly use the codes for billing. Conversely, the use of RVUs was a cause of negative reception from physical therapists and billers since there were instances where seemingly different procedures in terms of time spent and complexity had the same value. The negative reception and its impact on physical therapy practice prompted the APTA to make steps in finding a remedy to the problem.

Even with the intervention of the APTA, trying to find a solution to the problem was not an easy one. One of the issues uncovered was the coding did not work well and was not well received by practitioners who are non-physicians. But the APTA pushed on with ensuring that physical therapist's voice was heard on the table and given the chance to finally contribute to the process of revising the 97000 code to make sure that the value of using codes would be beneficial for the profession in general.

In January 1995, results of the work of the APTA proved to be successful when a 200% increase in payments was made to physical therapists that used the revised codes. The positive outcome of the efforts of the APTA pushed for attention to be given to an appropriate coding system physical therapists could use in terms of billing evaluation and reevaluation services for patients covered under Medicare Part B. One of the ways to better do this was to come up with a multi-level coding system describing most outpatient physical therapy services being billed. Due to its applicability, the CMS and Medicare in general were introduced to it, although some hesitation was expressed initially because of its efficiency and accuracy in the billing system. To solve the looming problem over a possible rejection of these codes, the APTA took the initiative to restructure the multi-level coding system into a single coding plan for both evaluation and reevaluation, leading to its final approval for use in April 1997 and subsequent implementation on January 1998.

In a final selection process that included weighing the options about the income potential in using a specific coding guideline, the flexibility and degree of freedom it gave for physical therapists to properly bill patients for the services that were provided, the APTA, together with the CMS and Medicare as well as other health care insurance agencies, decided to choose the use of the CPT codes for outpatient services. This created an impact on the practice of physical therapists since whatever system would be chosen, adopted and recognized by payers would contribute to earnings over a considerable length of time as well as the refining and development of this coding system for future use. The CPT was finally adopted for use in billing for services as part of the Correct Coding Initiative (CCI).

In Depth Look at CPT Codes

The Current Procedural Terminology codes, also known as CPT codes, are used to code procedures and services rendered by physicians. CPT codes usually consist of five-digit numbers that are assigned to a certain task or service a medical practitioner is performing on a patient. Insurers also use CPT codes to determine how much reimbursement is to be paid to providers. Using CPT codes ensures uniformity and accuracy in identifying procedures (CPT, 2004).

The provider must choose the name of a service that best describes the service that was rendered. In the event that there is no suitable code, a report needs to be made about the service using an unlisted procedure or service code. Subsequent supplementary procedures and other special services should also be listed. If needed, modifiers are also listed. Every service or procedure must have complete documentation. Modifiers are used if a service or a procedure has been modified by specific circumstances but still falls into the category of the code that has been assigned to that service or procedure.

Not all services and procedures have a corresponding CPT code. To report unlisted procedures, you can refer to specific code numbers that are used to report them. There are also services that are not often rendered because they are only used for rare conditions. These kinds of services may need a special report to determine if they are medically appropriate. An accurate description or definition of the service or procedure must be provided, along with its extent and the medical necessity. The time duration, equipment used, and the effort applied in providing the service is to be reported. Information about the nature of the symptoms, diagnostic conclusion, physical findings, diagnostic and therapeutic procedures, problems that exist alongside the condition and the plan for follow-up care can also be included in reporting the special service.

The physician may change a treatment plan written by a therapist. The therapist may only alter a written treatment plan following consultation with the physician, except in the case of an adverse reaction to the therapy by the patient.

The use of modalities as stand-alone treatments is rarely therapeutic, and usually not required or indicated as a sole treatment approach to a patient's condition. The use of exercise and activities has proven to be an essential part of a therapeutic program. Therefore, it is expected that a treatment plan consists not solely of modalities, but includes therapeutic procedures, such as therapeutic exercise, neuromuscular re-education, gait training and therapeutic activities. Examples of exceptions are wound care, or when a patient is unable to endure therapeutic procedures due to the acuteness of the condition. The standard treatment is up to 18 sessions within a six-week period. Services provided concurrently by a physical therapist and occupational therapist may be covered if separate and distinct goals are documented in the treatment plans.

When modalities, mechanical traction, and paraffin bath are used alone and solely to promote healing, relieve muscle spasm, reduce inflammation and edema, or as analgesia, one or two visits may be medically necessary to determine the effectiveness of treatment and for patient education. If effective, further treatment may be self-administered in the home as it is not medically necessary to continue "modality only" treatment by the therapist.

Generally, only one heating modality is coverable per session. Exceptions could include musculoskeletal pathology in which both superficial and deep structures are impaired. Documentation supporting the medical necessity for multiple heating codes such as paraffin bath, shortwave diathermy, microwave and ultrasound, on the same day, must be made available to Medicare upon request.

Generally, only one hydrotherapy modality is covered per session when the sole purpose is to relieve muscle spasm, inflammation, or edema. When treating wounds or other skin conditions, in addition to relieving muscle spasms, inflammation or edema, more than one may be reasonable and necessary. Documentation supporting the medical necessity for hydrotherapy modalities, such as whirlpool, Hubbard tank and aquatic exercise must be made available to Medicare upon request.

Modalities chosen to treat the patient's symptoms/conditions should be selected based on the most effective and efficient means of achieving the patient's functional goals. Use of more than two modalities on each visit date is unusual and should be carefully justified in the documentation.

When the symptoms that required the use of certain modalities begin to subside and function improves, the medical record should reflect the discontinuation of those modalities, so as to determine the patient's ability to self-manage any residual symptoms. As the patient improves, the medical record should reflect a progression of the other procedures of the treatment program (therapeutic exercise, therapeutic activities, etc.). In all cases, the patient and/or caregiver should be taught aspects of self-management of his/her condition from the start of therapy.

Coding for Procedures

Once the exact medical code for a patient's condition that calls for physical therapy services is known, the next thing to consider is the code for an intervention or a procedure that the physical therapist renders for the patients. This procedure coding includes evaluation assessment procedures, intervention procedures and even post-intervention assessment (Sculley, 2013).

At the start of the physical therapy session, where the initial evaluation takes place, an ICD-9-CM code is currently being used and correlated with a medical diagnosis of the patient. This entails the therapist comprehensively assessing the patient using the review of systems approach to determine the presence of a problem and its severity. This initial assessment then necessitates a plan of care to be drawn out and an intervention that needs another code to be input into a records system for processing. The plan to use ICD-10-CM codes has been in place since 2013, but the full implementation, as previously mentioned, will take place in 2015. The two year transition period was given for the billers, coders and physical therapists to adjust from using the former code guidelines to the newer one (Sculley, 2013; CMS, 2014; APTA, 2014; APTA 2015).

One of the more positive things about using a coding scheme for billing for procedures is that there can be a source document that can be created which contains the most common physical therapy services availed by patients. Documents of this type are usually given or created by the one who carries out the billing procedure and contains how the biller can encode the type of encounter with a given patient. An example of this would be the use of CPT Code 97001 when a patient and a physical therapist meet for the first time and an initial assessment or evaluation is made. After the initial evaluation, succeeding actions performed by the physical therapist on a patient are billed using other codes listed. To avoid confusion in billing, the most common activities performed by a therapist on a patient are usually presented together despite the medical diagnosis when making a source document. The more uncommon or least used therapies and interventions done on a patient are normally listed on the latter part of the document. This clustering allows for more efficient use of the coding system and faster referencing when billing is made (Sculley, 2013).

It is also worth noting that billing for patient care rendered by physical therapists extends beyond the initial evaluation and treatment. Different incidents leading to an injury, even if they receive the same treatment, would need to be billed according to their nature.

Another matter about billing with regard to procedures and treatments rendered by physical therapists is the need for the billers to know the correct CPT Code modifiers to use when preparing bills. There are instances in which Medicare does not make payments because of repeated encoding of a procedure or the wrong use of a CPT Code Modifier. The most common among these modifiers used in billing for physical therapy services are the procedural code modifiers. These consist of codes used based on the nature of the encounter between the patients and their physical therapists. When a 25 modifier (the most commonly used) is used for encoding, this means that the billers are submitting bills for patients who are in for the first time or are receiving periodic assessment of their conditions. They may also be ones who were in for counseling prior to discharge from their physical therapy treatment programs. The 21 Modifier, on the other hand, is used when patients are receiving care that is longer than what is normally allowed by their coverage plans. An example of this is when a patient is receiving physical therapy after a stroke. 21 Modifier codes require that the billers or the physical therapists use proper documentation when billing for it to justify its need.

The main feature of the CPT codes that initially proved to be challenging for most physical therapists to understand was the suffixes and superscripts used to relate it to the CCI modifiers. These modifier indicators are normally presented using the digits zero (0), nine (9) and (1), which are placed after each code number used. These three digits are used to denote the following:

- The numeral zero (0) indicates there is neither situation nor related conditions in which a specific modifier would be appropriate for use. This means that when this modifier is attached to a code or codes, these are not going to be paid separately by the payer.

- When one (1) is used, it denotes that there is a modifier that the therapist can refer to in order to differentiate among services provided to a client. If the code is correctly used and attached to a specific code, there is a basis for justification of billing of separate payments for services already provided.

- 9- Using nine (9) as a modifier code indicates that the codes with which it is used together may have been deleted at the same time with their relative effectivity dates. Simply stated, codes for which this modifier is used are no longer active and combinations may be billed without the need of modifiers for it to be considered valid.

The last of the most commonly used modifiers in billing for physical therapy procedures under Medicare Part B is the GP Modifier. This is mostly used when the services afforded to patients are performed on an outpatient basis such as those performed during physical therapist home visits or in community centers. This modifier needs to have a valid medical diagnosis and a reason for the need to do outpatient care.

Examples of CPT codes:

97110   Therapeutic exercises to develop strength and endurance, range of motion, and flexibility (15 minutes)

97140   Manual therapy techniques (e.g., connective tissue massage, joint mobilization and manipulation, and manual traction) (15 minutes)

97010   Hot or cold pack application

97014   Electrical stimulation (unattended)

97112   Neuromuscular re-education of movement, balance, coordination, kinesthetic sense, posture, and/or proprioception for sitting and/or standing activities (15 minutes)

97001   Physical therapy evaluation

97530   Dynamic activities to improve functional performance, direct (one-on-one) with the patient (15 minutes)

97035   Ultrasound (15 minutes)

97002   Physical therapy re-evaluation

97032   Electrical stimulation (manual) (15 minutes)

97116   Gait training (includes stair climbing) (15 minutes)

97012   Mechanical traction

97016   Vasopneumatic devices

97535   Self-care/home management training (e.g., activities of daily living [ADL] and compensatory training, meal preparation, safety procedures, and instructions in use of assistive technology devices/adaptive equipment), direct one-on-one contact (15 minutes)

97113   Aquatic therapy with therapeutic exercises (15 minutes)

97124   Massage, including effleurage, petrissage, and/or tapotement (stroking, compression, percussion) (15 minutes)

97033   Iontophoresis (15 minutes)

97150   Group therapeutic procedure(s) (two or more individuals)

97026   Infrared

97039   Unlisted modality (specify type and time if constant attendance)

97250   Myofascial release (no longer a CPT code, but billable under the California workers compensation system in lieu of 97140)

97018   Paraffin bath

97022   Whirlpool

98960   Education and training for patient self-management by a qualified, non-physician health care professional using a standardized curriculum, face-to-face with the individual patient (could include caregiver/family) (30 minutes)

29530   Knee strapping

98941   Chiropractic manipulative treatment (CMT) of the spine (three to four regions)

29540   Ankle and/or foot strapping

29240   Shoulder strapping (e.g., Velpeau)

97139   Unlisted therapeutic procedure (specify)

97750   Physical performance test or measurement (e.g., musculoskeletal, functional capacity), with written report (15 minutes)

95831   Extremity (excluding hand) or trunk muscle testing, manual (separate procedure) with report

90901   Biofeedback training by any modality

97799   Unlisted physical medicine/rehabilitation service or procedure

CPT codes are copyright 1995-2014 American Medical Association. All rights reserved.

Untimed CPT Codes

When a therapy treatment modality or procedure is not defined in the AMA CPT Manual by a specific time frame (such as "each 15 minutes"), the modality or procedure is considered an "untimed" service. Untimed services are billed based on the number of times the procedure is performed, often once per day. Untimed services billed as more than one unit will require significant documentation to justify treatment greater than one session per day per therapy discipline. See the section "CPT 97001 & 97003" for additional guidance on billing for evaluations that span more than one day. The minutes spent providing untimed services are reflected in the documentation under "Total Treatment Time" and are not included in the minutes for timed CPT codes when determining the number of timed-based units that may be billed.

Timed CPT Codes

Many CPT codes for therapy modalities and procedures specify that direct (one on one) time spent in patient contact is 15 minutes. The time counted is the time the patient is treated using skilled therapy modalities and procedures, and is recorded in the documentation as "Timed Code Treatment Minutes." Pre- and post-delivery services are not to be counted when recording the treatment time. The time counted is the "intra-service" care that begins when the qualified professional/auxiliary personnel is directly working with the patient to deliver the service. The patient should already be in the treatment area (e.g., on the treatment table or mat or in the gym) and prepared to begin treatment. The intra-service care includes assessment.

The first step when billing timed CPT codes is to total the minutes for all timed modalities and procedures provided to the patient on a single date of service for a single discipline. For example, a patient under a PT plan of care receives skilled treatment consisting of 20 minutes therapeutic exercise (CPT 97110) and 20 minutes self-care/home management training (CPT 97535). The total "Timed Code Treatment Minutes" documented will be 40 minutes. In addition, the combined time of 40 minutes will determine the total number of timed code PT units that shall be billed for the day. Whether a single timed code service is provided, or multiple timed code services, the skilled minutes documented in "Timed Code Treatment Minutes' will determine the number of units billed.

When the total Timed Code Treatment for the day is less than 8 minutes, the service(s) should not be billed.

It is important to allocate the total billable units for timed services to the appropriate CPT codes based upon the number of minutes spent providing each individual service. Any timed service provided for at least 15 minutes must be billed one unit. Any timed service provided for at least 30 minutes must be billed two units, and so on. When determining the allocation of units, it is easiest to separate out each service first into "15-minute time blocks." For example:

20 minutes of Therapeutic Exercise (CPT 97110) = one 15-minute block + 5 remaining minutes

- At least one unit must be allocated to this code.

38 minutes of Self-care/Home Management Training (97535) = two 15-minute blocks + 8 remaining minutes

- At least two units must be allocated to this code.

- If 38 minutes of CPT 97535 is the only treatment provided, then three units would be billed. However, as demonstrated in the examples below, there may be treatment sessions in which the correct billing would only allow two units, based on the "remaining minutes".

The "remaining minutes" (those minutes remaining after the "15-minute blocks" have been allocated) are considered when the total billable units for the day allow for an additional unit to be billed.

See the following example:

7 minutes of neuromuscular reeducation (CPT 97112)

7 minutes of therapeutic exercise (97110)

7 minutes of manual therapy (97140)

21 total Timed Code Treatment minutes

The clinician shall select which CPT code to bill since each service was performed for the same amount of time and only one unit is allowed. The correct coding is:

1 unit 97112

OR

1 unit 97110

OR

1 unit 97140

For treatment sessions with both timed and untimed services, the units and time documented for any untimed CPT codes should not be included in the counting of units and time for the timed CPT codes for a calendar day. The minutes for the timed codes are reflected in the Timed Code Treatment Minutes, with the units allocated as described above. The untimed minutes are reflected in the Total Treatment Time, which is a combination of the timed code minutes and the untimed code minutes. Per CMS, it is important that the total number of timed treatment minutes support the billing of units on the claim, and that the total treatment time reflects services billed as untimed codes. For example:

35 minutes PT evaluation (CPT 97001-untimed code)

25 minutes therapeutic exercise (CPT 97110)

8 minutes therapeutic activities (CPT 97530)

Total Timed Code Treatment minutes = 33 minutes

Total Treatment Time = 68 minutes

The evaluation, being an untimed code, is billable as one unit. Do not include the evaluation minutes in the total timed code treatment minutes when determining the appropriate number of units to bill for the timed codes. 33 total minutes of timed codes is billable as two units. To allocate the two timed code units, break out the 15-minute blocks first.

25 minutes 97110 = one 15-minute block + 10 remaining minutes; 8 minutes 97530 = zero 15-minute blocks + 8 remaining minutes

Since code 97110 has one 15-minute block, at least one unit of 97110 shall be billed. To determine which code shall be billed with the second unit, compare the remaining minutes. Since code 97110 has more remaining minutes, the second timed code unit shall be applied to this code. Correct coding for this session is:

One unit 97001 + two units 97110

The medical record documentation will note that the therapeutic activities were performed.

40 minutes PT evaluation (CPT 97001 (untimed))

20 minutes unattended electrical stimulation (CPT G0283 (untimed))

10 minute therapeutic exercise for home exercise program (CPT 97110)

Total Timed Code Treatment Minutes = 10 minutes

Total Treatment Time = 70 minutes

The untimed services are billable as one unit each. 10 minutes for the timed code is billable as one unit. The correct coding for this session is:

One unit 97001 + one unit G0283 + one unit 97110

Miscoded services may lead to improper payment, or if medically reviewed, denials of billed charges. Medical records must always support all HCPCS/CPT codes and units billed.

- Do not bill for documentation time separately (except for CPT code 96125).

- Do not code higher than what the procedure requires. Coding in this manner may allow the provider to collect inappropriate revenues without incurring additional costs.

- Do not select the HCPCS/CPT code based on the reimbursement amount associated with a particular HCPCS/CPT. Rather select the HCPCS/CPT based on the code that most accurately describes the service actually provided and/or the intention of the treatment to achieve the desired outcome/goal.

- Do not "unbundle" services/procedures. Unbundling refers to the practice of splitting a single payment code into two or more codes.

- Do not bill separately for supplies used to provide therapy services, such as electrodes, theraband, theraputty, etc.

- Therapists, or therapy assistants, working together as a "team" to treat a patient cannot each bill separately for the same or different service provided at the same time to the same patient. For example, if an OT and PT are co-treating a patient with sitting balance and ADL deficits for 30 minutes, then only two units total can be billed to the patient: either two units of OT only; two units of PT only; or one unit of OT and one unit of PT.

Utilization Guidelines and Maximum Billable Units per Date of Service

Rarely should therapy session length generally be greater than 30-60 minutes (the exception is during an evaluation). If longer sessions are required, documentation must support as medically necessary the duration of the session and the amount of interventions performed.

The following interventions should generally be reported no more than one unit per code per day per discipline:

97001, 97002, 97003, 97004, 97012, 97016, 97018, 97022, 97024, 97028, 97150, 97597, 97598, 97605, 97606, G0281, G0283, G0329.

The following timed modalities should generally be reported no more than two units per code per day per discipline:

97033, 97034, 97035, 97036.

The following interventions should be reported no more than four units per code per day per discipline; additional units will be denied:

97032, 97110, 97112, 97113, 97116, 97124, 97140, 97530, 97532, 97533, 97535, 97537, 97542, 97760, 97761, 97762.

0183T: Low Frequency, Non-Contact, Non-Thermal Ultrasound (MIST Therapy)

CPT/HCPCS code 0183T (Low frequency, non-contact, non-thermal ultrasound, including topical application(s) when performed, wound assessment, and instruction(s) for ongoing care, per day) describes a system that uses continuous low frequency ultrasonic energy to produce and propel a mist of liquid and deliver continuous low frequency ultrasound to the wound bed. This modality is often referred to as "MIST Therapy".

Low frequency, non-contact, non-thermal ultrasound (MIST Therapy) will be considered "reasonable and necessary" wound therapy only if provided two to three times per week and will be eligible for coverage by Medicare when provided as wound therapy for any of the following clinical conditions:

1. Acute or chronic painful venous stasis ulcers, which are too painful for sharp or excisional debridement.

2. Acute or chronic arterial/ischemic ulcers, which are too painful for sharp or excisional debridement.

3. Diabetic or neuropathic ulcers.

4. Radiation injuries or ulcers.

5. Patients with wounds or ulcers with documented contraindications to sharp or excisional debridement.

6. Burns that are painful and/or have significant necrotic tissue.

7. Wounds that have not demonstrated signs of improvement after 30 days of documented standard wound care.

8. Preparation of wound bed sites for application of bioengineered skin products or skin grafting.

Observable, documented improvements in the wound(s) should be evident after two weeks or six treatments. Improvements would include documented reduction in pain, necrotic tissue, or wound size or improved granulation tissue.

Medicare will cover up to six weeks or 18 treatments with documented improvements of pain reduction, reduction in wound size, improved and increased granulation tissue, or reduction in necrotic tissue. Continued treatments beyond 18 sessions per episode of treatment will be considered only upon individual consideration.

29065: Application of Casts and Strapping Codes

The casting and strapping procedures apply when the cast application or strapping is a replacement procedure used during or after the period of follow-up care, or when the cast application or strapping is an initial service performed without a restorative treatment or procedure(s) to stabilize or protect a fracture, injury, or dislocation and/or to afford comfort to a patient.

A clinician who applies the initial cast, strap or splint and also assumes all of the subsequent fracture, dislocation, or injury care cannot use the application of casts and strapping codes as an initial service, since the first cast/splint or strap application is included in the treatment of fracture and/or dislocation codes. A temporary cast/splint/strap is not considered to be part of the preoperative care.

General Guidelines for Casting (CPT codes 29065, 29075, 29085, 29086, 29345, 29355, 29365, 29405, 29425, and 29445):

Therapists typically do not utilize casting interventions for the treatment of fractures. However, casting techniques used by therapists for positioning and stretching are a covered service when an improvement can be noted in an individual's movement patterns and skills. For example, a spastic hand can be casted to facilitate relaxation of the fingers. Serial casting can be essential for individuals with traumatic brain injury-induced spasticity, CVA, and other conditions. Casting should not be utilized for basic contracture management issues. Casting goals should objectively indicate expectation of progress; whereas, the main function of contracture management is to decrease the risk of further contracture.

More than 8-10 visits for evaluation, treatment, modification and caregiver education would not be considered reasonable and necessary without significant documentation. These are untimed codes.

Special instructions for code 29580 (Strapping; Unna boot):

Strapping is not always synonymous with taping (such as McConnell taping or kinesiotaping). See additional information on taping under codes 97110 and 97112. See code 97140 for wrapping techniques for manual lymphatic drainage.

The application of Unna boot paste (zinc, gelatin, or other product) as a bandage or "cold" dressing, is applied to an extremity for the treatment of dermatological, vascular, and on occasion, other conditions. These dressings are often covered by an elastic bandage to give added support, hold the dressing in place and provide a protective cover. Unna boot application is appropriate in the treatment of ulcerations with and without inflammation due to stasis dermatitis produced by vascular insufficiency. The Unna boot is also appropriate for treating ligamentous injuries (sprains and strains) of the ankle. Unna boots need to be changed on a regular basis, depending on the exact type used and the indication. Bilateral Unna boots should be billed with modifier 50 (bilateral procedure). These are untimed codes.

Orthosis application differs from the purpose of an application of a cast or strapping device. Casting and strapping codes should not be reported for orthotics fitting and training. Splinting codes, though rarely used by therapists, may be appropriate for clinical situations (e.g., fracture, sprain, dislocation) where temporary immobilization/fixation is required until there is further treatment disposition. This example is based upon a clinical vignette in CPT Assistant-April 2002. Patient C is a 70-year-old female who presents to the outpatient orthopedic clinic following a left ankle injury when her foot became twisted in her dog's run chain. After the orthopedist evaluates the patient, radiologic views were obtained that substantiated the diagnosis of a sprained ankle ligament. A short-leg plaster posterior molded splint is applied by the physical therapist due to the degree of swelling (billable as CPT 29515). Upon return to the orthopedic clinic, the splint is removed, x-rays repeated, and based on those findings, a short-leg fiberglass non-walking cast is applied. These are untimed codes.

G0283: Electrical Stimulation (CPT G0283 or 97032)

Two codes for electrical stimulation (e-stim) are available under Medicare. 97014 is a valid CPT code, but not for Medicare. Denials of 97032 (direct one on one) occurred when 97032 was billed, but the documentation supported G0283 (supervised). The record should clearly indicate the type of e-stim provided for the reviewer to determine the correct code (G0283 vs. 97032). 97032 can be used if the patient is cognitively impaired and is not safe to be left alone. Electrodes are billed separately. This modality includes the following types of electrical stimulation: Transcutaneous Electrical Nerve Stimulation (TENS), Microamperage E-Stimulation (MENS), Percutaneous Electrical Nerve Stimulation (PENS), Electrogalvanic Stimulation (high voltage pulsed current), Functional Electrical Stimulation, and Interferential current/medium current.

Most electrical stimulation conducted via the application of electrodes is considered unattended electrical stimulation. Examples of unattended electrical stimulation modalities include Interferential Current (IFC), Transcutaneous Electrical Nerve Stimulation (TENS), cyclical muscle stimulation (Russian stimulation).

These types of electrical stimulation may be necessary during the initial phase of treatment, but there must be an expectation of improvement in function. Electrical stimulation must be utilized with appropriate therapeutic procedures to effect continued improvement. The equipment used to perform electrical stimulation must have an appropriate registration number from the Bureau of Medical Devices of the FDA. Electrical stimulation may be useful in reducing swelling and for pain control. It may also be used to accelerate wound healing. The types of electrical stimulation (ES) used for healing chronic venous and arterial wounds and pressure ulcers are pulsed current, such as high volt galvanic stimulation, or pulsed electromagnetic induction. The skills of a therapist are required to perform e-stim. A limited number of treatment sessions without a therapeutic procedure may be medically necessary for the treatment of muscle spasm and swelling. Standard treatment is up to 16 sessions within one month when used as adjunctive therapy or for muscle retraining. When e-stim is used for muscle strengthening or retraining, the nerve supply to the muscle must be intact. It is not medically necessary for motor nerve disorders in which there is complete denervation and no potential for recovery or restoration of function (Coverage Issues Manual, Sections 35–72 and 35–77).

Most non-wound care electrical stimulation treatment provided in therapy should be billed as G0283 as it is often provided in a supervised manner (after skilled application by the qualified professional/auxiliary personnel) without constant, direct contact required throughout the treatment.

97032 is a constant attendance electrical stimulation modality that requires direct (one on one) manual patient contact by the qualified professional/auxiliary personnel. Because the use of a constant, direct contact electrical stimulation modality is less frequent, documentation should clearly describe the type of electrical stimulation provided to justify billing 97032 versus G0283.

Types of electrical stimulation that may require constant attendance and should be billed as 97032 when continuous presence by the qualified professional/auxiliary personnel is required include the following examples.

Instructing a patient in the use of a home TENS unit:

- Once a trial of TENS has been done in the clinic over one to two visits and the patient has had a favorable response, the patient can usually be taught to use a TENS unit for pain control in one to two visits. Consequently, it is inappropriate for a patient to continue treatment for pain with a TENS unit in the clinic setting.

- Note that CPT code 64550 is for application of surface (transcutaneous) neurostimulator and is an operative/postoperative code. Use of this code would seldom fall under a therapy plan of treatment.

- Functional Electrical Stimulation (FES) or Neuromuscular Electrical Stimulation (NMES) while performing a therapeutic exercise or functional activity may be billed as 97032. Do not bill for CPT codes 97110, 97112, 97116 or 97530 for the same time period.

- Use for Walking in Patients with Spinal Cord Injury (SCI)

- The type of NMES that is used to enhance the ability to walk of SCI patients is commonly referred to as functional electrical stimulation (FES). See the section on CPT code 97116 for information on coverage for this use of NMES. (CMS Publication 100-03, Medicare National Coverage Determinations (NCD) Manual, section 160.12)

- Ultrasound with electrical stimulation provided concurrently (e.g., Medcosound, Rich-Mar devices), should be billed as ultrasound (97035). Do not bill for both ultrasound and electrical stimulation for the same time period.

- If providing an electrical stimulation modality that is typically considered supervised (G0283) to a patient requiring constant attendance for safety reasons due to cognitive deficits, do not bill as 97032. This type of monitoring may be done by non-skilled personnel.

- Non-Implantable Pelvic Floor Electrical Stimulation (CMS Publication 100-03, Medicare National Coverage Determinations (NCD) Manual, section 230.8.)

Non-implantable pelvic floor electrical stimulators provide neuromuscular electrical stimulation through the pelvic floor with the intent of strengthening and exercising pelvic floor musculature. Stimulation delivered by vaginal or anal probes connected to an external pulse generator may be billed as 97032. Stimulation delivered via electrodes should be billed as G0283.

The methods of pelvic floor electrical stimulation vary in location, stimulus frequency (Hz), stimulus intensity or amplitude (mA), pulse duration (duty cycle), treatments per day, number of treatment days per week, length of time for each treatment session, overall time period for device use, and between clinic and home settings. In general, the stimulus frequency and other parameters are chosen based on the patient's clinical diagnosis. Pelvic floor electrical stimulation with a non-implantable stimulator is covered for the treatment of stress and/or urge-based urinary incontinence in cognitively intact patients who have failed a documented trial of pelvic muscle exercise (PME) training.

The patient's medical record must indicate that the patient receiving a non-implantable pelvic floor electrical stimulator was cognitively intact, motivated, and had failed a documented trial of pelvic muscle exercise (PME) training.

Utilization of electrical stimulation may be necessary during the initial phase of treatment, but there must be an improvement in function. These modalities should be utilized with appropriate therapeutic procedures to effect continued improvement. Note: Coverage for this indication is limited to those patients where the nerve supply to the muscle is intact, including brain, spinal cord, peripheral nerves, and other non-neurological reasons for disuse are causing the atrophy (e.g., post-casting or splinting of a limb, and contracture due to soft tissue scarring).

Documentation must clearly support the medical necessity of electrical stimulation in more than 12 visits as adjunctive therapy or for muscle retraining.

Some patients can be trained in the use of a home muscle stimulator for retraining weak muscles. Only one to two visits should be necessary to complete the training. Once training is completed, this procedure should not be billed as a treatment modality in the clinic.

Non-covered Indications:

- Electrical Stimulation (CPT code 97032) used in the treatment of facial nerve paralysis, commonly known as Bell's palsy (CMS Manual 100-03, Medicare National Coverage Determinations (NOD) Manual, section 160.15)

- Electrical Stimulation (CPT code 97032) used to treat motor function disorders such as multiple sclerosis (CMS Manual 100-03, Medicare National Coverage Determinations (NOD) Manual, section 160.2)

- Electrical Stimulation (CPT code 97032) for the treatment of strokes when it is determined there is no potential for restoration of function

- Electrical Stimulation used when it is the only intervention utilized purely for strengthening of a muscle with at least Fair graded strength. Most muscle strengthening is more efficiently accomplished through a treatment program that includes active procedures such as therapeutic exercises and therapeutic activities.

Supportive Documentation Recommendations for 97032:

- Type of electrical stimulation used (do not limit the description to "manual" or "attended").

- Area(s) being treated.

- If used for muscle weakness, objective rating of strength and functional deficits.

- If used for pain, include pain rating, location of pain, and effect of pain on function.

Code G0283 is classified as a "supervised" modality, even though it is labeled as "unattended." A supervised modality does not require direct (one on one) patient contact by the provider. Most electrical stimulation conducted via the application of electrodes is considered unattended electrical stimulation. Examples of unattended electrical stimulation modalities include Interferential Current (IFC), Transcutaneous Electrical Nerve Stimulation (TENS), cyclical muscle stimulation (Russian stimulation).

If unattended electrical stimulation is used for control of pain and swelling, there should be documented objective and/or subjective improvement in swelling and/or pain within 6 visits. If no improvement is noted, a change in treatment plan (alternative strategies) should be implemented or documentation should support the need for continued use of this modality.

The charges for the electrodes are included in the practice expense portion of code G0283. Do not bill the Medicare contractor or the patient for electrodes used to provide electrical stimulation as a clinic modality.

Do not bill Medicare for unattended electrical stimulation using code 97014.

Electric Stimulation Therapy (CPT 97014) is not a Medicare recognized code. Use HCPCS code G0283 for electrical stimulation (unattended).

CPT G0281—Electrical stimulation, (unattended), to one or more areas, for chronic stage III and stage IV pressure ulcers, arterial ulcers, diabetic ulcers, and venous stasis ulcers not demonstrating measurable signs of healing after 30 days of conventional care, as part of a therapy plan of care

CPT G0329—Electromagnetic therapy, to one or more areas for chronic stage III and stage IV pressure ulcers, arterial ulcers, diabetic ulcers and venous stasis ulcers not demonstrating measurable signs of healing after 30 days of conventional care as part of a therapy plan of care.

G0261 code replaces code 97014, only where it applies to treatment of wounds, as defined in the code narrative.

Nationally Covered Indications (CMS Publication 100-03, Medicare National Coverage Determinations (NCD) Manual section 270.1): Electrical stimulation (ES) and electromagnetic therapy for the treatment of wounds are considered adjunctive therapies, and will only be covered for chronic Stage III or Stage IV pressure ulcers, arterial ulcers, diabetic ulcers, and venous stasis ulcers. Chronic ulcers are defined as ulcers that have not healed within 30 days of occurrence. ES or electromagnetic therapy will be covered only after appropriate standard wound therapy has been provided for at least 30 days and there are no measurable signs of healing. This 30-day period may begin while the wound is acute.

Standard wound care includes optimization of nutritional status, debridement by any means to remove devitalized tissue, maintenance of a clean, moist bed of granulation tissue with appropriate moist dressings, and necessary treatment to resolve any infection that may be present. Standard wound care based on the specific type of wound includes frequent repositioning of a patient with pressure ulcers (usually every two hours), offloading of pressure and good glucose control for diabetic ulcers, establishment of adequate circulation for arterial ulcers, and the use of a compression system for patients with venous ulcers.

Measurable signs of healing include a decrease in wound size (either surface area or volume), decrease in amount of exudates, and decrease in amount of necrotic tissue. ES or electromagnetic therapy must be discontinued when the wound demonstrates a 100% epithelialized wound bed. ES and electromagnetic therapy services can only be covered when performed by a therapist, a physician or incident to a physician's service. Evaluation of the wound is an integral part of wound therapy. When providing ES or electromagnetic therapy, the therapist must evaluate and frequently reassess the wound, contacting the treating physician if the wound worsens (do not bill a re-evaluation code for the wound assessment). If ES or electromagnetic therapy is being used, wounds must be evaluated at least monthly by the treating physician.

Per NCD 270.1 electrical stimulation (G0281) and electromagnetic therapy (G0329) are NOT COVERED for the treatment of:

- Stage I or stage II wounds.

- Electrical stimulation or electromagnetic therapy when used as an initial treatment modality.

- Continued treatment with ES or electromagnetic therapy if measurable signs of healing have not been demonstrated within any 30-day period of treatment.

- Wounds that demonstrate a 100% epithelialized wound bed.

CMS Publication 100-03, Medicare National Coverage Determinations (NCD) Manual, section 230.8 provides guidance on the use of non-implantable pelvic floor electrical stimulators to provide neuromuscular electrical stimulation through the pelvic floor with the intent of strengthening and exercising pelvic floor musculature. Pelvic floor electrical stimulation with a non-implantable stimulator is covered for the treatment of stress and/or urge-based urinary incontinence in cognitively intact patients who have failed a documented trial of pelvic muscle exercise (PME) training.

90911: Biofeedback Therapy

Biofeedback therapy provides visual, auditory or other evidence of the status of certain body functions so that a person can exert voluntary control over the functions, and thereby alleviate an abnormal bodily condition. Biofeedback therapy often uses electrical devices to transform bodily signals indicative of such functions as heart rate, blood pressure, skin temperature, salivation, peripheral vasomotor activity, and gross muscle tone into a tone or light, the loudness or brightness of which shows the extent of activity in the function being measured.

Biofeedback therapy differs from electromyography which is a diagnostic procedure used to record and study the electrical properties of skeletal muscle. An electromyography device may be used to provide feedback with certain types of biofeedback. Biofeedback therapy is covered under Medicare only when it is reasonable and necessary for the individual patient for muscle re-education of specific muscle groups or for treating pathological muscle abnormalities of spasticity, incapacitating muscle spasm, or weakness, and more conventional treatments (heat, cold, massage, exercise, and support) have not been successful. This therapy is not covered for treatment of ordinary muscle tension states or for psychosomatic conditions.

Biofeedback is covered for the treatment of stress and/or urge-based incontinence in cognitively intact patients who have failed a documented trial of pelvic muscle exercise (PME) training. Biofeedback is not a treatment, per se, but a tool to help patients learn how to perform PME. Biofeedback-assisted PME incorporates the use of an electronic or mechanical device to relay visual and/or auditory evidence of pelvic floor muscle tone, in order to improve awareness of pelvic floor musculature and to assist patients in the performance of PME.

Biofeedback therapy is covered under Medicare only when it is reasonable and necessary for the individual patient for muscle re-education of specific muscle groups or for treating pathological muscle abnormalities of spasticity, incapacitating muscle spasm, or weakness, and more conventional treatments (heat, cold, massage, exercise, and support) have not been successful. This therapy is not covered for treatment of ordinary muscle tension states or for psychosomatic conditions. (CMS Publication 100-03, Medicare National Coverage Determinations (NCD) Manual, Section 30.1)

Biofeedback for incontinence:

Medicare will allow biofeedback as an initial incontinence treatment modality only when, in the opinion of the physician, that approach is most appropriate, and there is documentation of medical justification and rationale for why a PME trial was not attempted first.

Patient selection is a major part of the process and the patient should be motivated, cognitively intact, and compliant. In addition, there must be assurance that the pelvic floor musculature is intact. Biofeedback therapy has proven successful for urinary incontinence when all three of the following conditions exist:

- The patient is capable of participation in the plan of care.

- The patient is motivated to actively participate in the plan of care, including being responsive to the care requirements (e.g., practice and follow-through by self or caregiver).

- The patient's condition is appropriately treated with biofeedback (e.g., pathology does not exist, preventing success of treatment).

When providing biofeedback procedures for urinary incontinence, use CPT 90901 when EMG and/or manometry are not performed.

CPT 90911 describes biofeedback that is more involved than conventional biofeedback measures (code 90901) and includes evaluations of the EMG activity of the pelvic muscles, urinary sphincter and/or anal sphincter by using sensors. This procedure can use manometry (measure of pressure of gases or liquids by use of a manometer) or EMG (electromyography; the recording of electrical activity initiated in the muscle tissue for testing purposes) to measure activity. The EMG activity is evaluated and provides objective information regarding the muscle activity and provides a basis for pelvic muscle rehabilitation utilizing biofeedback.

Biofeedback is not covered for:

- Home use of biofeedback therapy.

- Pelvic floor electrical stimulation lacking documentation of the failure of a trial of pelvic muscle exercise (PME) training, unless there is physician documentation justifying the need to initiate treatment with biofeedback before PME is attempted.

- Patients who do not have sufficient cognitive ability to adhere to and follow the PME protocol and/or cooperate in keeping a personal voiding diary.

Patients not showing improvement after six visits of retraining with biofeedback are not likely to improve with additional sessions. Additional documentation is necessary to justify biofeedback services beyond six visits.

The descriptor for codes 90901 and 90911 does not include a time element and therefore these codes should be billed as one unit.

Supportive Documentation Recommendations for 90901 and 90911

As noted in the NCD descriptions above, biofeedback is covered only when more conventional treatments such as heat, cold, massage, exercise (such as PME), and/or support have not been successful. Therefore, documentation must provide a clear history of the conventional treatments unsuccessfully tried before initiating biofeedback. Since biofeedback is only covered when there is a lack of response to other therapies, the lack of response to or contraindication to other therapies must be noted in the patient's record.

Additionally for the treatment of incontinence, include:

- Identification of the type and degree of incontinence, expectations from the treatment and the time frame in which an improvement is anticipated.

- Clear documentation of the formal instruction, monitoring and follow-up of a prescribed course of PME.

- Evidence of behavioral modification training including, but not limited to, bladder retraining and fluid intake modification.

- The use of a patient record-keeping system, such as a personal voiding diary, in evaluating and monitoring progress.

95851: Range of Motion Tests

Only a qualified therapist may perform range of motion tests and, therefore, such tests would constitute therapy. Range of motion exercises require the skills of a qualified therapist only when they are part of the active treatment of a specific disease which has resulted in a loss or restriction of mobility (as evidenced by therapy notes showing the degree of motion lost and the degree to be restored) and such exercises, either because of their nature or condition of the patient, may only be performed safely and effectively by or under the supervision of a qualified therapist.

CPT Codes 95831, 95832, 95833, 95834, 95851, and 95852—Muscle and Range of Motion Testing

For the typical patient, the evaluation (97001, 97002) and re-evaluation codes (97003, 97004) include all the necessary evaluation tools, including range of motion and manual muscle testing. Baseline measurements may be done with an initial evaluation, but are not separately billable in addition to the evaluation. In addition, assessments, which are separate from evaluations and re-evaluations, are included in the therapy treatment services and procedures and should be coded consistent with the intervention for which the assessment is necessary.

On rare occasions, it may be appropriate to perform a thorough range of motion or manual muscle test during the course of treatment that is separate from the evaluation/re-evaluation. Patients with complicated conditions may warrant specialized tests and measures with standardized reports. For example, a patient with an incomplete C5 quadriplegia at six months post-injury may need specialized testing for ROM or strength measurements to address specific deficits and goals.

Every muscle or joint in the affected extremity or trunk section, as described in the code descriptor, must be tested when coding these procedures. For example:

- Code 95831 is "Muscle testing, manual with report: extremity (excluding hand) or trunk". To use this code for extremity manual muscle testing, every muscle of at least one extremity would need to be tested, with documentation of why such a thorough assessment was warranted. It would not be appropriate to bill code 95831 if only hip strength needed to be tested.

- Code 95851 is "Range of motion measurements and report; each extremity (excluding hand) or trunk section (spine)". To use this code for extremity ROM testing, every joint of an extremity would need to be tested, with documentation of why such a thorough assessment was warranted. It would not be appropriate to bill code 95851 if only shoulder ROM needed to be tested.

It is not reasonable or necessary for these codes to be performed on a routine basis or to be routinely used for all patients (e.g., monthly or in the place of billing for a re-evaluation).

These codes are not covered on the same visit date as CPT codes 97001-97004 (due to CC edits).

Supportive Documentation Recommendations

These codes are typically consultative. It is expected that the administration of these tests will generate material that will be formulated into a report. That report should clearly indicate the purpose and rationale for the test, the test performed with results and how the information affects the treatment plan.

97001: Physical Therapy Evaluation

Evaluations are required prior to beginning therapy to determine the medical necessity of initiating rehabilitative or maintenance services. Patients must exhibit a significant change from normal functional ability to warrant an evaluation. The written evaluation must demonstrate the patient's need for skilled physical therapy based on functional diagnosis, prognosis, and positive prognostic indicators. The therapist must have an expectation that the patient will achieve the established goals. Initial evaluations from other therapy disciplines performed on the beneficiary may also be covered, provided the referral, evaluation, and plan of care are not duplicative.

97002: Physical Therapy Re-Evaluation

Therapy re-evaluations are separately payable if the documentation shows significant and unexpected change in the patient's condition that supports the need to perform a formal re-evaluation of the patient's status. When a patient exhibits a demonstrable change in physical functional ability, a re-evaluation is covered to re-establish appropriate treatment goals and interventions. Reassessments are considered a routine aspect of intervention and are not billed separately from the charge for the intervention. Re-evaluations are not routinely covered for purposes of updating the plan of care. The documentation should focus on assessing significant changes from the initial evaluation or progress toward treatment goals.

CMS Benefit Policy Manual 100-02 Chapter 15 Section 220.3 states a clinician may not merely supervise, but must apply the skills of a therapist by actively participating in the treatment of the patient during each Progress Report Period. The minimum Progress Report Period shall be at least once every 10 treatment days or at least once during each 30 calendar days, whichever is less. Verification of the clinician's required participation in treatment during the Progress Report Period shall be documented by the clinician's signature on the Treatment Note and/or on the Progress Report.

97010: Hot/Cold Packs

Heat treatments do not ordinarily require the skills of a qualified therapist; however, in a particular case, the skills, knowledge, and judgment of a qualified therapist might be required in such treatments or baths, e.g., where the patient's condition is complicated by circulatory deficiency, areas of desensitization, open wounds, or other complications. Also, if such treatments are given prior to but as an integral part of a skilled therapy procedure, they would be considered part of the therapy service. Services, which do not require the performance or supervision of the physician, are not considered reasonable or necessary therapy services even if they are performed or supervised by a physician.

Payment for hot/cold packs is bundled into payment for other related services. Separate payment is not allowed and providers cannot bill Medicare beneficiaries separately for this service. Hot or cold packs (including ice massage) applied in the absence of associated procedures or modalities, or used alone to reduce discomfort are not considered to require the unique skills of a therapist.

Code 97010 is bundled. It may be bundled with any therapy code. Regardless of whether code 97010 is billed alone or in conjunction with another therapy code, this code is never paid separately. If billed alone, this code will be denied.

Supportive Documentation Recommendations for 97010:

- The area(s) treated.
- The type of hot or cold application.

97012: Traction, Mechanical (to one or more areas)

Traction is generally limited to the cervical or lumbar spine with the expectation of relieving pain in or originating from those areas.

Specific indications for the use of mechanical traction include cervical and/or lumbar radiculopathy and back disorders such as disc herniation, lumbago, and sciatica.

This modality is typically used in conjunction with therapeutic procedures, not as an isolated treatment.

Documentation should support the medical necessity of continued traction treatment in the clinic for greater than 12 visits. For cervical conditions, treatment beyond one month can usually be accomplished by self-administered mechanical traction in the home. The time devoted to patient education related to the use of home traction should be billed under 97012.

Only one unit of CPT code 97012 is generally covered per date of service.

Equipment and tables utilizing roller systems are not considered true mechanical traction. Services using this type of equipment are non-covered.

The Medicare National Coverage Determinations (NCD) Manual, Chapter 1, Part 2, Section 160.16 states that vertebral axial decompression is performed for symptomatic relief of pain associated with lumbar disk problems. The treatment combines pelvis and/or cervical traction connected to a special table that permits the traction application. There is insufficient scientific data to support the benefits of this technique. Therefore, VAX-D is not covered by Medicare. There are various types of VAX-D devices including but not limited to: VAX-D, DRX-3000, DRX9000, Decompression Reduction Stabilization (DRS) System, IDD, MedX, Spina System, Accu-Spina System, SpineMED Decompression Table, Lordex Traction Unit, Triton DTS, and the Z-Grav. Regardless of the manufacturer of the device, VAX-D is not a covered service under the Medicare program.

97016: Vasopneumatic Devices (to one or more areas)

The use of vasopneumatic devices may be considered reasonable and necessary for the application of pressure to an extremity for the purpose of reducing edema or lymphedema.

Specific indications for the use of vasopneumatic devices include reduction of edema after acute injury or lymphedema of an extremity. Education on the use of a lymphedema pump for home use is covered when medically necessary and can typically be completed in three or fewer visits once the patient has demonstrated measurable benefit in the clinic environment.

Note: Further treatment of lymphedema by a vasopneumatic device rendered by a clinician after the educational visits is generally not reasonable and necessary unless the patient presents with a condition or status requiring the skills and knowledge of a physical or occupational therapist.

The use of vasopneumatic devices is generally not covered as a temporary treatment while awaiting receipt of ordered compression stockings.

See NOD 280.6 in CMS Publication 100-03, Medicare National Coverage Determinations (NOD) Manual for further coverage and use information on Pneumatic Compression Devices.

Supportive Documentation Recommendations for 97016:

- Area of the body being treated; location of edema.

- Objective edema measurements (1+, 2+ pitting, girth, etc.), comparison with uninvolved side.

- Effects of edema on function.

- Type of device used.

97018: Hot Wax/ Paraffin Treatment

Paraffin wax is primarily used for pain relief in chronic joint problems of the wrists, hands, or feet. For patients in a SNF with a chronic condition such as arthritis, coverage will be allowed until the treatment becomes maintenance in nature. For acute conditions and exacerbation of chronic conditions, it is reasonable to expect some other therapeutic procedure in conjunction with this modality. One or two treatments are usually sufficient to educate the patient in home-use and to evaluate effectiveness. Documentation supporting the medical necessity for additional treatments must be made available to Medicare upon request.

Paraffin bath treatments typically do not require the unique skills of a therapist. However, the skills, knowledge and judgment of a therapist might be required in the provision of such treatment or baths in a complicated case. Only in cases with complicated conditions will paraffin be covered, and then coverage is generally limited to educating the patient/caregiver in home use. Paraffin is contraindicated for open wounds or areas with documented desensitization.

Once a trial of monitored paraffin treatment has been done in the clinic over one or two visits and the patient has had a favorable response, the patient can usually be taught to use a paraffin unit in one or two visits. Consequently, it is inappropriate for a patient to continue paraffin treatment in the clinic setting. Only one unit of CPT code 97018 is generally covered per date of service. Documentation needs to support more than two visits to educate patient and/or caregiver in home use once effectiveness has been determined.

Supportive Documentation Recommendations for 97018:

- Rationale for requiring the unique skills of a therapist to apply and train the patient/caregiver, including the complicating factors.

- Area of body treated.

97022: Whirlpool

This involves the use of agitated water to relieve muscle spasms, improve circulation, or cleanse wounds (i.e., ulcers, exfoliative skin conditions). Site specific hydrotherapy such as power spray is not considered to be hydrotherapy. Patients with circulatory deficiency, areas of desensitization, impaired mobility or limitations in the positioning of a patient, or where there are concerns about safety should be supervised. Standard treatment is up to 16 sessions within one month. Documentation supporting the medical necessity for additional sessions must be made available to Medicare upon request. It is not medically necessary to have more than one form of hydrotherapy during a treatment session.

Whirlpool bath treatments typically do not require the unique skills of a therapist. However, therapist supervision of the whirlpool modality may be medically necessary for the following indications:

- A condition complicated by a circulatory deficiency or areas of desensitization.

- An open wound that is draining and/or has a foul odor, or necrotic tissue.

- Exfoliative skin impairments.

If greater than eight visits are needed for whirlpools that require the skills of a therapist, the documentation should support the medical necessity of the continued treatment.

Only one unit of CPT code 97022 should be billed per date of service.

Dry hydrotherapy massage (also known as aquamassage, hydromassage, or water massage) is considered investigational and is non-covered.

Whirlpool should not be separately billed when provided on the same date of service as debridement (97597-97598) for the same body part.

Fluidotherapy is a superficial dry heat modality consisting of a whirlpool of finely divided solid particles suspended in a heated air stream, with the mixture having the properties of a liquid. Use of fluidized therapy dry heat is covered as an acceptable alternative to other heat therapy modalities in the treatment of acute or sub-acute traumatic or non-traumatic musculoskeletal disorders of the extremities. (CMS Publication 100-03, Medicare National Coverage Determinations (NCD) Manual, Chapter 1, Section 150.8)

Supportive Documentation Recommendations for 97022:

- Rationale for requiring the unique skills of a therapist to apply, including the complicating factors.

- Area(s) being treated.

97024: Diathermy (i.e. microwave)

The objective of these treatments is to cause vasodilation and relieve pain from muscle spasm. Because heating is accomplished without physical contact between the modality and the skin, it can be used even if skin is abraded, as long as there is no significant edema.

Diathermy achieves a greater rise in deep tissue temperature than microwave. As diathermy is considered a deep heat treatment, careful consideration should be given to the size, location and depth of the tissue the diathermy is intended to heat.

Diathermy may be indicated when a large area of deep tissues requires heat. It would not be reasonable and necessary to perform both thermal ultrasound and diathermy to the same region of the body in the same visit as both are considered deep heat modalities.

Pulsed wave diathermy is covered for the same conditions and to the same extent as standard diathermy. (CMS Publication 100-03, Medicare National Coverage Determinations (NOD) Manual, Section 150.5)

Diathermy is not considered reasonable and necessary for the treatment of asthma, bronchitis, or any other pulmonary condition. (CMS Publication 100-03, Medicare National Coverage Determinations (NCD) Manual, Section 240.3) Microwave is not a covered service.

Only one unit of CPT code 97024 is covered per date of service. If no objective and/or subjective improvement are noted after six treatments, a change in treatment plan (alternative strategies) should be implemented, or documentation should include the therapist's rationale for continued diathermy. Documentation must clearly support the need for diathermy more than 12 visits.

Supportive Documentation Recommendations for 97024:

- Area(s) being treated.

- Objective clinical findings/measurements to support the need for a deep heat treatment.

- Subjective findings to include pain ratings, pain location, activities that increase or decrease pain, effect on function, etc.

97026: Infrared Therapy

The use of infrared and/or near-infrared light and/or heat, including monochromatic infrared energy (MIRE), is non-covered for the treatment, including symptoms such as pain arising from these conditions, of diabetic and/or non-diabetic peripheral sensory neuropathy, wounds and/or ulcers of the skin and/or subcutaneous tissues in Medicare beneficiaries. Infrared (to one or more areas) including Anodyne and any related accessories are not reasonable and necessary. The use of infrared and/or near-infrared light and/or heat, including monochromatic infrared energy, is non-covered for the treatment, including the symptoms such as pain arising from these conditions, of diabetic and/or non-diabetic peripheral sensory neuropathy, wounds and/or ulcers of the skin and/or subcutaneous tissues. See OMS Publication 100-03 Medicare National Coverage Determinations (NOD) Manual, section 270.6 and Publication 100-04, Medicare Claims Processing Manual, Chapter 5, section 20.4.

97028: Ultraviolet (to one or more areas)

Treatment of this type is generally used for patients requiring the application of a drying heat. For example, this treatment would be considered reasonable and necessary for the treatment of severe psoriasis where there is limited range of motion.

Only one unit of CPT code 97028 is covered per date of service.

Supportive Documentation Recommendations for 97028:

- Area(s) being treated.

- Objective clinical findings/measurements to support the need for ultraviolet.

- Minimal erythema dosage.

97033: Iontophoresis

Iontophoresis is covered only for intractable, disabling primary focal hyperhidrosis. Denials occur when iontophoresis is billed without an appropriate ABN when the diagnosis is for anything but primary focal hyperhidrosis. Good hygiene measures, extra-strength antiperspirants (for axillary hyperhidrosis), and topical aluminum chloride should initially be tried. This must be billed on a separate demand claim.

Iontophoresis is the introduction into the tissues, by means of an electric current, of the ions of a chosen medication. This modality is used to reduce pain and edema caused by a local inflammatory process in soft tissue, e.g., tendonitis, bursitis.

The evidence from published, peer-reviewed literature is insufficient to conclude that the iontophoretic delivery of non-steroidal anti-inflammatory drugs (NSAID5) or corticosteroids is superior to placebo when used for the treatment of musculoskeletal disorders. Therefore, iontophoresis will not be covered for these indications.

Iontophoresis will be allowed for treatment of intractable, disabling primary focal hyperhidrosis that has not been responsive to recognized standard therapy. Good hygiene measures, extra-strength antiperspirants (for axillary hyperhidrosis), and topical aluminum chloride should initially be tried.

97034: Contrast Baths (to one or more areas)

Contrast baths are a form of therapeutic heat and cold applied to distal extremities in an alternating pattern. The effectiveness of contrast baths is thought to be due to reflex hyperemia produced by the alternating exposure to heat and cold.

Hot and cold baths ordinarily do not require the skills of a therapist. However, the skills, knowledge and judgment of a therapist might be required in the provision of such treatments in a particular case, e.g., where the patient's condition is complicated by circulatory deficiency, areas of desensitization, open wounds, fracture or other complication.

Documentation must indicate the presence of these complicating factors for reimbursement of this code. If there are no complicating factors requiring the skills of a therapist, this modality is non-covered.

CPT Code 97034 is not covered when the services provided are hot and cold packs.

This modality should be used in conjunction with therapeutic procedures, not as an isolated treatment.

No more than two visits will generally be covered to educate the patient and/or caregiver in home use, and to evaluate effectiveness. Documentation must support the medical necessity of continued use of this modality for greater than two visits.

This is a constant attendance code requiring direct, one on one patient contact by the provider. Only the actual time of the provider's direct contact with the patient is to be billed.

Supportive Documentation Recommendations for 97034:

- Rationale requiring the unique skills of a therapist to apply, including the complicating factors.

- Area(s) being treated.

- Subjective findings to include pain ratings, pain location, effect on function.

97035: Ultrasound (to one or more areas)

Therapeutic ultrasound is a deep heating modality that produces a sound wave of 0.8 to 3.0 MHz. In the human body, ultrasound has several pronounced effects on biologic tissues. It is attenuated by certain tissues and reflected by bone. Thus, tissues lying immediately next to bone may receive as much as 30% greater dosage of ultrasound than tissue not adjacent to bone. Because of the increased extensibility ultrasound produces in tissues of high collagen content, combined with the close proximity of joint capsules, tendons, and ligaments to cortical bone where tissue may receive a more intense irradiation, ultrasound is an ideal modality for increasing mobility in those tissues.

Covered ultrasound may be pulsed or continuous width and should be used in conjunction with therapeutic procedures, not as an isolated treatment.

Specific indications for the use of ultrasound application include but are not limited to:

- Limited joint motion that requires an increase in extensibility.

- Symptomatic soft tissue calcification.

- Neuromas.

Ultrasound application is not considered reasonable and necessary for the treatment of:

- Asthma, bronchitis, or any other pulmonary condition.

- Wounds.

Phonophoresis (the use of ultrasound to enhance the delivery of topically applied drugs) will be reimbursed as ultrasound, billable using CPT 97035. Separate payment will not be made for the contact medium or drugs.

Ultrasound with electrical stimulation provided concurrently (e.g., Medcosound, Rich-Mar devices), should be billed as ultrasound (97035). Do not bill for both ultrasound and electrical stimulation for the same time period.

If no objective and/or subjective improvement are noted after six treatments, a change in treatment plan (alternative strategies) should be implemented, or documentation should support the need for continued use of ultrasound. Documentation must clearly support the need for ultrasound more than 12 visits.

Supportive Documentation Recommendations for 97035:

- Area(s) being treated.

- Frequency and intensity of ultrasound.

- Objective clinical findings such as measurements of range of motion and functional limitations to support the need for ultrasound.

- Subjective findings to include pain ratings, pain location, effect on function.

97036: Hubbard Tank (to one or more areas)

This modality involves the patient's immersion in a tank of agitated water in order to relieve muscle spasm, improve circulation, or cleanse wounds, ulcers, or exfoliative skin conditions.

Qualified professional/auxiliary personnel providing one-on-one supervision of the patient are required. If the level of care does not require the skills of a therapist, then the service is not covered.

Hubbard tank treatments more than 12 visits require clear documentation supporting the medical necessity of continued use of this modality.

It is not medically necessary to have more than one form of hydrotherapy during a visit (CPT codes 97022, 97036)

- Rationale requiring the unique skills of a therapist to apply, including the complicating factors.

- Area(s) being treated.

97110: Therapeutic Exercises

Therapeutic exercises are movement to correct impairment and improve musculoskeletal function. These types of exercises can help ambulation and mobilize joints and muscles. They also improve circulation, coordination, balance, and muscle strength (Lieberman et. al., 2009). The following are examples to document the approaches used for therapeutic exercises: progressive resistance exercises, open chain exercises, closed chain exercises, gymnastic ball or theraband for resistance exercises, quad sets, squats, heel raises, ankle pumps, hip abduction, straight leg raises, and upper extremity (UE) and lower extremity (LE) range of motion exercises on all planes. Document measurable indicators such as functional loss of joint motion or muscle strength, as well as the impact of these limitations to the patient's daily function. Demonstrate how the improvement in one or more of these measures improves function.

If an exercise is taught to a patient and performed for the purpose of restoring functional strength, range of motion, endurance training, and flexibility, CPT code (97110) is the appropriate code. If the focus is not strength, range of motion, endurance or flexibility, then it is likely that a different CPT code is more appropriate.

Many therapeutic exercises require the unique skills of a therapist to evaluate the patient's abilities, design the program, and instruct the program. More than two to four visits to develop and train the patient or caregiver in performing PROM, exercises to promote overall fitness, flexibility, and endurance (in absence of a complicated patient condition), aerobic conditioning, weight reduction, and maintenance exercises to maintain range of motion and/or strength are non-covered. In addition, exercises that do not require, or no longer require, the skilled assessment and intervention of qualified professional/auxiliary personnel are not covered.

NGS LCD 26884 Outpatient Physical and Occupational Therapy Services provide the following example of when a service that is initially skilled becomes non-skilled: "as part of the initial therapy program following total knee arthroplasty (TKA), a patient may start a session on the exercise bike to begin gentle range of motion activity. Initially the patient requires skilled progression in the program from pedal-rocks, building to full revolutions, perhaps assessing and varying the seat height and resistance along the way. Once the patient is able to safely exercise on the bike, no longer requiring frequent assessment and progression, even if set up is required, the bike now becomes an 'independent' program and is no longer covered by Medicare. While the qualified professional/auxiliary personnel may still require the patient to 'warm up' on the bike prior to other therapeutic interventions, it is considered a non-skilled, unbillable service and should not be included in the total timed code treatment minutes."

Supportive Documentation Recommendations for 97110:

- Objective measurements of loss of strength and range of motion (with comparison to the uninvolved side) and effect on function.

Repetitive type exercises often can be taught to the patient or a caregiver as part of a self-management, caregiver or nursing program that includes passive-only exercise. Include the following in your documentation:

- If used for pain, include pain rating, location of pain, and effect of pain on function.
- Analysis of substitutions.
- Progressions/downgrades.
- Techniques used to ensure proper performance.
- Instruction in HEP or caregivers.
- Emphasize why therapist was important in therapeutic exercise.

Exercises to promote overall fitness, flexibility, endurance (in absence of a complicated patient condition), aerobic conditioning, weight reduction, and maintenance exercises to maintain range of motion and/or strength are non-covered. In addition, exercises that do not require, or no longer require, the skilled assessment and intervention of qualified professional/auxiliary personnel are non-covered. Repetitive type exercises often can be taught to the patient or a caregiver as part of a self-management, caregiver or nursing program.

Documentation should describe new exercises added, or changes made to the exercise program to help justify that the services are skilled. Documentation must also show that exercises are being transitioned as clinically indicated to an independent or caregiver-assisted exercise program ("home exercise program" (HEP)). An HEP is an integral part of the therapy plan of care and should be modified as the patient progresses during the course of treatment.

If an exercise is taught to a patient and performed for the purpose of restoring functional strength, range of motion, endurance training, and flexibility, CPT code 97110 is the appropriate code. For example, a gym ball exercise used for the purpose of increasing the patient's strength should be considered as therapeutic exercise when coding for billing. Also, the minutes spent taping, such as McConnell taping, to facilitate a strengthening intervention would be counted under 97110.

Lack of exercise equipment at home does not make continued treatment in the clinic skilled or reasonable and necessary. The home program may need to be carried out through community resources.

Documentation must clearly support the need for continued therapeutic exercise greater than 12-18 visits.

For many patients a passive-only exercise program should not be used more than two to four visits to develop and train the patient or caregiver in performing PROM. Documentation would be necessary to support services beyond this level (such as PROM where these is an unhealed, unstable fracture, or new rotator cuff repair, requiring the skills of a therapist to ensure that the extremity is maintained in proper position and alignment during the PROM).

Supportive Documentation Recommendations for 97110:

- Objective measurements of loss of strength and range of motion (with comparison to the uninvolved side) and effect on function.

- If used for pain, include pain rating, location of pain, and effect of pain on function.

Document specific exercises that are performed, purpose of exercises as related to function, instructions given, and/or assistance needed to perform exercises to demonstrate that the skills of a therapist were required.

When skilled cardiopulmonary monitoring is required, include documentation of pulse oximetry, heart rate, blood pressure, perceived exertion, etc.

97110 –Therapeutic Exercises to develop strength and endurance, range of motion and flexibility (one or more areas, each 15 minutes) may require the unique skills of a therapist to evaluate the patient's abilities, design the program, and instruct the patient or caregiver in safe completion of the special technique. However, after the teaching has been successfully completed, repetition of the exercise and monitoring for the completion of the task, in the absence of additional skilled care, is non-covered. Documentation should include not only measurable indicators such as functional loss of joint motion or muscle strength, but also information on the impact of these limitations on the patient's life and how improvement in one or more of these measures leads to improved function. For many patients, a passive-only exercise program should not be used more than two to four visits to develop and train the patient or caregiver in performing PROM.

97112: Neuromuscular Re-education

People afflicted with restrained movements because of conditions such as cerebrovascular accident can benefit from neuromuscular reeducation. The objective is for the patient to regain the functioning of the affected part of the body. This is to help the patient be more independent and carry on with his or her daily life. The following are examples of neuromuscular reeducation activities:

- BAPS (Biomechanical Ankle Platform System) board.

- Bobath techniques; coordination techniques.

- Desensitization techniques.

- Proprioceptive Neuromuscular Facilitation.

- Lumbar stabilization exercises.

- Feldenkrais; neuromuscular development techniques (NDT).

- Object placement and release techniques.

- Postural control.

- Reflex integration techniques.

- Techniques for inhibition of abnormal reflex activity.

- Visual feedback techniques.

In the 2009 Medicare Physician Fee Schedule final rule, CMS created CPT code 95992 describing canalith repositioning procedures. This procedure is bundled into an Evaluation and Management services and therefore not paid separately. However, since therapists also provide this service and they cannot bill for E/M services, they should continue to bill 97112 for this service.

If an exercise/activity is taught to the patient and performed for the purpose of restoring functional balance, motor coordination, kinesthetic sense, posture, or proprioception for sitting or standing activities, CPT 97112 is the appropriate code. When therapy is instituted because there is a history of falls or a falls screening has identified a significant fall risk, documentation should indicate:

- Specific fall dates and/or hospitalization(s) and reason for the fall(s), if known.

- Most recent prior functional level of mobility, including assistive device, level of assist, frequency of falls or "near-falls".

- Functional loss due to the recent change in condition.

- Balance assessments (preferably standardized), lower extremity range of motion and muscle strength testing.

- Patient and caregiver training.

- Carry-over of therapy techniques to objectively document progress.

This therapeutic procedure is provided to improve balance, coordination, kinesthetic sense, posture, and proprioception (i.e., proprioceptive neuromuscular facilitation, Feldenkreis, Bobath, BAP's boards, and desensitization techniques). The procedure may be reasonable and medically necessary for impairments that affect the body's neuromuscular system (i.e., poor static or dynamic sitting/standing balance loss of gross and fine motor coordination, hypo/hypertonicity).

CPT 97112 – Neuromuscular Re-education of movement, balance, coordination, kinesthetic sense, posture, and/or proprioception for sifting and/or standing activities (one or more areas, each 15 minutes).

This therapeutic procedure is provided for the purpose of restoring balance, coordination, kinesthetic sense, posture, and proprioception (e.g., proprioceptive neuromuscular facilitation (PNF), BAP's boards, vestibular rehabilitation, desensitization techniques, balance and posture training).

This procedure may be reasonable and necessary for restoring prior function, which has been affected by:

- Loss of deep tendon reflexes and vibration sense accompanied by paresthesia, burning, or diffuse pain of the feet, lower legs, and/or fingers.

- Nerve palsy; such as peroneal nerve injury causing foot drop.

- Muscular weakness or flaccidity as result of a cerebral dysfunction, a nerve injury or disease or having had a spinal cord disease or trauma.

- Poor static or dynamic sitting/standing balance.

- Postural abnormalities.

- Loss of gross and fine motor coordination.

- Hypo/hypertonicity.

It may not be reasonable and necessary to extend visits for a patient with falls, or any patient receiving therapy services, if the purpose of the extended visits is to:

- Remind the patient to ask for assistance.

- Offer close supervision of activities due to poor safety awareness.

- Remind a patient to slow down.

- Offer routine verbal cues for compensatory or adaptive techniques already taught.

- Remind a patient to use an assistive device.

- Train multiple caregivers.

- Begin a maintenance program.

In these instances, once the appropriate cues have been determined by the qualified professional/ auxiliary personnel, training of caregivers can be provided and the care should be turned over to supportive personnel or caregivers since repetitive cues and reminders do not require the skills of a therapist.

Documentation must clearly support the need for continued neuromuscular reeducation greater than 12-18 visits.

Supportive Documentation Recommendations for 97112:

- Objective loss of ADLs, mobility, balance, coordination deficits, hypo- and hypertonicity, posture and effect on function.

- Specific exercises/activities performed (including progression of the activity), purpose of the exercises as related to function, instruction given, and/or assistance needed, to support that the skills of a therapist were required.

97112 – Neuromuscular Re-education of movement, balance, coordination, kinesthetic sense, posture, and/or proprioception for sitting and/or standing activities (one or more areas, each 15 minutes) would be used if PNF or techniques for tone reduction are delivered.

97113: Aquatic Therapy with Therapeutic Exercise

This procedure uses the therapeutic properties of water (e.g. buoyancy, resistance) to facilitate improvement in function. When therapy services may be furnished appropriately in a community pool by a clinician in a physical therapy private practice or physician office, the practice/office or provider shall rent or lease the pool, or a specific portion of the pool. The use of that part of the pool during specified times should be restricted to the patients of that practice or provider.

Aquatic therapy refers to any therapeutic exercise, therapeutic activity, neuromuscular re-education, or gait activity that is performed in a water environment including whirlpools, hubbard tanks, underwater treadmills and pools. Exercises in the water environment to promote overall fitness, flexibility, improved endurance, aerobic conditioning, weight reduction, or for maintenance purposes are non-covered.

Documentation must show objective loss of joint motion, strength, or mobility (i.e., degrees of motion, strength grades, and levels of assistance). This code should not be used in situations where no exercise is being performed in the water environment (i.e., debridement of ulcers). This procedure may be medically necessary for training patients whose walking abilities have been impaired by neurological, muscular, or skeletal abnormalities or trauma. This procedure is not reasonable or medically necessary when the patient's walking ability is not expected to improve. Repetitive walking for feeble or unstable patients to increase endurance does not require skilled supervision and will be deemed by Medicare as not reasonable and necessary.

This code should not be used in situations where no exercise is being performed in the water environment (e.g., debridement of ulcers).

If continued aquatic exercise is needed, the patient should be instructed in a home program during these visits. Lack of pool facilities at home does not make continued treatment skilled or reasonable and necessary. The home program may need to be carried out through community resources. Documentation must clearly support the need for aquatic therapy greater than eight visits.

Consider the following points when providing aquatic therapy services:

- Does your patient require the skills as a therapist, or could the patient achieve functional improvement through a community-based aquatic exercise program?

- There are a limited number of therapeutic exercises generally performed in the water. These exercises become repetitive quickly. Once a patient can demonstrate an exercise safely, you may no longer bill Medicare for the time it takes the patient to perform this now independent exercise. If the same exercise is performed over a number of sessions, the documentation must describe the skilled nature of the qualified professional's/auxiliary personnel's intervention during the therapeutic exercise to support the ongoing medical necessity.

- The aquatic therapy treatment minutes counted toward the total timed code treatment minutes should only include actual skilled exercise time that required direct one on one patient contact by the qualified professional/auxiliary personnel. Do not include minutes for the patient to dress/undress, get into and out of the pool, etc.

- Do not bill for the water modality used to provide the aquatic environment, such as whirlpool (97022), in addition to 97113.

See CPT 97150 Group Therapy for guidelines when treating more than one patient at the same time in the aquatic environment.

97116: Gait Training

Gait evaluation and training rendered to a patient whose ability to walk has been impaired by neurological, muscular, or skeletal abnormality requires the skills of a qualified therapist. However, if gait evaluation and training cannot reasonably be expected to significantly improve the patient's ability to walk, such services would not be considered reasonable and necessary.

Repetitive exercises to improve gait or maintain strength and endurance, and assistive walking, such as provided in support for feeble or unstable patients, are appropriately provided by supportive personnel such as aides or nursing personnel and do not require the skills of a qualified therapist.

This procedure may be reasonable and necessary for training patients and instructing caregivers in ambulating patients whose walking abilities have been impaired by neurological, muscular, or skeletal abnormalities or trauma.

Indications for gait training include, but are not limited to:

- Musculoskeletal trauma, requiring ambulation reeducation.
- A chronic, progressively debilitating condition for which safe ambulation has recently become a concern.
- An injury or condition that requires instruction in the use of a walker, crutches, or cane.
- A condition that requires retraining in stairs/steps or other uneven surfaces appropriate to home and community function (ramps, inclines, curbs, grass, etc.).
- Instructing a caregiver in appropriate guarding and assistive techniques.

Gait training is not considered reasonable and necessary when the patient's walking ability is not expected to improve.

Antalgic gait alone does not support the need for ongoing skilled gait training. Antalgic gait refers to a gait pattern assumed in order to avoid or lessen pain. Limited gait training may be appropriate, when supported as medically necessary in the documentation, to teach the patient improved gait patterns to reduce the stress on the painful area. In most circumstances, as the pain decreases (with or without skilled therapy intervention) the gait will improve spontaneously without the need for skilled gait training intervention.

Documentation must clearly support the need for continued gait training beyond 12-18 visits within a four to six week period.

Neuromuscular Electrostimulation—is used for Walking in patients with Spinal Cord Injury (SCI) (CPT code 97116). The type of NMES that is used to enhance the ability of SCI patients to walk is commonly referred to as functional electrical stimulation (FES). These devices are surface units that use electrical impulses to activate paralyzed or weak muscles in precise sequence. Coverage for the use of NMES/FES is limited to SCI patients, for walking, who have completed a training program, which consists of at least 32 physical therapy sessions with the device over a period of three months. The trial period of physical therapy will enable the physician treating the patient for his or her spinal cord injury to properly evaluate the person's ability to use these devices frequently and for the long-term. Physical therapy necessary to perform this training must be directly performed by the physical therapist as part of a one on one training program.

The goal of physical therapy must be to train SCI patients on the use of NMES/FES devices to achieve walking, not to reverse or retard muscle atrophy.

Coverage for NMES/FES for walking will be covered in SCI patients with all of the following characteristics:

1. Persons with intact lower motor units (L1 and below) (both muscle and peripheral nerve).

2. Persons with muscle and joint stability for weight bearing at upper and lower extremities that can demonstrate balance and control to maintain an upright support posture independently.

3. Persons that demonstrate brisk muscle contraction to NMES and have sensory perception [of] electrical stimulation sufficient for muscle contraction.

4. Persons that possess high motivation, commitment and cognitive ability to use such devices for walking.

5. Persons that can transfer independently and can demonstrate independent standing tolerance for at least three minutes.

6. Persons that can demonstrate hand and finger function to manipulate controls.

7. Persons with at least 6-month post recovery spinal cord injury and restorative surgery.

8. Persons with/without hip and knee degenerative disease and no history of long bone fracture secondary to osteoporosis.

9. Persons that have demonstrated a willingness to use the device long-term.

(From CMS Publication 100-03, Medicare National Coverage Determinations (NCD) Manual, section 160.12)

ICD-9-CM diagnosis code 344.1 must be present for payment to be made. However, while paraplegia of lower limbs is a necessary condition for coverage, the nine criteria above are also required.

97116 is the only code to be billed. It must be used for one on one face-to-face service provided by the physician or therapist.

In documenting gait training, the reason for providing the gait training must be present in the medical records. These include adjustment of center of mass over base of support, facilitation of righting reactions, facilitation of symmetrical stance, training in compensatory strategies with gait on varying surfaces, training in correct hand and foot placement during gait, training strategies to compensate for inadequate (B) hip/knee flexion during stance and training strategies to safely maneuver around obstacles. Gait training locations can be in the following areas: on level and uneven surfaces, outdoors, in hallway, throughout nursing facility, and on inclines. An important long-term goal of therapists is to have patients move around and walk independently with minimum pain and assistance.

97124: Massage, including effleurage, petrissage and/or tapotement (stroking, compression, percussion) (one or more areas, each 15 minutes)

Massage may be medically necessary as adjunctive treatment to another therapeutic procedure on the same day, which is designed to reduce edema, improve joint motion, or relieve muscle spasm. Massage chairs, aqua-massage tables and roller beds are not considered massage. These services are non-covered. Massage is not covered as an isolated treatment.

Documentation must clearly support the need for continued massage beyond eight visits, including instruction, as appropriate, to the patient and caregiver for continued treatment.

This code is not covered on the same visit date as CPT code 97140 (manual therapy techniques).

Do not bill 97124 for percussion for postural drainage.

Supportive Documentation Recommendations for 97124:

- Area(s) being treated.
- Objective clinical findings such as measurements of range of motion, description of muscle spasms and effect on function.
- Subjective findings including pain ratings, pain location and effect on function.

97140: Manual Therapy

This CPT code became effective January 1, 1999, and covers the following previous CPT codes: 97122, 97250, 97260, 97261, and 97265, which were discontinued (not accepted for payment) March 31, 1999. Several different modalities, all with different indications, are included under HCPCS code 97140. For example: Manual traction is not indicated for rheumatoid arthritis, while joint mobilization is indicated for rheumatoid arthritis. Because of this, each modality included under code 97140 has different limited coverage. Documentation of the exact modality used must be kept in the patient's medical records. It may include soft tissue mobilization, myofascial release, joint mobilization techniques, manual edema mobilization, stretching of shortened connective tissue, manual lymphatic drainage, manipulation techniques, and manual traction.

For cervical radiculopathy, patients in a SNF will be covered until symptoms have stabilized and no further improvement is possible. The necessity for continued coverage in a SNF should be supported by documentation in the medical records. Myofascial Release/Soft Tissue Mobilization may be medically necessary for the treatment of restricted motion of soft tissues involving the extremities, neck, and/or trunk. Skilled manual techniques (active and/or passive) are applied to effect changes in the soft tissues, articular structures, neural, or vascular systems. It may be medically necessary to perform this procedure prior to therapeutic exercises up to 16 sessions within one month.

Manual traction may be considered reasonable and necessary for cervical dysfunctions such as cervical pain and cervical radiculopathy.

Joint Mobilization (peripheral and/or spinal) may be considered reasonable and necessary if restricted or painful joint motion is present and documented. It may be reasonable and necessary as an adjunct to therapeutic exercises when loss of articular motion and flexibility impedes the therapeutic procedure.

Myofascial release/soft tissue mobilization, one or more regions, may be reasonable and necessary for treatment of restricted motion of soft tissues in involved extremities, neck, and trunk. Skilled manual techniques (active or passive) are applied to soft tissue to effect changes in the soft tissues, articular structures, and neural or vascular systems.

Manipulation, which is a high-velocity, low-amplitude thrust technique or Grade V thrust technique, may be reasonable and necessary for treatment of painful spasm or restricted motion in the periphery, extremities or spinal regions.

Manual lymphatic drainage/complex decongestive therapy is indicated for both primary and secondary lymphedema. Lymphedema in the Medicare population is usually secondary lymphedema, caused by known precipitating factors. Common causes include surgical removal of lymph nodes, fibrosis secondary to radiation, and traumatic injury to the lymphatic system.

Both primary and secondary lymphedemas are chronic and progressive conditions, which can be brought under long-term control with effective management. By maintaining control of the lymphedema, patients can:

- Restore a normal, or near-normal, shape.

- Reduce the potential for complications (e.g., cellulitis, lymphangitis, deformity, injury, fibrosis, lymphangiosarcoma (rare), etc.).

- Reduce functional deficits to resume activities of daily living.

Manual lymphatic drainage/complex decongestive therapy consists of skin care, manual lymph drainage, compression wrapping, and therapeutic exercises. Coverage of Manual lymphatic drainage/complex decongestive therapy would only be allowed if all of the following conditions have been met:

- There is a physician-documented diagnosis of lymphedema (primary or secondary).

- The patient has documented signs or symptoms of lymphedema.

- The patient or patient's caregiver has the ability to understand and comply with the continuation of the treatment regimen at home.

The goal of treatment is to reduce lymphedema of an extremity by routing the fluid to functional pathways, preventing backflow as the new routes become established, and to use the most appropriate methods to maintain such reduction of the extremity after therapy is complete. This therapy involves intensive treatment to reduce the volume by a combination of manual decongestive therapy and serial compression bandaging, followed by an exercise program. Ultimately the plan must be to transfer the responsibility of care from the therapist to management by the patient, patient's family, or patient's caregiver.

In moderate-severe lymphedema, daily visits may be required for the first week. Education should be provided to the patient and/or caregiver on the correct application of the compression bandage.

The therapeutic exercise component for Manual lymphatic drainage/complex decongestive therapy is covered under CPT code 97110.

Manual lymphatic drainage/complex decongestive therapy is not covered for:

- Conditions reversible by exercise or elevation of the affected area.

- Dependent edema related to congestive heart failure or other cardiomyopathies.

- Patients who do not have the physical and cognitive abilities, or support systems, to accomplish self-management in a reasonable time.

- Continuing treatment for a patient non-compliant with a program for self-management.

Documentation must clearly support the need for continued manual therapy treatment beyond 12-18 visits. When the patient and/or caregiver has been instructed in the performance of specific techniques, the performance of these same techniques should not be continued in the clinic setting and counted as minutes of skilled therapy.

CPT code 97124 (massage) is not covered on the same visit as this code.

Supportive Documentation Recommendations for 97140:

- Area(s) being treated.

- Soft tissue or joint mobilization technique used.

- Objective and subjective measurements of areas treated (may include ROM, capsular end-feel, pain descriptions and ratings,) and effect on function.

Supportive documentation should include:

- Medical history related to onset.

- Exacerbation and etiology of the lymphedema.

- Comorbidities.

- Prior treatment.

- Cognitive and physical ability of patient and/or caregiver to follow self-management techniques.

- Pain/discomfort descriptions and ratings.

- Limitation of function related to self-care, mobility, ADLs and/or safety.

- Prior level of function.

- Limb measurements of affected and unaffected limbs at start of care and periodically throughout treatment.

- Description of skin condition, wounds, infected sites, scars.

CPT code 97140-Manual Therapy Techniques (e.g., mobilization/manipulation, manual lymphatic drainage, manual traction), one or more regions, each 15 minutes.

97150: Group Therapy Services

Contractors pay for therapy services provided simultaneously to two or more individuals by a practitioner as group therapy services. The individuals can be, but need not be performing the same activity. The physician or therapist involved in group therapy services must be in constant attendance, but one on one patient contact is not required. Code 97150 must be reported for each member of the group.

Group therapy consists of therapy treatment provided simultaneously to two or more patients who may or may not be doing the same activities. If the therapist is dividing attention among the patients, providing only brief, intermittent personal contact, or giving the same instructions to two or more patients at the same time, one unit of CPT code 97150 is appropriate per patient.

Supervision of a previously taught exercise program or supervising patients who are exercising independently is not a skilled service and is not covered as group therapy or as any other therapeutic procedure. Supervision of patients exercising on machines or exercise equipment, in the absence of the delivery of skilled care, is not a skilled service and is not covered as group therapy or as any other therapeutic procedure.

Non-covered as group therapy:

- Groups directed by a student, therapy aide, rehabilitation technician, nursing aide, recreational therapist, exercise physiologist, or athletic trainer.

- Routine (i.e., supportive) groups that are part of a maintenance program, nursing rehabilitation program, or recreational therapy program.

- Groups using biofeedback for relaxation.

- Viewing video recordings, listening to audio recordings.

- Group treatment that does not require the unique skills of a therapist.

If group therapy is billed on a given day, it must be listed in the Treatment Note. The minutes of this untimed code must be added to the Total Treatment Time for that day. Further documentation describing the skilled nature of the group session documented in the progress report or the treatment note may assist in supporting the medical necessity of the service.

Supportive Documentation Recommendations for 97150:

- The purpose of the group and the number of participants in the group.

- Description of the skilled activity provided in the group setting, such as instruction in proper form, or upgrading the difficulty of the activity for an individual.

Group therapy on the same day: You may duplicate CPT codes in the same day as long as the interventions you are providing are not duplicative in nature, and your documentation can support the provision of both groups. Using the same code twice or more on the same day may be flagged by the intermediary as duplication of services or a billing error.

In 2002, the Medicare program was targeted with issues and concerns related to the use of codes. This has been given special attention by physical therapists because use of codes affects how billing is done for outpatient services provided. Two of the most common areas of concern identified are use of one-on-one code and the use of a group code. Through the support shown by the APTA among its members in the position of having clearer interpretation of the codes used for outpatient group physical therapy, the CMS has clarified their definitions in the Carriers Manual Transmittal 1753 (Sculley, 2013; CMS, 2014).

Despite the agreement of the APTA with how the CMS interprets one-on-one codes and group codes, the organization also believes that the CMS should take the needed steps in making sure there is a proper organization of group codes when they are used for reimbursement for services provided. This is borne out of the fact that, despite the use of codes, there is still a considerable number of payers contracted by the CMS that has little knowledge of the 97150 code. This means that when 97150 is used in making payment claims, these contractors refuse to pay the biller if the said code is put in the same bill as a one-on-one code (Coding and Billing APTA, 2014).

The use of one-on-one codes was first introduced to billing and making payments claims in 1994 when it was first published in the Federal Register. This introduction of the codes included the appropriate description of the one-on-one codes and how to best use them. To ensure that physical therapists, billers and other concerned parties were well aware of this, another publication appeared two years after, in 1996. However, despite this, confusion still occurred, prompting the CMS to further clarify the use of the codes in May of 2002 when it published Carriers Manual Transmittal 1753 (APTA: Coding, 2014).

It is established here that CPT Code 97150 is one of the codes causing confusion to billers and therapists. In its essence, it can be used to bill for procedures done on groups of patients by a single therapist, or two or more practitioners treating a single patient. If one of the practitioners is an assistant, then it is necessary that he be under the direction of a physical therapist during the performance of the procedure. On the other hand, if the group is being treated by a single physical therapist, the therapist should be present the whole time that the group is being treated. An example of this is a group of patients being given therapy for muscle weakness after prolonged bed confinement who need active range of motion exercises. The therapist would be the one to provide the instructions on how the exercises will be performed but should remain present while the said exercises are being performed to assess patients and to validate the group billing code used.

The use of one-on-one and group codes when needed is one of the most effective ways for billing. Due to this, the APTA expresses its support for moves in coming up with how to best interpret these codes and how physical therapists can use them to bill for individual and group therapies as long as other required documents are appropriately included in the billing. Moreover, the time that the group therapy lasted for which a group code is used should be sufficient for the provision of professional services. This is due to the fact that the code is not timed, and therefore can be used with other procedures performed on a particular patient within the same day. When doing this, however, modifier codes may be required for correct billing and coding for claims.

97545: Work Hardening (97545, 97546)

These services are related solely to specific work skills and will be denied as not medically necessary for the diagnosis or treatment of an illness or injury.

CPT 97545– Work hardening/conditioning (initial 2 hours) and CPT 97546 (each additional hour).

These services are related solely to specific work skills and will be denied as not medically necessary for the diagnosis or treatment of an illness or injury.

97530: Therapeutic Activities

Therapeutic activities can help patients of a long-term care facility improve their cognitive skills and physical skills. These would also help them resolve behavioral problems and improve their emotional well-being and self-esteem. The following are therapeutic activities that patients can undergo:

- Bed mobility training.
- Bilateral manipulation.
- Buttoning, zipping and hooking clothing fasteners to improve fine motor coordination.
- Crossing midline to facilitate independence in functional skill performance.
- Dexterity tasks.
- Dynamic functional activities.
- Facilitation of position in space.
- Facilitation of postural control.
- Fine and gross motor coordination training.
- Overhead activities, balance and dynamic task performance.
- Static and dynamic balance activities during sitting and standing.
- Techniques to facilitate body awareness.
- Techniques to facilitate proprioception.
- Theraputty techniques.
- Throwing/catching.

- Training in rolling, scooting, bridging.

- Transfer training.

- Visual motor reintegration and training.

Write a rationale for the activity that is functional—in other words, to increase functional skills, to increase range and flexibility.

Therapeutic activities are considered reasonable and necessary for patients needing a broad range of rehabilitative techniques that involve movement. Movement activities can be for a specific body part or could involve the entire body. This procedure involves the use of functional activities (e.g., bending, lifting, carrying, reaching, catching, pushing, pinching, grasping, transfers, bed mobility and overhead activities) to restore functional performance in a progressive manner. The activities are usually directed at a loss or restriction of mobility, strength, balance, or coordination. They require the skills of the therapist to design the activities to address a specific functional need of the patient and to instruct the patient in their performance. These dynamic activities must be part of an active treatment plan and must be directed at a specific outcome.

Use of these procedures requires the qualified professional/auxiliary personnel to have direct (one on one) patient contact. Only the actual time of direct contact with the patient providing a service, which requires the skills of a therapist, is considered for coverage. Supervision of a previously taught exercise or exercise program, patients performing an exercise independently without direct contact by the qualified professional/auxiliary personnel, or use of different exercise equipment without requiring the intervention/skills of the qualified professional/ auxiliary personnel are not covered. The patient may be in the facility for a longer period of time, but only the time the qualified professional/ auxiliary personnel is actually providing direct, one on one, patient contact which requires the skills of a therapist is considered covered time for these procedures, and only those minutes of treatment should be recorded.

Under Medicare, time spent in documentation of services (medical record production) is part of the coverage of the respective CPT code; there is no separate coverage for time spent on documentation (except for CPT Code 96125).

In order for therapeutic activities to be covered, the following requirements must be met:

- The patient has a documented condition for which therapeutic activities can reasonably be expected to restore or improve functioning.

- There is a clear correlation between the type of therapeutic activity performed and the patient's underlying medical condition.

- The patient's condition is such that he/she is unable to perform the therapeutic activities without the skilled intervention of the qualified professional/auxiliary personnel.

Documentation must clearly support the need for continued therapeutic activity treatment beyond 10-12 visits.

Supportive Documentation Recommendations for 97530:

- Objective measurements of loss of ADLs, balance, strength, coordination, range of motion, mobility and effect on function.

- Specific activities performed and amount and type of assistance to demonstrate that the skills and expertise of the therapist was required.

97532: Development Of Cognitive Skills To Improve Attention, Memory, Problem Solving, (includes compensatory training) direct (one on one) patient contact by the provider, each 15 minutes

This activity is designed to improve attention, memory, and problem-solving, including the use of compensatory techniques. Cognitive skill training may be medically necessary for patients with acquired cognitive deficits resulting from head trauma, or acute neurologic events including cerebrovascular accidents. Impaired functions may include but are not limited to:

- Ability to follow simple commands.

- Attention to tasks, problem-solving skills, memory, ability to follow numerous steps in a process and perform in a logical sequence, and ability to compute.

Conditions without potential for improvement or restoration, such as chronic progressive brain conditions, would not be appropriate. Evidence-based reviews indicate that cognitive rehabilitation (and specifically memory rehabilitation) is not recommended for patients with severe cognitive dysfunction. Cognitive skill training should be aimed towards improving or restoring specific functions, which were impaired by an identified illness or injury, and expected outcomes, should be reasonably attainable by the patient as specified by the plan of care.

Cognitive skills are an important component of many tasks, and the techniques used to improve cognitive functioning are integral to the broader impairment being addressed. Cognitive therapy techniques are most often covered as components of other therapeutic procedures and are typically better reported using other codes (such as 97535).

Activities billed as cognitive skills development include only those that require the skills of a therapist and must be provided with direct (one on one) contact between the patient and the qualified professional/auxiliary personnel. Those services that a patient may engage in without a skilled therapist qualified professional/auxiliary personnel are not covered under the Medicare benefit.

Supportive Documentation Recommendations for 97532:

- Objective assessment of the patient's cognitive impairment and functional abilities.

- Prognosis for recovery of the specific impaired cognitive abilities (remediation).

- A determination of a range of compensatory strategies that the individual can realistically utilize to improve daily functioning in a meaningful way.

- Specific cognitive activities performed, amount of assistance, and the patient's response to the intervention, to demonstrate that the skills and expertise of the therapist were required.

CPT 97533—Sensory integrative techniques to enhance sensory processing and promote adaptive responses to environmental demands, direct (one on one) patient contact by the provider, each 15 minutes

Sensory integrative techniques are performed to enhance sensory processing and promote adaptive responses to environmental demands. These treatments are performed when a deficit in processing input from one of the sensory systems (e.g., vestibular, proprioceptive, tactile, visual or auditory) decreases an individual's ability to make adaptive sensory, motor and behavioral responses to environmental demands. Individuals in need of sensory integrative treatments demonstrate a variety of problems, including sensory defensiveness, over- reactivity to environmental stimuli, attention difficulties, and behavioral problems.

Utilization of this service should be infrequent for Medicare patients. Supportive Documentation Recommendations for 97533:

- Objective assessments of the patient's sensory integration impairments and functional limitations.

- Describe the treatment techniques used that will improve sensory processing and promote adaptive responses to environmental demands, and the patient's response to the intervention, to support that the skills of a therapist were required.

97535: Self–Care/Home Management Training

This code should be used for skilled therapy services addressing activities of daily living (ADL), IADLs, compensatory training for ADLs/IADLs, safety procedures, and instructions in the use of adaptive equipment and assistive technology for use in the home environment. The documentation must support that the patient has a condition for which self-care/home management training is reasonable and necessary. This is supported by objective documentation of functional limitations and functional goals based on the identified limitations. Supportive Documentation Recommendations for 97535 include:

- Objective measurements of the patient's activity of daily living (ADL)/instrumental activity of daily living (IADL) impairment to be addressed.

- Specific ADL and/or compensatory training provided.

- Specific safety procedures addressed.

- Specific adaptive equipment/assistive technology utilized.

- Instruction given and assist required (verbal or physical).

- Progression in technique to more complex or less patient dependence.

A common billing mistake is to bill all education under CPT code 97535, self-care/home management. However, proper coding is to use the CPT code that best describes the focus of the educational activity. For example, if the instruction given is for exercises to be done at home to improve ROM or strength use 97110; if instructing the patient in balance or coordination activities at home, use 97112; if instructing the patient on using a sock aide for dressing, use 97535; if teaching tub transfers use 97530, and if instructing in a home electrical stimulation unit, use 97032.

Self-care/home management training (e.g., activities of daily living (ADL) and compensatory training, meal preparation, safety procedures, and instructions in use of assistive technology devices/adaptive equipment) requires direct one on one contact by provider, each 15 minutes.

This procedure is reasonable and necessary only when it requires the skills of a therapist, is designed to address specific needs of the patient, and is part of an active treatment plan directed at a specific outcome.

The patient must have a condition for which self-care/home management training is reasonable and necessary. The training should be focused on a functional limitation(s) in which there is potential for improvement in a functional task that will be meaningful to the patient and the caregiver. The patient and/or caregiver must have the capacity and willingness to learn from instructions. Documentation must relate the training to expected functional goals that are attainable by the patient.

This code should be used for activities of daily living (ADL) and compensatory training for ADL, safety procedures, and instructions in the use of adaptive equipment and assistive technology for use in the home environment.

Many ADL/IADL impairments may require the unique skills of a therapist to evaluate the patient's abilities and to design the program and instruct the patient or caregiver in safe completion of the special technique. However, repetitious completion of the activity, once taught and monitored, is non-covered care.

As the patient progresses through an episode of care involving self-care/home management training, documentation needs to clearly support that the skills of a therapist continue to be necessary. Documentation that demonstrates progression in the technique to more complex or less patient dependence will assist in demonstrating that the technique remains skilled. It is important that documentation demonstrates that the skills of a therapist are needed and that the patient is not merely practicing techniques that have already been taught.

Supportive Documentation Recommendations for 97535:

- Objective measurements of the patient's activity of daily living (ADL)/instrumental activity of daily living (IA DL) impairment to be addressed.

- The specific ADL and/or compensatory training provided, specific safety procedures addressed, specific adaptive equipment/assistive technology utilized, instruction given and assist required (verbal or physical), and the patient's response to the intervention, to support that the services provided required the skills and expertise of a therapist.

97537: Community/Work Reintegration Training (e.g., shopping, transportation, money management, avocational activities and/or work environment (modification analysis, work task analysis) direct one on one contact by provider, each 15 minutes)

For wheelchair management/propulsion training use 97542

This training may be medically necessary when performed in conjunction with a patient's individual treatment plan aimed at improving or restoring specific community functions which were impaired by an identified illness or injury and when realistically expected outcomes are specified in the plan. This code should be utilized when a patient is trained in the use of assistive technology to assist with mobility, seating systems and environmental control systems for use in the community.

General activity programs, and all activities which are primarily social in nature, will be denied because the professional skills of a therapist are not required. Services must be necessary for medical treatment of an illness or injury rather than related solely to specific leisure or employment opportunities, work skills or work settings.

Coverage beyond six visits for community training should be justified by documentation to prove the medical necessity of treatment of this length.

Supportive Documentation Recommendations for 97537:

- Objective measurements of the patient's community IADL impairment to be addressed.

- Specific training provided, amount of assist required (verbal or physical), and the patient's response to the intervention, to support that the services rendered required the skills of a therapist.

97542: Wheelchair Management

Wheelchair management evaluation services include:

- Assessment, fitting, and training; analysis of patient's body alignment and functional skills in new or existing wheelchair.

- Measurement/design of new wheelchair to enable functional independence.

- Instruction in proper body alignment in wheelchair to facilitate skin integrity.

- Training in wheelchair propulsion/maneuvering within patient's environment.

- Training in safely removing wheelchair arm/leg rests.

- Training in locking/unlocking brakes to facilitate safety.

- Training in maneuvering around obstacles and instruction with emphasis on safe wheelchair mobility up and down curbs.

When utilized for wheelchair adjustments, describe the specific adaptations. When used for training, document the established goals. If multiple seating issues are identified, treat them concurrently.

This procedure is medically necessary only when it requires the professional skills of a therapist, is designed to address specific needs of the patient, and must be part of an active treatment plan directed at a specific goal. The patient must have the capacity to learn from instructions. Documentation of medical necessity must be available on request for an unusual frequency or duration of training sessions. Typically up to four sessions within one month are sufficient. When billing 97542 for wheelchair propulsion training, documentation must relate the training to expected functional goals that are attainable by the patient.

This code is used to reflect the skilled wheelchair management intervention clinicians provide related to the assessment, fitting and/or training for patients who must utilize a wheelchair for mobility. This service trains the patient, family and/or caregiver in functional activities that promote safe wheelchair mobility and transfers. Patients who are wheelchair bound may occasionally need skilled input on positioning to avoid pressure points, contractures, and other medical complications.

A wheelchair assessment may include but is not limited to the patient's strength, endurance, living situation, capacity for transferring in and out of the chair, level of independence, weight, skin integrity, muscle tone, and sitting balance. Following verification of the patient's need, patient measurements are taken prior to ordering equipment to ensure accuracy of sizing wheelchair components. This measurement may also involve testing the patient's abilities with various chair functions including propulsion, transferring from the chair to other surfaces (bed, toilet, car), and use of the chair's locking mechanism on various types of equipment for optimal determination of the appropriate equipment by the patient and caregiver.

There may be circumstances where a patient may be seen one time for a wheelchair assessment. If it is not necessary to complete a full patient evaluation, but only an assessment related to specific wheelchair needs, this one-time only session may be billed under 97542 with the appropriate units reflecting the time spent in the assessment.

For many patient situations, a full evaluation is needed to develop the appropriate treatment plan in addition to wheelchair fitting and training. In these situations, it may be appropriate to bill the initial evaluation code (97001), with the minutes spent for the evaluation/assessment assigned to 97001. On the day that the evaluation code is billed, the minutes assigned to 97542 should only be related to any wheelchair fitting and training provided, as 97542 is a timed code. For example, if a physical therapist spends 35 minutes gathering the patient history, prior functional status, current functional status, social considerations, range of motion, strength, sensation, balance, and transfers, this time would be assigned to the PT initial evaluation code 97001. As the session continues, the PT spends 45 minutes assessing the patient in a variety of wheelchair set ups, trying a variety of adaptations to best meet the patient's comfort and functional needs, and initiates training with the patient and family. These 45 minutes would be assigned to code 97542.

Typically up to four dates of service should be sufficient to train the patient/caregiver in wheelchair management. Coverage beyond this utilization should have supportive documentation.

Documentation for a skilled wheelchair assessment should include the following:

- The recent event that prompted the need for a skilled wheelchair assessment.

- Any previous wheelchair assessments have been completed, such as during a Part A SNF stay.

- Most recent prior functional level.

- If applicable, any previous interventions was that have been tried by nursing staff, caregivers or the patient that may have failed, prompting the initiation of skilled therapy intervention.

- Functional deficits due to poor seating or positioning.

- Objective assessments of applicable impairments such as range of motion (ROM), strength, sitting balance, skin integrity, sensation and tone.

- The response of the patient or caregiver to the fitting and training.

When billing CPT code 97542 for wheelchair management/training, documentation must relate the training to expected functional goals that are attainable by the patient and/or caregiver.

Describe the interventions to show that the skills of a therapist were required. For example, describe the various wheelchair adaptations trialed and the patient's response to the intervention. If training is provided, describe the type of training, the amount of assistance required and the patient response to the training.

97597: Selective Debridement

Selective Debridement is used to remove devitalized tissue and promote healing. It is indicated when necrotic tissue is present in an open wound. It may be indicated in cases of abnormal wound healing or repair. Wounds of any size with tunneling may require this. Only one unit is billed per session regardless of the number or complexity of the wounds treated. It includes removal and application of dressings to the wound.

CPT 97597—Removal of devitalized tissue from wound(s), selective debridement, without anesthesia (e.g., high pressure water jet with/without suction, sharp selective debridement with scissors, scalpel and forceps), with or without topical application(s), wound assessment, and instruction(s) for ongoing care, may include use of a whirlpool, per session; total wound(s) surface area less than or equal to 20 square centimeters

CPT 97598—Total wound(s) surface area greater than 20 square centimeters

CPT 97602—Removal of devitalized tissue from wound(s), non-selective debridement, without anesthesia (e.g., wet-to-moist dressings, enzymatic, abrasion), including topical application(s), wound assessment, and instruction(s) for ongoing care, per session

Do not report 97597-97602 in conjunction with 11040-11044

Active wound care procedures are performed to remove devitalized tissue and promote healing and involve selective and non-selective debridement techniques. Debridement is indicated whenever necrotic tissue is present in an open wound. Debridement may also be indicated in cases of abnormal wound healing or repair. Debridement will not be considered a reasonable and necessary procedure for a wound that is clean and free of necrotic tissue.

The wound care performed must be in accordance with accepted standards of medical practice. If debridement is performed, the type of debridement should be appropriate to the type of wound and the devitalized tissue, and the patient's condition. Not all wounds require debridement at each session or the same level of debridement at each session. It is unusual to debride more than one time per week for more than three months. A greater frequency or duration of selective debridement should be justified in the documentation. Most very small wounds do not require selective debridement. Ulcers that may require selective debridement are typically larger than two centimeters square. Wounds with tunneling, regardless of size, may require selective debridement. Selective debridement is usually not reasonable and necessary for blisters; ulcers smaller than those described above and uninfected ulcers with clear borders.

Documentation for each treatment must include a detailed description of the procedure and the method (e.g., scalpel, scissors, 4x4 gauze, wet-to-dry, enzyme) used when billing 97597, 97598 and 97602. Because the correct debridement code is dependent on type of debridement and wound size, documentation should include frequent wound measurements. The documentation should also include a description of the appearance of the wound (especially size, but also depth, stage, bed characteristics), as well as the type of tissue or material removed. The documentation must meet the criteria of the code billed.

Medicare coverage for wound care on a continuing basis for a particular wound requires documentation in the patient's record that the wound is improving in response to the wound care being provided. It is not medically reasonable or necessary to continue a given type of wound care if evidence of wound improvement cannot be shown.

Evidence of improvement includes measurable changes (decreases) in at least some of the following:

- Drainage.

- Inflammation.

- Swelling.

- Pain.

- Wound dimensions (diameter, depth).

- Necrotic tissue/slough.

Such evidence must be documented periodically (e.g. weekly.) A wound that shows no improvement after 30 days requires a new approach, which may include a physician/non-physician practitioner reassessment of underlying infection, metabolic, nutritional, or vascular problems inhibiting wound healing, or a new treatment approach.

In rare instances, the goal of wound care provided in outpatient settings may only be to prevent progression of the wound, which, due to severe underlying debility or other factors such as inoperability, is not expected to improve. If this is the case, documentation should clearly indicate this rationale for continued skilled wound care.

Examples of Selective Debridement (without anesthesia) (CPT codes 97597, 97598):

- Conservative Sharp Debridement: Conservative sharp debridement is a minor procedure that requires no anesthesia. Scalpel, scissors, forceps, or tweezers may be used and only clearly identified devitalized tissue is removed. Generally, there is no bleeding associated with this procedure.

- High Pressure Water Jet Lavage: (non-immersion hydrotherapy) is an irrigation device, with or without pulsation used to provide a water jet to administer a shearing effect to loosen debris, within a wound.

Some electric pulsatile irrigation devices include suction to remove debris from the wound after it is irrigated.

Examples of Non-Selective Debridement (without anesthesia) (CPT 97602) include the following items.

- Blunt debridement: Blunt debridement involves the removal of necrotic tissue by cleansing or scraping (abrasion. It may also involve the cleaning and dressing of small or superficial lesions.

- Enzymatic debridement: Debridement with topical proteolytic enzymes is used as an adjunctive therapy in treating chronic wounds. The manufacturers' product insert contains indications, contraindications, precautions, dosage and administration guidelines; it is the clinician's responsibility to comply with those guidelines. Wet-to-moist dressings: Wet-to-moist dressings may be used with wounds that have a high percentage of necrotic tissue, and should be used cautiously as maceration of surrounding tissue may hinder healing. Autolytic and chemical debridement.

- Maggot Debridement Therapy (MDT): Biosurgery, or the use of maggots, is another effective method of debridement. The larvae produce enzymes to break down dead tissue without harming healthy tissue.

These codes are not timed.

Do not bill for more than one unit per session, regardless of the number or complexity of the wounds treated.

Do not bill for both 97597/97598 and 97602 for the same wound.

Use the 59 modifier to indicate nonselective and selective debridement provided in a single encounter at different anatomical sites.

Application and removal of dressings to the wound are included in the work and practice expenses of 97597, 97598 and 97602 and should not be billed separately under a therapy plan of care. Charges for dressings, gauze, tape, sterile water for irrigation, tweezers, scissors, Q-tips, and medications used in the wound care treatment will be denied even if the wound care service is found to be medically reasonable and necessary. Payment for dressings applied to the wound is included in HCPCS codes 97597, 97598 and 97602, and they are not to be billed separately. If a simple dressing change is performed without any active wound procedure as described by these codes, do not bill these codes to describe the service.

For wound assessment, it is not appropriate to bill therapy re-evaluation codes (97002, 97004) along with codes the 97597, 97598 and 97602 codes. The assessment, including measurements of the wound and a written report, is considered a part of the 9 759 7, 97598 and 97602 codes.

97022 (whirlpool) and codes 97597/97598 (selective wound debridement) should not be billed together as the whirlpool treatment is a component of the selective wound debridement code (unless there is a separately identifiable condition being treated and documentation supports this treatment).

Patient and caregiver instructions are included in codes 97597, 97598 and 97602. Do not bill separately under any other code for instructing the patient/care giver in care of the wound.

These codes represent "sometimes therapy" services and will be paid under the OPPS when (a) the service is not performed by a therapist, and (b) it is inappropriate to bill the service under a therapy plan of care. Nurses performing debridement (where allowed by state scope of practice acts) described by codes 97597, 97598 and 97602 may bill these codes using revenue codes other than the therapy revenue codes 42x (PT) and 43x (OT).

Payment for 97602, when performed by qualified professional/auxiliary personnel under a therapy plan of care, is recognized as a bundled service under the Medicare Physician Fee Schedule (MPFS). Regardless of whether billed alone or in conjunction with another therapy code, separate payment is never made for 97602.

Evaluation and management services should not be billed along with the debridement service unless a significant, separately identifiable evaluation and management service, correctly identified with modifier 25 on the claim, was also provided to the patient during the same encounter (therapists should not use the evaluation and management codes at any time.)

Documentation for a Selective Debridement (without anesthesia) includes the following:

- Etiology and duration of wound.

- Prior treatment by a physician, non-physician practitioner, nurse and/or therapist.

- Stage of wound.

- Description of wound: length, width, depth, grid drawing and/or photographs.

- Amount, frequency, color, odor, type of exudate.

- Evidence of infection, undermining, or tunneling.

- Nutritional status.

- Comorbidities (e.g., diabetes mellitus, peripheral vascular disease).

- Pressure support surfaces in use.

- Patient's functional level.

- Skilled plan of treatment, including specific frequency, modalities and procedures.

- Type of debridement performed, including instrument used, to support the debridement code billed.

- Changing plan of treatment based on clinical judgment of the patient's response or lack of response to treatment.

- Frequent skilled observation and assessment of wound healing are recommended daily or weekly to justify the skilled service.

At a minimum, the Progress Report must document the continuing skilled assessment of wound healing as it has progressed since the evaluation or last Progress Report.

Note: While debridement is considered a covered service for appropriately selected wounds, the following services are considered non-covered for the treatment of wounds"

- Topical application of oxygen (CMS Publication 11-03, Medicare National Coverage Determinations (NCD) Manual, section 270.4)

- Ultrasound.

- Infrared and/or near-infrared light and/or heat, including monochromatic infrared energy (MIRE) (CMS Publication 11-03, Medicare National Coverage Determinations (NCD) Manual, section 270.6).

- Low-level Laser Treatment (LLLT).

- Magnet therapy.

- Autologous blood-derived products for chronic, non-healing wounds (CMS Publication 11-03, Medicare National Coverage Determinations (NCD) Manual, section 270.3).

- Routine dressing changes.

- Non-Contact Normothermic Wound Therapy (NNWT) (CMS Publication 11-03, Medicare National Coverage Determinations (NCD) Manual, section 270.2).

97605: Negative Pressure Wound Therapy (e.g., vacuum assisted drainage collection), including topical application(s), wound assessment, and instruction(s) for ongoing care, per session: total wound(s) surface area less than or equal to 50 square centimeters

97606—Total wound(s) surface greater than 50 square centimeters

Negative pressure wound therapy (NPWT) involves negative pressure to the wound bed to manage wound exudates and promote wound healing. NPWT consists of a sterile sponge held in place with transparent film, a drainage tube inserted into the sponge, and a connection to a vacuum source.

NPWT is indicated for use as an adjunct to standard treatment in carefully selected patients who have failed all other forms of treatment. NPWT may be indicated for wounds such as:

- Stage III or IV pressure ulcers.

- Neuropathic (for example, diabetic) ulcers.

- Chronic arterial or venous insufficiency ulcers.

- Complications of surgically created or traumatic wounds.

NPWT is not covered for:

- Stage 1 or II pressure ulcers.

- Wounds with eschar if debridement is not attempted.

- Untreated osteomyelitis within the vicinity of the wound.

- Cancer present in the wound.

- Active bleeding.

- The presence of a fistula to an organ or body cavity within the vicinity of the wound. Additional guidance for NP WT codes.

These codes are not timed.

Do not bill for more than one unit per session, regardless of the number or complexity of the wounds treated.

Patient and caregiver instructions are included in codes 97605/97606. Do not bill separately under any other code for instructing the patient/caregiver in care of the wound.

It is not appropriate to bill the therapy re-evaluation code (97002) along with 97605-97606. The assessment, including measurements of the wound and a written report, is considered a part of 97605-97606.

Supportive Documentation Recommendations for 97605 and 97606:

- Etiology and duration of wound.

- Prior treatment by a physician, non-physician practitioner, nurse and/or therapist.

- Stage of wound.

- Description of wound: length, width, depth, grid drawing and/or photographs.

- Amount, frequency, color, odor, type of exudate.

- Evidence of infection, undermining, or tunneling.

- Nutritional status.

- Comorbidities (e.g., diabetes mellitus, peripheral vascular disease).

- Pressure support surfaces in use.

- Patient's functional level.

- Skilled plan of treatment, including specific frequency, modalities and procedures.

- Changing plan of treatment based on clinical judgment of the patient's response or lack of response to treatment.

- Frequent skilled observation and assessment of wound healing are recommended daily or weekly to justify the skilled service. At a minimum, the Progress Report must document the continuing skilled assessment of wound healing as it has progressed since the evaluation or last Progress Report.

97750: Physical Performance Testing

CPT code 97750, physical performance testing, may be reasonable and necessary for patients with neurological, musculoskeletal, or pulmonary conditions. Examples of physical performance tests or measurements include isokinetic testing, Functional Capacity Evaluation (FCE), six minute walk test (with a computerized report of the patient's oxygen saturation levels with increasing stress levels, performed under a PT plan of care on pulmonary rehabilitation patients), and Tinetti or other balance tests. There must be written evidence documenting the problem requiring the test, the specific test performed, and a separate measurement report. CPT code 97750 is not covered on the same day as CPT codes 97001-97002 (due to CCI edits).

The therapy evaluation and re-evaluation codes are for a comprehensive review of the patient including, but not limited to, history, systems review, current clinical findings, establishment of a therapy diagnosis, and estimation of the prognosis and determination and/or revision of further treatment. CPT 97750 is intended to focus on patient performance of a specific activity or group of activities (CPT Assistant, December 2003).

There must be written evidence documenting the problem requiring the test, the specific test performed, and a separate measurement report. This report may include torque curves and other graphic reports with interpretation.

It is not reasonable and necessary for the test to be performed and billed on a routine basis (i.e., monthly or instead of billing a re-evaluation) or to be routinely performed on all patients treated. 97750 should not be used to bill for patient assessments/re-assessments such as ROM testing or manual muscle testing completed at the start of care (as this is typically part of the examination included in the initial evaluation) and/or as the patient progresses through the episode of treatment.

CPT code 97750 is not covered on the same day as CPT codes 97001-97002 (due to CC/edits).

Supportive Documentation Recommendations for 97750:

- Problem requiring the test and the specific test performed.

- Separate measurement report, including any graphic reports.

- Application to functional activity.

- How the test impacts the plan of care.

97755: Assistive Technology Assessment (e.g., to restore, augment or compensate for existing function, optimize functional tasks and/ or maximize environmental accessibility), direct one on one contact by provider, with written report, each 15 minutes

The provider performs an assessment of the suitability and benefits of acquiring any assistive technology device or equipment that will help restore, augment, or compensate for existing functional ability in the patient (e.g., provision of large amounts of rehabilitative engineering).

Coverage is specifically for assessment of mobility, seating and environmental control systems that require high-level adaptations, not for routine seating and mobility systems (e.g., manual/power wheelchair evaluations).

This is an assessment code, per each 15 minutes, and must be accompanied by a written report explaining the nature and complexity of the assistive technology needed by the patient. This can include testing multiple components/systems to determine optimal interface between client and technology applications, and determining the appropriateness of commercial (off the shelf) or customized components/systems. This assessment may require more than one patient visit due to the complexity of the patient's condition and his/her decreased tolerance for activity at one session.

Training for use in assistive technology in the home environment is coded as 97535 and for use in the community as 97537.

CPT code 97755 is not covered on the same day as CPT codes 97001-97002 (due to CCI edits). Utilization of this service should be infrequent.

Supportive Documentation Recommendations for 97755:

- The goal of the assessment.

- The technology/component/system involved.

- A description of the process involved in assessing the patient's response.

- The outcome of the assessment.

- Documentation of how this information affects the treatment plan.

97760: Orthotic Management & Training

This code is to be used when educating the patient in the use of the orthotic and is not appropriate when issuing pre-fabricated lumbar rolls, positioning supports, or cone shaped forms for hand contractures. Document the specific orthotic and the date issued, why the patient needs it, description of the training provided and the patient's response.

CPT code 97760 is time-based and reported at 15-minute intervals. If the splint has a Level II HCPCS code (usually an L-code), this code is reported for the orthotic and for the evaluation and fitting of the orthotic. CPT code 97760 is appropriate for reporting any training time necessary for the patient to use the orthotic. The documentation must support reporting both codes, including specific information to support reporting training with CPT code 97760.

The orthotic and prosthetic management codes are time-based and intended for reporting once for each 15-minute increment. Materials and supplies may be reported separately with an appropriate supply or material code (e.g., CPT code 99070 or HCPCS Level II code). HCPCS L-codes for orthotics include the evaluation and fitting components of the service. However, any training time associated with using the orthotic may be reported using CPT code 97760. The time reported must be only for time that the patient is present.

CPT code 97760 includes additional orthotic management and training during follow-up visits, including:

- Exercises performed in the orthotic.

- Instruction pertaining to skin care and orthotic wearing time.

- Time associated with modification of the orthotic due to healing of tissues, change in edema, or interruption in skin integrity.

If a HCPCS II code (e.g., an L-code) is reported for an orthotic, the provider may only use CPT code 97760 to describe the services associated with training, as described in the preceding clinical scenario. Assessment and fitting of the orthotic are included in the L-code. The health care practitioner's documentation should reflect the services provided and support reporting either the CPT code or the HCPCS II code. CPT code 97760 remains a 15-minute timed code

Code 97760 should not be reported with 97116 for the same extremity.

An orthotic is a brace that includes rigid and semi-rigid components that are used for the purpose of supporting a weak or deformed body member or restricting or eliminating motion in a diseased or injured part of the body. (Elastic stockings, garter belts, neoprene braces and similar devices do not come within the scope of the definition of a brace.) HCFA Ruling 96-1 clarifies that the "orthotics" benefit is limited to leg, arm, back, and neck braces that are used independently rather than in conjunction with, or as components of, other medical or non-medical equipment.

When consideration is made for a patient to require an orthotic, the therapist targets the problems in performance of movements or tasks, or identifies a part that requires immobilization, and selects the most appropriate orthotic device, then fits the device, and trains the patient and/or caregivers in its use and application. The goal is either to promote indicated immobilization or to assist the patient to function at a higher level by decreasing functional limitations or the risk of further functional limitations.

The complexity of the patient's condition is to be documented to show the medical necessity of skilled therapy to assess, fit, and instruct in the use of the orthotic.

An orthotic may be prefabricated or custom-fabricated.

A prefabricated orthotic is one that is manufactured in quantity and then modified with a specific patient in mind. A prefabricated orthotic may be trimmed, bent, molded (with or without heat), or otherwise modified for use by a specific patient (i.e., custom fitted). An orthotic that is assembled from prefabricated components is considered prefabricated.

A custom fabricated orthotic is one that is individually made for a specific patient starting with basic materials including, but not limited to, plastic, metal, leather, or cloth, from the patient's individualized measurements.

A molded-to-patient model orthotic is a particular type of custom fabricated orthotic in which an impression of the specific body part is made and the impression is then used to make a positive model. The orthotic is molded from the patient-specific model.

Outpatient hospital therapy departments, comprehensive outpatient rehabilitation facilities (CORFs), outpatient rehabilitation facilities, nursing homes (limited to patients covered under a Medicare Part B stay); and home health agencies (limited to patients not under a HH plan of care) bill the Fiscal Intermediary for the orthotic utilizing the relevant HCPCS Level II L code and revenue code 274 on the claim form. These settings do not require a DME supplier-billing enrollment to bill and be reimbursed for the L codes.

A physical therapist in private practice or a physician/non-physician practitioner is considered by Medicare to be a "supplier" and must bill the Durable Medical Equipment Medicare Administrative Contractor (DME MAC) for orthotics. Any supplier that issues orthotics must be enrolled as a supplier of Durable Medical Equipment, Prosthetics, Orthotics, or Supplies (DMEPOS) prior to billing the DME MAC. Follow the directions, from the DME MAC when billing for orthotics (utilizing an L code). Note: Therapists in private practice and physicians/non-physician practitioners should follow the guidance below for billing CPT 97760 to the Medicare carrier.

Payment for prosthetics and orthotics is made on the basis of a fee schedule whether it is billed to the DME MAC or the Fl.

The L codes for orthotics provide a brief description of the device and describe whether the device needs to be molded to a patient model, custom fabricated, custom fitted, or have no fitting specifications. Select the appropriate L code based on the description of the brace provided.

The Medicare payment for the L codes includes the following items.

- Assessment of the patient regarding the orthotic.

- Measurement and/or fitting.

- Supplies to fabricate or modify the orthotic.

- Time associated with making the orthotic.

CPT 97760 should be used for orthotic "training" completed by qualified professionals/auxiliary personnel. CPT 97760 may be used in conjunction with the L code only for the time spent training the patient in the use of the orthotic. Orthotic training may include teaching the patient regarding a wearing schedule, placing and removing the orthosis, skin care and performing tasks while wearing the device. To avoid duplicate billing, the time spent assessing, measuring and/or fitting, fabricating or modifying, or making the orthotic may not be included in calculating the number of units to bill for CPT 97760 when also billing the appropriate L code. CPT 97760 is a "timed" code and only minutes actually spent in the training of the patient should be counted when determining units to bill when an L code is also billed.

There may be circumstances where a patient is only going to be seen for a brief therapy episode for issuance of an orthotic. If it is not necessary to complete a full, comprehensive patient evaluation, but only an assessment related to determining the specific orthotic, does not bill an initial therapy evaluation code in addition to the L code.

For other patient situations, however, a full patient initial evaluation is needed to develop the appropriate treatment plan in addition to an assessment related to determining the specific orthotic. In these situations, it may be appropriate to bill the initial evaluation code (97001), with the minutes spent for the evaluation assigned to 97001. For example, a patient is referred to physical therapy for an ankle-foot orthotic with possible continued therapy. The PT spends 35 minutes evaluating the patient, which includes the history, subjective complaints, prior and current functional levels, ROM, strength, gait, skin integrity, and ADL assessment. This time would be assigned to the PT evaluation code 97001. The PT then begins the assessment of the patient for the orthotic, which includes determining the need for the orthotic and the type of orthotic, subsequently fabricating the appropriate device and fitting it to the patient. This time, which takes 45 minutes, would be reimbursed under the L code. The PT spends an additional 20 minutes training the patient in the wearing schedule of the orthotic, skin care and exercises to be performed while the orthotic is in place. These 20 minutes would be assigned to code 97760, billable as one unit for the training component.

Per CPT Assistant, February 2007 "Code 97760 includes additional orthotic management and training during follow-up visits including exercises performed in the orthotic, instruction in skin care and orthotic wearing time, and time associated with modification of the orthotic due to healing of tissues, change in edema, or interruption in skin integrity."

For an orthotic to be billed, it must be medically necessary for the patient's condition. To bill for training the patient to use the orthotic (CPT 97760), the documentation must justify the need for a skilled qualified professional/auxiliary personnel to train the patient in the use and care of the orthotic. When the management of the orthotic can be turned over to the patient, the caregiver or nursing staff, the services of the therapist will no longer be covered.

An orthotic provided for positioning and/or increasing range of motion in a non-functional extremity must include documentation that the unique skills of a therapist are required to fit and manage the orthotic and that the orthotic is medically necessary for the patient's condition.

For uncomplicated conditions, the following services would not be considered reasonable and necessary, as they would not require the unique skills of a therapist:

- Issuing off-the-shelf splints for foot drop or wrist drop.
- Issuing off-the-shelf foot or elbow cradles for routine pressure relief (these are not considered orthotics).
- Issuing "carrots" (i.e., cylindrical, cone-shaped forms) or towel rolls for hand contractures for hygiene purposes.
- Bed positioning (e.g., pillows, wedges, rolls, foot cradles to relieve potential pressure areas).

Repetitive range of motion prior to placing an orthotic/positioner to maintain the range of motion is not reasonable and necessary when the therapeutic intent is primarily to maintain range of motion within a chronic condition.

Ongoing therapy visits for increasing wearing time are generally not reasonable and necessary when patient problems related to the orthotic have not been observed.

Ongoing visits by the qualified professional/auxiliary personnel to apply the device would be considered monitoring. Once the initial fit is established, any further visits should be used for specific documented problems and modifications that require skilled therapy; these are billed with CPT 97762. It is reasonable and necessary to require 1-3 visits to fit and educate the patient or caregiver. The medical necessity of any further visits must be supported by documentation in the medical record.

Coverage under CPT code 97760 is not for prefabricated/commercial (i.e., off the shelf) components such as, but not limited to a lumbar roll, non-customized foam supports/wedges (e.g., heel cushions), or multi-podus boots. Such components do not require the skills of a therapist and are non-covered. Minor modifications to prefabricated orthotics do not constitute a customized orthotic.

It is not appropriate to bill CPT 97760 for measurements taken to obtain custom fitted burn or pressure garments. These garments do not fit the definition of an orthotic.

Supportive Documentation Recommendations for 97760:

- A description of the patient's condition (including applicable impairments and functional limitations) that necessitates an orthotic.

- Any complicating factors.

- The specific orthotic provided and the date issued.

- A description of the skilled training provided.

- Response of the patient to the orthotic.

97761: Prosthetic Training, upper and/or lower extremity(s), each 15 minutes

Prosthetic training is the professional instruction necessary for a patient to properly use an artificial device that has been developed to replace a missing body part.

Prosthetic training includes preparation of the stump, skin care, modification of prosthetic fit (revisions to socket liner or stump socks), and initial mobility and functional activity training. Once a patient begins gait training with the prosthesis, use code 97116.

Supportive Documentation Recommendations for 97761:

- Type of prosthesis, extremity involved.

- Specific training provided and amount of assistance needed.

- Any complicating factors and specific description of these (with objective measurements), such as pain, joint restrictions/contractures, strength deficits, etc.

97762: Checkout For Orthotic/Prosthetic Use, established patient, each 15 minutes

These assessments are intended for established patients who have already received their orthotic or prosthetic device.

These assessments of the response to wearing the device may be reasonable and necessary when patients experience a loss of function directly related to the device (e.g., pain, skin breakdown, and falls). According to CPT Assistant—February 2007, code 97762 includes patient's response to wearing the device, whether the patient is donning/doffing the device correctly, patient's need for padding, underwrap, or socks, and of the patient's tolerance to any dynamic forces being applied.

If the checkout assessment resulted in the need for further training in the use of the orthotic/prosthetic, codes 97760/97761 would be appropriate for the training.

These assessments may not be considered reasonable and necessary when a device is newly issued or when a device is reissued or replaced after normal wear and no modifications are needed.

Documentation must clearly support the need for more than two visits for the checkout assessment. CPT code 97762 is not covered on the same date as CPT codes 97001-97002.

Supportive Documentation Recommendations for 97762:

- Reason for assessment.

- Findings from the assessment.

- Specific device, modifications made, instruction given.

97799: Unlisted Physical Medicine/Rehabilitation Service Or Procedure, not timed (97799, 97139 or 97039)

If an existing CPT code does not describe the service performed, an unlisted CPT code may be used. When reporting such a service, the appropriate unlisted code may be used to indicate the service, identifying it by "Special Report" as described below.

All therapy unlisted codes are now carrier-priced. When unlisted codes are used, the provider/supplier must submit information, for the contractor's review, to describe the "unspecified" modality(s) or therapeutic procedure(s) performed. The "Special Report" is used to assist in determining the medical appropriateness of the treatment and the appropriateness of the unlisted code billed.

"Special Report" documentation is required to support the medical necessity and appropriate payment of this code. In addition to a detailed service description, information in the medical record and on the claim submitted to the contractor must specify the type of modality utilized and, if the modality requires the constant attendance of the qualified professional/auxiliary personnel, the time spent by the qualified professional/auxiliary personnel, one on one with the beneficiary. This information should be included on the "Remarks Page" of the online claim to assist in processing this code.

Note: Low-level/cold laser light therapy (LLLT) is considered not reasonable and necessary under SSA 1862(a)(1)(A) and is not payable by Medicare. This procedure is considered non-covered billed under any HCPCS/CPT codes, including S8948 and 97039.

Miscellaneous Services (Non-covered)

The following are non-covered as skilled therapy services. This is not an all-inclusive list:

- Iontophoresis.
- Anodyne.
- Low-level laser treatment (LLLT)/cold laser therapy.
- Hydrotherapy massage (e.g., aquamassage, hydromassage, or water massage).
- Massage chairs or roller beds.
- Interactive metronome therapy.
- Loop reflex training.
- Vestibular ocular reflex training.
- Continuous passive motion (CPM) device setup and adjustments.
- Craniosacral therapy.
- Electro-magnetic therapy, except as indicated for chronic wounds.
- Work-hardening programs.
- Pelvic floor dysfunction (not including incontinence).

Due to the lack of peer reviewed evidence concerning the effect on patient health outcomes, skilled therapy interventions (e.g., ultrasound, electrical stimulation, soft tissue mobilization, and therapeutic exercise) for the treatment of the following conditions is considered investigational and thus non-covered:

- Pelvic floor congestion.
- Pelvic floor pain not of spinal origin.
- Hypersensitive clitoris.
- Prostatitis.
- Cystourethrocele.

- Enterocele rectocele vulvodynia.

- Vulvar vestibulitis syndrome (VVS).

Bill Type Codes

Contractors may specify Bill Types to help providers identify those Bill Types typically used to report this service. Absence of a Bill Type does not guarantee that the policy does not apply to that Bill Type. Complete absence of all Bill Types indicates that coverage is not influenced by Bill Type and the policy should be assumed to apply equally to all claims.

Modifiers

Modifiers are used to modify payment of a procedure code, assist in determining appropriate coverage or otherwise identify the detail on the claim. The use of modifiers becomes more important every day when reporting services to ensure appropriate reimbursement from Medicare. These codes should be entered in item 24d of the CMS-1500 claim form or the electronic equivalent.

Therapy Modifiers

Modifiers are used to identify therapy services when financial limitations are in effect. Providers/suppliers must continue to report one of these modifiers for any therapy code on the list of applicable therapy codes. Therapy modifiers should never be used with codes that are not on the list of applicable therapy codes. This includes the codes for the Physician Quality Reporting System (PQRS).

The claim must include the following modifier to distinguish the discipline of the plan of care under which the service is delivered.

Outpatient Therapy

GP   Services delivered under an outpatient PT plan of care

KX   Requirements specified in the medical policy have been met

When the beneficiary qualifies for a therapy cap exception, the provider shall add a KX modifier to the therapy HCPCS subject to the cap limits. The KX modifier shall not be added to any line of service that is not a medically necessary service; this applies to services that, according to a Local Coverage Determination by the contractor, are not medically necessary services. The KX modifier is in addition to the GP therapy modifier and is added to each line of the claim that contains a service that exceeds the cap.

By appending the KX modifier, the provider is attesting that the services billed:

- Are reasonable and necessary services that require the skills of a therapist.

- Are justified by appropriate documentation in the medical record.

- Qualify for an exception using the automatic process exception.

If this attestation is determined to be inaccurate, the provider/supplier is subject to sanctions resulting from providing inaccurate information on a claim. When the KX modifier is appended to a therapy HCPCS code, the contractor will override the CWF system, reject for services that exceed the caps and pay the claim if it is otherwise payable. Providers and suppliers shall continue to append national correct coding initiative (NCCI) HCPCS modifiers under current instructions.

If a claim is submitted without KX modifiers and the cap is exceeded, those services will be denied. If it is brought to their attention, contractors may reopen and/or adjust a claim in cases where appending the KX modifier would have been appropriate.

The codes subject to the therapy cap tracking requirements for a given calendar year are listed at: www. cms.hhs.gov/TherapyServices/05_Annual_Therapy_Update.asp#TopOfPage.

Claims containing any of the "always therapy" codes should have the GP therapy modifier appended. When any code on the list of therapy codes is submitted with specialty codes 65 (physical therapist), 67 (occupational therapist), or 15 (speech-language pathologist) they always represent therapy services, because they are provided by therapists. Contractors shall return claims for these services when they do not contain therapy modifiers for the applicable HCPCS codes.

CMS identifies certain codes listed at the above website as "sometimes therapy" services, regardless of the presence of a financial limitation. Claims from physicians (all specialty codes) and non-physician practitioners, including specialty codes 50 (nurse practitioner), 89 (clinical nurse specialist), and 97 (physician assistant) may be processed without therapy modifiers when they are not therapy services. On review of these claims, "sometimes therapy" services that are not accompanied by a therapy modifier must be documented, reasonable and necessary, and payable as physician or non-physician practitioner services, and not services that the contractor interprets as therapy services.

Modifier 25: Significant, Separately Identifiable Evaluation and Management Service by the Same Physician on the Same Day of the Procedure or Other Service

The physician may need to indicate that on the day a procedure or service identified by a CPT code was performed, the patient's condition required a significant, separately identifiable E/M service above and beyond the other service provided or beyond the usual preoperative and postoperative care associated with the procedure performed. The E/M service may be prompted by the symptom or condition for which the procedure and/or service was provided. As such, different diagnoses are not required for reporting of the E/M services on the same date. This circumstance may be reported by adding the modifier 25 to the appropriate level of E/M service.

Modifier 76: Repeat Procedure by Same Provider

The provider may need to indicate that a service was repeated subsequent to the original service on the same day. In regard to therapy services, if the same procedure for a different diagnosis is rendered on the same day, modifier 76 will be indicated on the subsequent service.

Modifier 59: Distinct Procedural Service

The provider may need to indicate that a service was distinct or separate from other services performed on the same day. This may be:

- A different session or patient encounter.
- A different site.
- A separate injury.

Caution:

Modifier 59 relates to the National Correct Coding Initiative (NCCI) and should not be used for code combinations that are not subject to CCI. This modifier should only be used when no other modifier is appropriate. The medical record must reflect that the modifier is being used appropriately to describe separate services. The documentation should be maintained in the patient's medical record and must be made available upon request.

The CPT Manual defines modifier 59 as the following:

"Under certain circumstances, the physician may need to indicate that a procedure or service was distinct or independent from other services performed on the same day. Modifier 59 is used to identify procedures [and/or] services that are not normally reported together, but are appropriate under the circumstances. This may represent a different session or patient encounter, different procedure or surgery, different site or organ system, separate incision/excision, separate lesion, or separate injury (or area of injury in extensive injuries) not ordinarily encountered or performed on the same day by the same physician. However, when another already established modifier is appropriate, it should be used rather than modifier 59. Only if no more descriptive modifier is available, and the use of modifier 59 best explains the circumstances, should modifier 59 be used."

The National Correct Coding Initiative (NCCI) has created "edit pairs" based on the most common procedures therapists perform together. Billing a CPT code that is paired with another code allows payment of only one of the codes. The therapist needs to determine if a service provided is linked or completely separate and bill accordingly.

The example used on the CMS website follows:

"For example, let's look at one of the more common codes billed: 97140 (manual therapy techniques like mobilization/manipulation, manual lymphatic drainage, or manual traction on one or more regions, each for 15 minutes). For this code, NCCI states 95851, 95852, 97002, 97004, 97018, 97124, 97530, 97750, and 99186 are all linked services when billed in combination with 97140. So, if you bill any of these codes with 97140, you'll receive payment for only 97140. "

According to CMS, modifier 59 is appropriate only if the therapist performs two procedures in discernably different 15 minute blocks of time within the same session when billing a 97140 and 97530 (therapeutic activities; direct, one-on-one patient contact by the provider; or use of dynamic activities to improve functional performance, each for 15 minutes). Therefore, two codes cannot be reported together if performed during the same 15-minute time interval.

If treatment performed truly holds up to that standard, a modifier 59 can be added to 97530 to indicate it was a wholly separate service and should be reimbursed along with the 97140. This is consistent for billing 97140 with 95851, 95852, 97002, 97004, 97018, 97530, or 97750. However, 97124 can never be billed with a 97140—CMS deems these codes as "mutually exclusive procedures."

Below is an edited version of a table with the common CCI edit pairs related to physical therapy, courtesy of PT compliance expert Rick Gawenda, owner of Gawenda Seminars Consulting. Look for the primary CPT code to be billed in Column 1. If billing any of the codes in Column 2, they will be considered mutually exclusive or linked. If the code in Column 2 has a "y" next to it, a modifier 59 can be added; if there's an "n," then the code should not be billed in combination with the code in Column 1.

Note that this is the CCI edit list from Medicare. Most government payers—like Medicare, Tricare, and Medicaid—use this same list. However, private payers often create their own edit pairs; therefore, there is no guarantee they will pay, even with an applied modifier 59.

CCI 20.1 Correct Coding Initiative (CCI) Edits

The CCI or Correct Coding Initiative was first implemented January 1st, 1996, when the CMS made efforts to have a standardized coding system for efficient billing and payments collections. The CCI has promoted and helped physicians and other practitioners use the proper codes for the billing made for services provided. After all, the CCI was developed to correct problems with bundling and unbundling of services being billed by practitioners under Medicare Part B. An independent private company in

Indiana developed CCI after being contracted by CMS to come up with the system. However, it is still the CMS that has final and full authority to implement the CCI among all stakeholders.

In the CCI, an approximate number of 80,000 codes are used and edited. Codes usually consist of two separate CPT codes, which cannot be put together in one bill. This prohibition may stem from the codes being exclusive in their own rights, or that these paired codes are considered to be a part of another more encompassing code. If either condition happens, the code combinations are then verified, resulting in the payment of only one between the combined codes.

Errors often occur when electronic means are used to facilitate claim or payment submissions for physical therapy services rendered. When such errors occur and there is a need to screen and catch these errors, the process is known as editing. Editing is a product of the CCI that suggests services rendered by physical therapists not be placed together in a single bill. The CCI requires that claims regarding physical therapy services filed under Medicare undergo editing to ensure that the correct codes are used according to a procedure performed frequently. In some instances, editing is done manually to be able to accommodate codes that are not usually done at the same time on the same patient. When using the CCI, there is an increased efficiency in billing and payment claims (CMS: National Correct Coding Initiative, 2014).

As of April 2012, the CMS no longer published the Mutually Exclusive edit file and made it unavailable for the practitioners and outpatient hospitals that were using it as guide for billing. File edits, whether

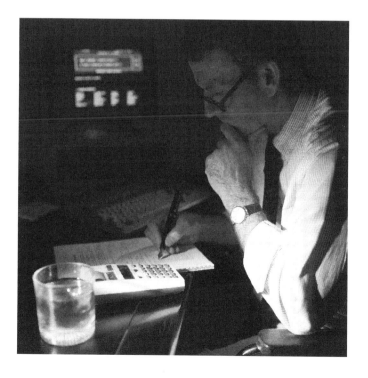

Starting your Own Practice from Scratch

active or deleted, were transferred into the Column One/Column Two Correct Coding edit file on the website. This new file contains all the previously edited codes from the now discontinued Mutually Exclusive edit file (CMS: National Correct Coding Initiative Edits, 2014).

Because of this change, a considerable number of edited original codes (that were developed by the CMS hired contractor for CCI) being used by practitioners became inconsistent with the correct interpretation as per the 97000 series codes based on the CPT. As a response to the confusion this created for billers and payers, the APTA instructed its contractor about the paired codes used in edits and which ones are appropriate and inappropriate in actual practice of rehabilitation medicine and physical therapy.

In keeping up with the ever changing and dynamic health care profession, the CCI is also evolving continually to ensure that proper codes are used and implemented for efficient billing of services. It would not be unusual therefore to find that codes are going to be added, modified or even deleted in manuals issued by the CMS regarding CCI quarterly. CPT codes communicate uniform information about medical services and procedures among healthcare payers. The difference is that on claim forms, CPT codes identify services rendered rather than patient diagnoses.

Most Commonly Used CCI Edits for PT Private Practice Settings

Current as of March 2015

CPT Code	Description	Timed?	Column 2 (n=modifier not allowed)
90911	Biofeedback for Incontinence	N	90901n; 97032y; 97110y; 97112y; 97530y; 97535y; 97550y
G0451	Developmental testing	N	96125y
95831	Muscle testing, extremity (excluding hand) or trunk	N	95851n; 97140y
95832	Muscle testing, hand	N	95852n; 97140y
95833	Muscle testing, total eval body, excluding hands	N	95831n; 95832n; 95851n; 97140y
95834	Muscle testing, total eval body, including hands	N	95831n; 95832n; 95833n; 95851n; 95852n; 97140y
95992	Canalith Re-positioning	N	97110y; 97112y; 97140y; 97530y
96110	Developmental testing, limited	N	96125y
96111	Developmental testing, extended	N	96125y; G0451n, G0459n

(Continued)

CPT Code	Description	Timed?	Column 2 (n=modifier not allowed)
97001	PT Eval	N	96105y; 96125y; 97750n; 97755n; 97762n 95831n; 95832n; 95833n; 95834n; 95851n; 95852n
97002	PT Re-eval	N	96105y; 96125y; 97001n; 97750n; 97755n; 97762n 95831n; 95832n; 95833n; 95834n; 95851n; 95852n
97012	Mechanical Traction	N	97002y; 97004y; 97018y; 97140y
G0281	Electrical Stimulation - Stage 3-4 Wounds	N	97002y; 97004y; 97032y; G0283y
G0283	Electrical Stimulation - Other Than Wound Care	N	97002y; 97004y; 97032y
97016	Vasopneumatic device	N	97002y; 97004y; 97018y; 97026y
97018	Paraffin Bath	N	97002y; 97004y; 97022y
97022	Whirlpool	N	97002y; 97004y
97024	Diathermy	N	97002y; 97004y; 97018y; 97026y
97026	Infrared	N	97002y; 97004y; 97018y; 97022y
97028	Ultraviolet	N	97002y; 97004y; 97018y; 97022y; 97026y
97032	Electrical Stimulation	Y	64550y; 97002y; 97004y
97033	Electrical Current	Y	97002y; 97004y
97034	Contrast Bath	Y	97002y; 97004y
97035	Ultrasound	Y	97002y; 97004y
97036	Hubbard Tank	Y	97002y; 97004y
97039	Physical Therapy Treatment	Y	97002y; 97004y
97110	Therapeutic Exercises	Y	97002y; 97004y
97112	Neuromuscular Re Education	Y	97002y; 97004y; 97022y; 97036y
97113	Aquatic Therapy/Exercises	Y	97002y; 97004y; 97022y; 97036n; 97110y
97116	Gait Training	Y	97002y; 97004y
97124	Massage	Y	97002y; 97004y

(Continued)

CPT Code	Description	Timed?	Column 2 (n=modifier not allowed)
97139	Physical Medicine Procedure	Y	97002y; 97004y
97140	Manual Therapy	Y	95851y; 95852y; 97002y; 97004y; 97018y; 97124n; 97530y; 97750y
97150	Group Therapeutic Procedures	N	97002y; 97004y; 97110y; 97112y; 97113y; 97116y; 97124y; 97140y; 97530y; 97532y; 97533y; 97535y; 97537y; 97542y; 97760y; 97761y
97530	Therapeutic Activities	Y	95831n; 95832n; 95833n; 95834n; 95851n; 95852n; 97002y; 97004y; 97113y; 97116y; 97532y; 97533y; 97535y; 97537y; 97542y; 97750y
97532	Cognitive Skills Development	Y	97002y; 97004y
97533	Sensory Integration	Y	97002y; 97004y
97535	Self Care Management Training	Y	97002y; 97004y
97537	Community/work Reintegration	Y	97002y; 97004y
97542	Wheelchair Management Training	Y	97002y; 97004y
97545	Work Hardening	Y	97002y; 97004y; 97140n
97546	Work Hardening Add On	Y	
97597	Wound Care Selective First 20 sq centimeters	N	29105y; 29125y; 29130y; 29260y; 29345y; 29405y; 29425y; 29445y; 29515y; 29540y; 29550y; 29580y; 29581y; 29582y; 29584y; 97002y; 97022y; 97602n; 97605y; 97606y; 97610y
97598	Wound Care Selective; Each additional 20 sq centimeters	N	29580y; 29581y; 29582y; 97002y; 97022y; 97602n; 97605y; 97606y; 97610y
97602	Wound Care Non-Selective	N	29580y; 29581y; 97002y

(Continued)

CPT Code	Description	Timed?	Column 2 (n=modifier not allowed)
97610	Low Frequency, Non-Contact, Non-Thermal Ultrasound	N	97035y; 97602n
97750	Physical Performance Test	Y	95831n; 95832n; 95833n; 95834n; 95851n; 95852n; 97150n
97755	Assistive Technology Assessment	Y	97035y; 97110y; 97112y; 97140y; 97530y; 97532y; 97533y; 97535y; 97537y; 97542y; 97545y; 97750n; 97760y; 97761y; 97762n
97760	Orthotic Management Training	Y	29105y; 29125y; 29126y; 29130y; 29131y; 29200y; 29240y; 29260y; 29280y; 29505y; 29515y; 29520y; 29530y; 29540y; 29550y; 29580y; 29581y; 29582y; 29583y; 29584y; 97002y; 97004y; 97016y; 97110y; 97112y; 97116y; 97124y; 97140y; 97662y
97761	Prosthetic Training	Y	97002y; 97004y; 97016y; 97110y; 97112y; 97116y; 97124y; 97140y; 97760y; 97762y
97762	Orthotic/Prosthetic Check Out	Y	

5
CHAPTER

SERVICE UNITS AND THERAPY CERTIFICATIONS

Timed and Untimed Codes

When reporting service units for HCPCS codes where the procedure is not defined by a specific timeframe ("untimed" HCPCS), the provider enters "1" in the field labeled units. For untimed codes, units are reported based on the number of times the procedure is performed, as described in the HCPCS code definition (often once per day).

Several CPT codes used for therapy modalities, procedures, and tests and measurements specify that the direct (one-on-one) time spent in patient contact is 15 minutes. Providers report procedure codes for services delivered on any single calendar day using CPT codes and the appropriate number of 15-minute units of service.

Counting Minutes for Timed Codes in 15-Minute Units

For any single timed CPT code in the same day measured in 15-minute units, providers bill a single 15-minute unit for treatment greater than or equal to 8 minutes through and including 22 minutes. If the duration of a single modality or procedure in a day is 23 minutes, but not more than 37 minutes, then 2 units should be billed.

Time intervals for 1 through 8 units are as follows:

- 8–22 minutes = 1 unit

- 23–37 minutes = 2 units

- 38–52 minutes = 3 units

- 53–67 minutes = 4 units

- 68–82 minutes = 5 units

- 83–97 minutes = 6 units

- 98–112 minutes = 7 units

- 113–127 minutes = 8 units

The pattern remains the same for treatment times in excess of two hours.

If a service represented by a 15-minute timed code is performed in a single day for at least 15 minutes that service shall be billed for at least one unit. If the service is performed for at least 30 minutes, that service shall be billed for at least two units, etc. It is not appropriate to count all minutes of treatment in a day toward the units for one code if other services were performed for more than 15 minutes.

When more than one service represented by 15-minute timed codes is performed in a single day, the total number of minutes of service (as noted on the chart above) determines the number of timed units billed.

If any 15-minute timed service that is performed for seven minutes or less than seven minutes on the same day as another 15-minute timed service that was also performed for 7 minutes or less and the total time of the two is eight minutes or greater than eight minutes, then bill one unit for the service performed for the most minutes. This is correct because the total time is greater than the minimum time for one unit. The same logic is applied when three or more different services are provided for seven minutes or less than seven minutes.

The expectation (based on the work values for these codes) is that a provider's direct patient contact time for each unit will average 15 minutes in length. If a provider has a consistent practice of billing less than 15 minutes for a unit, the Contractor may request medical records.

If more than one 15-minute timed CPT code is billed during a single calendar day, then the total number of timed units that can be billed is constrained by the total treatment minutes for that day.

The amount of time for each specific intervention/modality provided to the patient is not required to be documented in the treatment note. However, the total number of timed minutes must be documented. These examples indicate how to count the appropriate number of units for the total therapy minutes provided.

Example:

   24 minutes of neuromuscular reeducation, code 97112

   23 minutes of therapeutic exercise, code 97110

   Total timed code treatment time was 47 minutes

   The 47 minutes falls within the range for 3 units = 38 to 52 minutes.

Appropriate billing for 47 minutes is only three timed units. Each of the codes is performed for more than 15 minutes, so each shall be billed for at least one unit. The correct coding is two units of code 97112 and one unit of code 97110, assigning more timed units to the service that took the most time.

Example:

   18 minutes of therapeutic exercise (97110),

   13 minutes of manual therapy (97140),

   10 minutes of gait training (97116),

   8 minutes of ultrasound (97035),

   49 Total timed minutes

Appropriate billing is for three units. Bill the procedures you spent the most time providing. Bill one unit each of 97110, 97116, and 97140. You are unable to bill for the ultrasound because the total time of timed units that can be billed is constrained by the total timed code treatment minutes (i.e., you may not bill four units for less than 53 minutes regardless of how many services were performed). You would still document the ultrasound in the treatment notes.

Note: The above schedule of times is intended to provide assistance in rounding time into 15-minute increments. It does not imply that any minute until the eighth should be excluded from the total count. The total minutes of active treatment counted for all 15 minute timed codes includes all direct treatment time for the timed codes. Total treatment minutes–including minutes spent providing services represented by untimed codes–are also documented.

Ref: (http://www.cms.gov/Regulations-and-Guidance/Guidance/Manuals/Downloads/bp102c15.pdf)

Medicare Part B pays for physical therapy, speech-language pathology, and occupational therapy services provided simultaneously to two or more individuals by a practitioner as group therapy services (97150). The individuals can be, but need not be, performing the same activity. The physician or therapist involved in group therapy services must be in constant attendance, but one on one patient contact is not required (Maxwell & Baseggio, 2001).

Student Supervision

Effective October 1, 2011, students are no longer required to be under the line-of-sight supervision of a therapist or therapy assistant. However the SNF's supervising therapists and assistants are expected to exercise their own judgment regarding the level of supervision a particular student may require. The student is considered an extension of the therapist. In order to code for individual therapy a therapist or student is treating one patient. The therapist cannot treat or supervise any other patient.

Line-of-sight supervision for students is no longer required. Providers must still exercise discretion over which students are prepared to operate independently.

Billing Scenarios for Medicare Part B
Scenario 1

Therapist A treated Patient A one on one for 11 minutes of therapeutic activities, 10 minutes of gait training, and 9 minutes of neuromuscular re-education.

Part B:

Therapeutic Activities = one unit

Gait training = one unit

Do not bill for neuromuscular re-education, since the total treatment minutes is 30. Maximum unit allowed is two. (Two units=23–37 minutes).

CPT Codes Clarification

It is important to recognize that CPT codes were intended for use with the outpatient population, and not for long-term care patients. Therefore, the codes associated with the services provided to long-term care population may not be as "black and white" as one would like.

CPT codes that do not have a time associated with them should be used only once, regardless of the amount of time taken to provide that service. The only time that you would use one of these codes twice in one day is if you have a BID order for that treatment modality. All other "time oriented" codes should be used according to the amount of time taken to provide the service.

Codes for services such as functional maintenance programs should reflect the nature of the therapy services provided.

For example, when developing a functional maintenance program for self-feeding, the code associated with those sessions should be Self-Care/Home Management Training (code 97535), and should be recorded for each 15 minutes of service provided. Therefore, a 45-minute ADL session would be recorded as 97535 x 3.

Caregiver/family training: code used should be reflective of the topic of training.

For example, if the therapist is teaching the nursing staff proper guarding techniques for gait on a patient with THR precautions, the service is to be recorded as gait training, code 97116. All caregiver/family training must occur with the patient present and participating in the training as part of his/her direct care.

Wheelchair seating or positioning: If the patient is not currently on your caseload, the appropriate code for an initial evaluation would be 97001 (PT initial eval). If the patient is currently on caseload, then use 97112 (neuromuscular reeducation of movement, balance, coordination, kinesthetic sense, posture, and proprioception). This code is also appropriate for balance and fine/gross motor activities. Use the code 97542 (wheelchair management and propulsion training, including assessment, fitting) for teaching the patient use of the equipment and how to perform activities with it. Self-care/home management (97535) or community re-integration (97537) may also be appropriate depending on the services being provided as part of the wheelchair positioning intervention. Finally, the PT re-evaluation code may be used if an adjustment in the plan of care is indicated for a patient already on caseload.

Bed mobility and transfer training: The most reasonable code to use for this is 97530 (therapeutic activities, direct (one on one) patient contact by the provider use of dynamic activities to improve functional performance).

AROM and AAROM exercises for strengthening and endurance: The most reasonable code to utilize for this is 97110 (therapeutic exercises to develop strength, endurance, range of motion and flexibility).

Fabricating a splint: 97760 (orthotics fitting and training, upper and/or lower extremities). After the splint has been made, the code 97762 (checkout for orthotic/prosthetic use) is used to check on the fit of a splint, how well it facilitates function, etc.

Unlisted therapeutic procedure: this code has a higher likelihood of being flagged for review. It should only be used if there are no other appropriate codes. Also, if the fee screen attached to that code is higher than the more appropriate code, inappropriate use may be construed as billing fraud. The therapist's documentation should be able to support how the services billed by the same code are different, for instance how the OTs therapeutic exercises are different than the PTs.

Test and measurement codes on the same day as an evaluation: Test and measurement codes should not be used on the same day as an evaluation. If a specialized test is needed, it should be done on another day during the treatment period. In addition, a separate, stand-alone report of the test/measurement finding that is comprehensive in and of itself must be generated to justify the use of the separate test and measurement codes.

Therapy Certifications

The Centers for Medicare and Medicaid Services (CMS) included a provision in the Medicare Physician Fee Schedule Final Rule of 2008 that extended the therapy plan of care recertification period from 30 to 90 days for Medicare beneficiaries seen on or after January 1, 2008. The plan of care must be reviewed and re-certified by the physician/non-physician practitioner at least every 90 days unless the physician specifies a shorter time frame. The 90-day period begins on the date of the initial therapy treatment session.

The physician or non-physician practitioner (if it is within his or her scope of practice) must certify the plan of care. Certification requires a dated signature on the plan of care or some other document that indicates approval of the plan of care. The therapist should forward the plan to the physician/non-physician practitioner as soon as it is established, and obtain certification (dated signature) "as soon as possible." In other words, the physician/non-physician practitioner shall certify the plan as soon as it is obtained or within the first 30 days after the initial therapy treatment session.

The physician must certify, and then periodically recertify, the need for extended care services in the skilled nursing home. The initial certification affirms that the patient meets the existing SNF level of care definition, or validates via written statement that the beneficiary's assignment to one of the upper RUG-IV (Top 52) groups is correct. Recertification is used to document the continued need for skilled extended care services.

Certification requires a dated signature on the plan of care or some other document that indicates approval of the plan of care. It is not appropriate for a physician/non-physician practitioner to certify a plan of care if the patient was not under the care of some physician/non-physician practitioner at the time of the treatment or if the patient did not need the treatment. Since delayed certification is allowed, the date the certification is signed is important only to determine if it is timely or delayed. The certification must relate to treatment during the interval on the claim.

The format of all certifications and recertifications and the method by which they are obtained are determined by the individual practitioner. Acceptable documentation of certification may be, for example, a physician's progress note, a physician/non-physician practitioner order, or a plan of care that is signed and dated during the interval of treatment by a physician/non-physician practitioner, and indicates the physician/non-physician practitioner is aware that therapy service is or was in progress and the physician/non-physician practitioner makes no record of disagreement with the plan when there is evidence the plan was sent (e.g., to the office) or is available in the record (e.g., of the institution that employs the physician/non-physician practitioner) for the physician/non-physician practitioner to review.

The certification should be retained in the clinical record and made readily available if requested by the contractor.

Initial Certification

The physician's/non-physician practitioner's certification of the plan (with or without an order) satisfies all of the certification requirements noted above for the duration of the plan of care, or 90 calendar days from the date of the initial treatment, whichever is less. The initial treatment includes the evaluation that resulted in the plan.

Timing of Initial Certification

The provider should obtain certification as soon as possible after the plan of care is established, unless the requirements of delayed certification are met. "As soon as possible" means that the physician/non-physician practitioner shall certify the initial plan as soon as it is obtained, or within 30 days of the initial therapy treatment.

Since payment may be denied if a physician does not certify the plan, the therapist should forward the plan to the physician as soon as it is established. Evidence of diligence in providing the plan to the physician may be considered by the Medicare contractor during review in the event of a delayed certification.

Timely certification of the initial plan is met when physician/non-physician practitioner certification of the plan for the first interval of treatment is documented, by signature or verbal order, and dated in the 30 days following the first day of treatment (including evaluation). If the order to certify is verbal, it must be followed within 14 days by a signature to be timely. A dated notation of the order to certify the plan should be made in the patient's medical record.

Recertification is not required if the duration of the initially certified plan of care is more than the duration (length) of the entire episode of treatment.

Review of Plan and Recertification

The timing of recertification changed on January 1, 2008. Certifications signed on or after January 1, 2008, follow the rules in this section. Certifications signed on or prior to December 31, 2007, follow the rule in effect at that time, which required recertification every 30-calendar day.

Payment and coverage conditions require that the plan must be reviewed, as often as necessary but at least whenever it is certified or re-certified to complete the certification requirements. It is not required that the same physician/non-physician practitioner who participated initially in recommending or planning the patient's care certifies and/or recertifies the plans.

Recertification that documents the need for continued or modified therapy should be signed whenever a significant modification of the plan is needed or at least 90 days after initiation of treatment under that plan, unless they are delayed.

Physician/Non-physician Practitioner Options for Certification

A physician/non-physician practitioner may certify or recertify a plan for whatever duration of treatment the physician/non-physician practitioner determines it is appropriate, up to a maximum of 90 calendar days. Many episodes of therapy treatment last less than 30 calendar days. Therefore, it is expected that the physician/non-physician practitioner should certify a plan that appropriately estimates the duration of care for the individual, even if it is less than 90 days. If the therapist writes a plan of care for a duration that is more or less than the duration approved by the physician/non-physician practitioner, then the physician/non-physician practitioner would document a change to the duration of the plan and certify it for the duration the physician/non-physician practitioner finds appropriate (up to 90 days). Treatment beyond the duration certified by the physician/non-physician practitioner requires that a plan be re-certified for the extended duration of treatment. It is possible that patients will be discharged by the therapist before the end of the estimated treatment duration because some will improve faster than estimated and/or some were successfully progressed to an independent home program.

Physicians/non-physician practitioners may require that the patient make a physician/non-physician practitioner visit for an examination if, in the professional's judgment, the visit is needed prior to certifying the plan, or during the planned treatment. Physicians/non-physician practitioners should indicate their requirement for visits, preferably on an order preceding the treatment, or on the plan of care that is certified.

If the physician wishes to restrict the patient's treatment beyond a certain date when a visit is required, the physician should certify a plan only until the date of the visit. After that date, services will not be considered reasonable and necessary due to lack of a certified plan. Physicians/non-physician practitioners should not sign a certification if they require a visit and a visit was not made. However, Medicare does not require a visit unless a National Coverage Determination (NCD) for a particular treatment requires it.

Restrictions on Certification

Certifications and recertifications by doctors of podiatric medicine must be consistent with the scope of the professional services provided by a doctor of podiatric medicine as authorized by applicable state law. Optometrists may order and certify only low vision services. Chiropractors may not certify or recertify plans of care for therapy services.

Delayed Certification

Certifications are required for each interval of treatment based on the patient's needs, not to exceed 90 calendar days from the initial therapy treatment. Certifications are timely when the initial certification (or certification of a significantly modified plan of care) is dated within 30 calendar days of the initial treatment under that plan. Delayed certification and recertification requirements shall be deemed satisfied where, at any later date, a physician/non-physician practitioner makes a certification accompanied by a reason for the delay. Certifications are acceptable without justification for 30 days after they are due. Delayed certification should include one or more certifications or recertifications on a single signed and dated document.

Delayed certifications should include any evidence the provider or supplier considers necessary to justify the delay. For example, a certification may be delayed because the physician did not sign it, or the original was lost. In the case of a long delayed certification (over 6 months), the provider or supplier may choose to submit with the delayed certification some other documentation (e.g., an order, progress notes, telephone contact, requests for certification or signed statement of a physician/non-physician practitioner) indicating need for care and that the patient was under the care of a physician at the time of the treatment. Such documentation may be requested by the contractor for delayed certifications if it is required for review.

It is not intended that needed therapy be stopped or denied when certification is delayed. The delayed certification of otherwise covered services should be accepted unless the contractor has reason to believe that there was no physician involved in the patient's care, or treatment did not meet the patient's need (and therefore, the certification was signed inappropriately).

Denials Due to Certification

Denial for payment that is based on absence of certification is a technical denial, which means a statutory requirement has not been met. Certification is a statutory requirement in SSA 1835(a)(2)- ('periodic review" of the plan). For example, if a patient is treated and the provider/supplier cannot produce (on contractor request) a plan of care (timely or delayed) for the billed treatment dates certified by a physician/non-physician practitioner, then that service might be denied for lack of the required certification. If an appropriate certification is later produced, the denial shall be overturned.

In the case of a service furnished under a provider agreement as described in 42CFR489.21, the provider is precluded from charging the beneficiary for services denied as a result of missing certification.

However, if the service is provided by a supplier in the office of the physician/non-physician practitioner, or therapist, a technical denial due to absence of a certification results in beneficiary liability. For that reason, it is recommended that the patient be made aware of the need for certification and the consequences of its absence.

A technical denial decision may be reopened by the contractor or reversed on appeal as appropriate, if delayed certification is later produced.

Exceptions for Medically Necessary Services

Clinicians may utilize the automatic process for exception for any diagnosis or condition for which they can justify services exceeding the cap. Regardless of the diagnosis or condition, the patient must also meet other requirements for coverage.

Codes representing the medical condition that caused the treatment are used when there is no code representing the treatment. Complicating conditions are preferably used in non-primary positions on the claim and are billed in the primary position only in the rare circumstance that there is no more relevant code.

The condition or complexity that caused treatment to exceed caps must be related to the therapy goals and must either be the condition that is being treated or a complexity that directly and significantly impacts the rate of recovery of the condition being treated such that it is appropriate to exceed the caps. Documentation for an exception should indicate how the complexity (or combination of complexities) directly and significantly affects treatment for a therapy condition.

It is very important to recognize that most conditions would not ordinarily result in services exceeding the cap. Use the KX modifier only in cases where the condition of the individual patient is such that services are **APPROPRIATELY** provided in an episode that exceeds the cap. Routine use of the KX modifier for all patients with these conditions will likely show up on data analysis as aberrant and invite inquiry. Be sure that documentation is sufficiently detailed to support the use of the modifier.

In justifying exceptions for therapy caps, clinicians and contractors should not only consider the medical diagnoses and medical complications that might directly and significantly influence the amount of treatment required but also other variables (such as the availability of a caregiver at home) that affect appropriate treatment. Factors that influence the need for treatment should be supportable by published research, clinical guidelines from professional sources, and/or clinical or common sense. See Pub. 100-02, chapter 15, section 220.3 for information related to documentation of the evaluation, and section 220.2 on medical necessity for some factors that complicate treatment.

Note: The patient's lack of access to outpatient hospital therapy services alone does not justify excepted services. Patients of skilled nursing facilities prevented by consolidated billing from accessing hospital services, debilitated patients for whom transportation to the hospital is a physical hardship, or lack of therapy services at hospitals in the beneficiary's county may or may not qualify as justification for continued services above the caps. The patient's condition and complexities might justify extended services, but their location does not.

Appeals Related to Disapproval of Cap Exceptions

When a service beyond the cap is determined to be medically necessary, it is covered and payable. But, when a service provided beyond the cap (outside the benefit) is determined to be NOT medically necessary, it is denied as a benefit category denial. Contractors may review claims with KX modifiers to determine whether the services are medically necessary, or for other reasons. Services that exceed therapy caps but do not meet Medicare criteria for medically necessary services are not payable even when clinicians recommend and furnish these services.

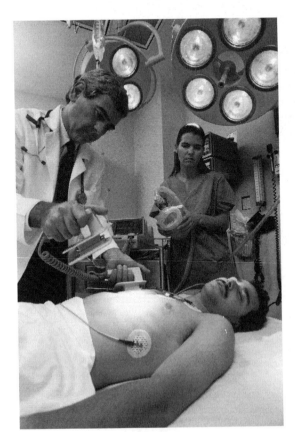

Services without a Medicare benefit may be billed to Medicare with a GY modifier for the purpose of obtaining a denial that can be used with other insurers.

Appeals

If a beneficiary whose exception services do not meet the Medicare criteria for medical necessity elects to receive such services, and a claim is submitted for such services, the resulting determination would be subject to the administrative appeals process.

Application of New Coding Requirements

The functional data reporting and collection system will be described in detail later in the next chapter of this book. The system was put into effect for therapy services with dates of service on and after January 1, 2013. A testing period from January 1, 2013, through June 30,

2013, allowed providers to use the new coding requirements in order to assure the systems work. During that time, period claims without G-codes and modifiers were processed; however, claims without the functional G-code modifier were then returned or rejected as of July 1, 2013.

In order to implement use of these G-codes for reporting function data on January 1, 2013, a new status indicator of "Q" was created for the Medicare Physician Fee Schedule Database (MPFSDB). This new status indicator identifies codes being used exclusively for functional reporting therapy services. These functional G-codes have been added to the MPFSDB with the new "Q" status indicator, but since these are non-payable G-codes, there are no Relative Value Units or payment amounts for these codes. The new "Q" status code indicator reads, as follows:

Status Code Indicator "Q"–"Therapy functional information code, used for required reporting purposes only." (http://www.cms.gov/Regulations-and-Guidance/Guidance/Transmittals/Downloads/R165BP.pdf)

Services Affected

The reporting and collection requirements of beneficiary functional data apply to all claims for services furnished under the Medicare Part B outpatient therapy benefit and the PT services furnished under the Comprehensive Outpatient Rehabilitation Facility (CORF) benefit.

Providers and Practitioners Affected

These reporting requirements apply to the therapy services furnished by the following providers: hospitals, Critical Access Hospitals (CAHs), Skilled Nursing Facilities (SNFs), Comprehensive Outpatient Rehabilitation Facilities (CORFs), rehabilitation agencies, and Home Health Agencies (HHAs) (when the beneficiary is not under a home health plan of care). It also applies to the following practitioners: Therapists in Private Practice (TPPs), physicians, and non-physician practitioners as noted above.

6
CHAPTER

FUNCTIONAL LIMITATION REPORTING, G-CODES AND PQRS

As required by the Middle Class Tax Relief Jobs Creation Act of 2012, CMS began collecting data on claim forms about patient functional status for patients receiving outpatient physical therapy, speech therapy, and occupational therapy as of January 1, 2013. Therapists are required to report new G-codes accompanied by modifiers on the claim form that convey information about a patient's functional limitations and goals at initial evaluation, every 10 visits, and at discharge. This data is for informational purposes not reimbursement. Until July 1, 2013, claims were processed regardless of the inclusion of functional limitation codes. Since July 1, 2013, all claims have had to include the functional limitation codes in order to be paid by Medicare.

The Middle Class Tax Relief Act of 2012 included a mandate that CMS collect information on Medicare Part B claims regarding the beneficiaries' function and condition, therapy services furnished, and outcomes achieved. CMS intends to utilize this information in the future to reform payment for outpatient therapy services. The policy applies to physical therapy, occupational therapy, and speech therapy services furnished in hospitals, Critical Access Hospitals (CAH's), Skilled Nursing Facilities (SNF's), Comprehensive Outpatient Rehabilitation Facilities (CORFs), rehabilitation agencies, home health agencies (when the beneficiary is not under a home health plan of care), and in private offices of therapists, physicians and non-physician practitioners. The reporting of the functional limitations on the claim form was implemented on January 1, 2013, tested for a smooth transition until July 1, 2013, and then enforced with claims being returned unpaid after July 1, 2013 if the appropriate G-codes and modifiers were missing.

Under this new rule, non-payable G-codes and modifiers are included on the claim form to capture data on the beneficiary's functional limitations. This occurs (a) at the outset of the therapy episode; (b) at a minimum every 10th visit; (c) when an evaluative or re-evaluative procedure is done; (d) at discharge; (e) when a particular functional limitation is ended and there is a need for further therapy, and (f) when reporting begins for a new or different functional limitation within the same episode of care. In addition, the therapist's projected goal for functional status at the end of treatment is reported on the first claim for services and at the end of the episode. Modifiers indicate the extent of the severity/complexity of the functional limitation (APTA 2015).

Functional Reporting Codes — G-codes

So, what exactly is a G-code? G-codes are the functional limitation codes that represent a beneficiary's functional limitation. Current status, projected goal status, and discharge status each need a G-code associated with it. The 42 functional G-codes consist of 14 functional code sets with three types of codes in each set. Physical therapists need to be familiar with the six G-code sets generally applicable for PT and OT functional limitations. The other eight G-code sets are for speech therapy functional limitations.

A G-code set is chosen by providers and practitioners based on which code corresponds most closely with the primary functional limitation being treated or the code that is the primary reason for treatment.

Functional Reporting Codes — Severity/Complexity Modifiers

Severity modifiers indicate how bad the functional limitation is for the beneficiary based on a percentage of functional impairment, which is determined by the practitioner providing therapy. Each non-payable G-code requires a severity/complexity modifier to denote the level of severity for that functional limitation. The beneficiary's current status, projected goal status, and discharge status are reported with a G-code and the appropriate severity modifiers.

Modifier	Impairment limitation restriction
CH	0 percent impaired, limited or restricted
CI	At least 1 percent but less than 20 percent impaired, limited or restricted
CJ	At least 20 percent but less than 40 percent impaired, limited or restricted
CK	At least 40 percent but less than 60 percent impaired, limited or restricted
CL	At least 60 percent but less than 80 percent impaired, limited or restricted
CM	At least 80 percent but less than 100 percent impaired, limited or restricted
CN	100 percent impaired, limited or restricted

For the complete list of Functional Reporting G-codes and Severity/Complexity Modifiers, refer to the Functional Reporting Quick Reference Chart found on the CMS website: Functional Reporting - Centers for Medicare & Medicaid Services. The relevant G-code sets for physical therapy are laid out in the next section of this chapter. For a complete understanding of how to properly select a functional limitation and determine a severity level, refer to the links within the "Resources for Functional Reporting" section of the CMS website (CMS 2015).

Function-related G-codes

The functional limitations categories selected by CMS are from the International Classification of Functioning, Disability and Health (ICF). The ICF is a classification of health and health-related domains. The ICE model acknowledges that every human being can experience some level of "disability" and views functioning and disability as an interaction between health, the environment, personal and social factors. For more information on the ICE, please see the APTA ICF web site. The way that CMS is using the term "functional limitation" is within the context of the areas of the ICF relating to "activity limitations" and "participation restrictions".

The definitions of the terms described below come from the International Classification of Functioning, Disability and Health, World Health Organization, 2001, Geneva.

The following Healthcare Common Procedure Coding System (HCPCS) G-codes are used to report the status of a beneficiary's functional limitations:

Mobility G-code Set:

Mobility: Moving by changing body position or location or by transferring from one place to another, by carrying, moving or manipulating objects, by walking, running or climbing, and by using various forms of transportation.

   a. Walking: Moving along a surface on foot, step by step, so that one foot is always on the ground, such as when strolling, sauntering, walking forwards, backwards, or sideways. Inclusions: walking short or long distances, walking on different surfaces, walking around obstacles.

   b. Moving Around: Moving the whole body from one place to another by means other than walking, such as climbing over a rock or running down a street, skipping, scampering, jumping, somersaulting or running around obstacles. Inclusions: crawling, climbing, running, jogging, jumping, and swimming.

   c. Moving around in different locations: Walking and moving around in various places and situations, such as walking between rooms in a house, within a building, or down the street of a town. Inclusions: moving around within the home, crawling or climbing within the home, walking or moving within buildings other than the home, and outside the home and other buildings.

d. Moving around using equipment: Moving the whole body from place to place, on any surface or space, by using specific devices designed to facilitate moving or create other ways of moving around, such as with skates, skis, or scuba equipment, or moving down the street in a wheelchair or a walker.

e. Moving around using transportation: Using transportation to move around as a passenger, such as being driven in a car or on a bus, rickshaw, jitney, animal-powered vehicle, or private or public taxi, bus, train, tram, subway, boat or aircraft. Inclusions: using human-powered transportation, using private motorized or public transportation

   • G8978, Mobility current status: walking & moving around functional limitation, current status, at therapy episode outset and at reporting intervals.

   • G8979, Mobility goal status: walking & moving around functional limitation, projected goal status, at therapy episode outset, at reporting intervals, and at discharge or to end reporting.

   • G8980, Mobility D/C status: walking & moving around functional limitation, discharge status, at discharge from therapy or to end reporting.

Changing & Maintaining Body Position G-code set:

Changing body position: Getting into and out of a body position and moving from one location to another, such as getting up out of a chair to lie down on a bed, and getting into and out of positions of kneeling or squatting. Inclusion: changing body position from lying down, from squatting or kneeling, from sitting or standing, bending and shifting the body's center of gravity

a. Maintaining a body position: Staying in the same body position as required, such as remaining seated or remaining standing for work or school. Inclusions: maintaining a lying, squatting, kneeling, sitting and standing position.

b. Transferring oneself: Moving from one surface to another, such as sliding along a bench or moving from a bed to a chair, without changing body position. Inclusion: transferring oneself while sitting or lying.

   • G8981, Body pos current status: Changing & maintaining body position functional limitation, current status, at therapy episode outset and at reporting intervals.

   • G8982, Body pos goal status: Changing & maintaining body position functional limitation, projected goal status, at therapy episode outset, at reporting intervals, and at discharge or to end reporting

   • G8983, Body pos D/C status: Changing & maintaining body position functional limitation, discharge status, at discharge from therapy or to end reporting.

Carrying, Moving & Handling Objects G-code Set

Lifting and carrying objects: Raising up an object or taking something from one place to another, such as when lifting a cup or carrying a child from one room to another. Inclusions: lifting, carrying in the hands or arms, or on shoulders, hip, back or head; putting down

a. Moving objects with lower extremities: Performing coordinated actions aimed at moving an object by using the legs and feet, such as kicking a ball or pushing pedals on a bicycle. Inclusions: pushing with lower extremities, kicking.

b. Fine hand use: Performing the coordinated actions of handling objects, picking up, manipulating and releasing them using one's hand, fingers and thumb, such as required to lift coins off a table or turn a dial or knob. Inclusions: picking up, grasping, manipulating and releasing.

c. Hand and arm use: Performing the coordinated actions required to move objects or to manipulate them by using hands and arms, such as when turning door handles or throwing or catching an object Inclusions: pulling or pushing objects, reaching, turning or twisting the hands or arm, throwing, catching.

- G8984, Carry current status: Carrying, moving & handling objects functional limitation, current status, at therapy episode outset and at reporting intervals.

- G8985, Carry goal status: Carrying, moving & handling objects functional limitation, projected goal status, at therapy episode outset, at reporting intervals, and at discharge or to end reporting.

- G8986, Carry D/C status: Carrying, moving & handling objects functional limitation, discharge status, at discharge from therapy or to end reporting.

Self-Care G-code Set

Self-Care: caring for oneself, washing and drying oneself, caring for one's body and body parts, dressing, eating and drinking, and looking after one's health.

a. Washing oneself: Washing and drying one's whole body, or body parts, using water and appropriate cleaning and drying materials or methods, such as bathing, showering, washing hands and feet, face and hair, and drying with a towel. Inclusions: washing body parts, the whole body; and drying oneself.

b. Caring for body parts: Looking after those parts of the body, such as skin, face, teeth, scalp, nails and genitals, that require more than washing and drying. Inclusions: caring for skin, teeth, hair, finger and toe nails.

c. Toileting: Planning and carrying out the elimination of human waste (menstruation, urination and defecation), and cleaning oneself afterwards. Inclusions: regulating urination, defecation and menstrual care.

d. Dressing: Carrying out the coordinated actions and tasks of putting on and taking off clothes and footwear in sequence and in keeping with climatic and social conditions, such as by putting on, adjusting and removing shirts, skirts, blouses, pants, undergarments, saris, kimono, tights, hats, gloves, coats, shoes, boots, sandals and slippers. Inclusions: putting on or taking off clothes and footwear and choosing appropriate clothing.

e. Looking after one's health: Ensuring physical comfort, health and physical and mental well-being, such as by maintaining a balanced diet, and an appropriate level of physical activity, keeping warm or cool, avoiding harms to health, following safe sex practices, including using condoms, getting immunizations and regular physical examinations. Inclusions: ensuring one's physical comfort; managing diet and fitness; maintaining one's health.

- G8987, Self-care current status: Self-care functional limitation, current status, at therapy episode outset and at reporting intervals.

- G8988, Self-care goal status: Self-care functional limitation, projected goal status, at therapy episode outset, at reporting intervals, and at discharge or to end reporting.

- G8989, Self-care D/C status: Self-care functional limitation, discharge status, at discharge from therapy or to end reporting.

Other PT/OT Primary G-code Set:

- G8990, Other PT/OT current status: Other physical or occupational primary functional limitation, current status, at therapy episode outset and at reporting intervals.

- G8991, Other PT/OT goal status: Other physical or occupational primary functional limitation, projected goal status, at therapy episode outset, at reporting intervals, and at discharge or to end reporting: MM8005 Related.

- G8992, Other PT/OT D/C status: Other physical or occupational primary functional limitation, discharge status, at discharge from therapy or to end reporting.

Other PT/OT Subsequent G-code Set:

- G8993, Sub PT/OT current status: Other physical or occupational subsequent functional limitation, current status, at therapy episode outset and at reporting intervals.

- G8994, Sub PT/OT goal status: Other physical or occupational subsequent functional limitation, projected goal status, at therapy episode outset, at reporting intervals, and at discharge or to end reporting.

- G8995, Sub PT/OT D/C status: Other physical or occupational subsequent functional limitation, discharge status, at discharge from therapy or to end reporting.

Documentation Requirements

Providers must document the functional G-codes and severity modifiers that are used to report the patient's current, projected goal, and discharge status in the patient's medical record. Modifiers must be selected based on long term goals, because the modifier should not change throughout the course of treatment with only some rare exceptions. Severity modifiers require a description of how the provider determined the modifier. This documentation applies to each date of service for which the reporting is done.

To determine the severity of a beneficiary's functional limitation, therapists must use a valid, reliable objective measure and/or assessment tool to quantify the functional limitation and provide appropriate supporting documentation. Therapists need to document in the medical record how they selected the modifier so the same process can be followed at succeeding assessment intervals. Sometimes more than one assessment tool is needed to determine the patient's functional limitation severity. It is also acceptable for professional judgment of the therapist to guide the selection of the appropriate modifier.

It is important to know what needs to be submitted to Medicare when reporting the functional limitation. Along with documenting the G-code descriptor and related modifier in the medical record, documentation of relevant objective and subjective information used to determine the overall percentage of functional limitation to select the severity modifier should also be included in the record. The corresponding therapy modifier (GP for physical therapy) must also accompany the reporting of the functional limitation G code. In addition, for each line on the institutional claim submitted by hospitals, SNFs, rehabilitation agencies, CORFs and HHAs, a charge of one cent, $0.01, is added. For each line on the professional claim submitted by private practice therapists and physician/non-physician practitioners, a charge of $0.00 is added.

Currently, only one functional limitation can be reported and documented, even if the patient has more than one functional limitation. The primary functional limitation is reported to Medicare for each patient. Reporting on more than one functional limitation may be required for some patients when treatment continues after the goal is achieved, as reporting on another functional limitation is then required. Two limitations cannot occur simultaneously; therefore, once reporting on the primary functional limitation is finished, the therapist can begin reporting on the next functional limitation using another set of G-codes.

Functional limitation reporting is required at discharge. However, if the beneficiary does not pursue the entire course of treatment and discontinues therapy prior to the anticipated discharge visit, discharge reporting is not required. Medicare realizes there simply is no G-code to report if a patient expires prior to the end of the therapy, either (CMS 2015).

G-Codes Examples and Clarification

As noted above, functional reporting coincides with the progress reporting frequency, which is on or before every 10th treatment day. In the example below, the G-codes for the mobility functional limitation (G8978-8980) are used to illustrate the timing of the functional reporting.

At the outset of therapy, the DOS the evaluative procedure is billed or the initial therapy services are furnished:

- G8978-CL to report the functional limitation (Mobility with current mobility limitation of at least 60% but less than 80percent impaired, limited or restricted').

- G8979-CT to report the projected goal for a mobility restriction of "at least 1% but less than 20% impaired, limited or restricted".

At the end of each progress reporting period - on the claim for the DOS when the services related to the progress report (which must be done at least once each 10 treatment days) are furnished, the clinician will report the same two G-codes but the modifier for the current status may be different.

- G8978 and G8979, along with the related severity modifiers, are used to report the current status and projected goal status of the mobility functional limitation.

At the time the beneficiary is discharged from the therapy episode—the DOS the discharge progress report services are furnished:

- G8979 and G8980, along with the related severity modifiers, are used to report the projected goal and discharge status of the mobility functional limitation.

In this example, the clinician determines that the beneficiary's mobility restriction is the most clinically relevant functional limitation and selects the Mobility G-code set (G8978-G8980) to represent the beneficiary's functional limitation. The clinician also determines the severe complexity of the beneficiary's functional limitation and selects the appropriate modifier. In this example, the clinician determines that the beneficiary has a 75% mobility restriction for which the CL modifier is applicable. The clinician expects that at the end of therapy the beneficiaries will have only a 15% mobility restriction for which the CI modifier is applicable. When the beneficiary attains the mobility goal, therapy continues to be medically necessary to address a functional limitation for which there is no categorical G-code. The clinician reports this using (G8990- G8992).

G8978 with the appropriate modifier are reported to show the beneficiary's current status as of this DOS. So if the beneficiary has made no progress, this claim will include G8978-CL if the beneficiary made progress and now has a mobility restriction of 65% CL would still be the appropriate modifier for 65percent, and G8978-CL would be reported in this case. If the beneficiary now has a mobility restriction of 45%, G8978-CK would be reported.

G8979-CI would be reported to show the expected goal. This severity modifier would not change unless the clinician adjusts the beneficiary's goal.

This step is repeated as necessary and clinically appropriate, adjusting the current status modifier used as the beneficiary progresses through therapy.

At the time the beneficiary is discharged from the therapy episode - the final claim for therapy episode will include two G-codes.

G8980-CI would be reported if the beneficiary attained the 15% mobility goal. Alternatively, if the beneficiary's mobility restriction only reached 25%, G8980-CJ would be reported.

To end reporting of one functional limitation: As noted above, functional reporting is required to continue throughout the entire episode of care. Accordingly, when further therapy is medically necessary after the beneficiary attains the goal for the first reported functional limitation, the clinician would end reporting of the first functional limitation by using the same G-codes and modifiers that would be used at the time of discharge. Using the mobility example, to end reporting of the mobility functional limitation, G8979-CI and G8980-CI would be reported on the same DOS that coincides with end of that progress-reporting period.

To begin reporting of second functional limitation: At the time reporting is begun, file a new and different functional limitation within the same episode of care (i.e., after the reporting of the prior functional limitation is ended). Reporting on the second functional limitation, however, is not begun until the DOS of the next treatment day—which is day one of the new progress-reporting period. When the next functional limitation to be reported is NOT defined by one of the other three PT/OT categorical codes, the G-code set (G8990- G8992) for the "other PT/OT primary" functional limitation is used, rather than the G-code set for the "other PT/OT subsequent"—because it is the first reported "other PT/OT" functional limitation. This reporting begins on the DOS of the first treatment day following the mobility "discharge" reporting, which is counted as the initial service for the "other PT/OT primary "functional limitation and the first treatment day of the new progress reporting period. In this case, G8990 and G8991, along with the corresponding modifiers, are reported on the claim for therapy services.

In the above example, if further therapy is medically necessary once reporting for the mobility functional limitation has ended, the therapist begins reporting on another functional limitation using a different set of G-codes. Reporting of the next functional limitation is required on the DOS of the first treatment day after the reporting was ended for the mobility functional limitation.

When functional reporting is required on a claim for therapy services, two G-codes will generally be required. Two exceptions exist:

1. Therapy services under more than one therapy POC. Claims may contain more than two non-payable functional G-codes when in cases where a beneficiary receives therapy services under multiple POCs (PT, OT, and/or SLP) from the same therapy provider.

2. One-Time Therapy Visit. When a beneficiary is seen and future therapy services are either not medically indicated or are going to be furnished by another provider, the clinician reports on the claim for the DOS of the visit, all three G-codes in the appropriate code set (current status, goal status and discharge status), along with corresponding severity modifiers.

Each reported functional G-code must also contain the following essential line of service information:

- Functional severity modifier in the range CH-CN.

- Therapy modifier indicating the discipline of the POC—GP, GO or GN—for PT, OT, and SLP services, respectively.

- Date of the corresponding billable service.

Required Tracking and Documentation of Functional G-codes and Severity Modifiers

The reported functional information is derived from the beneficiary's functional limitations set forth in the therapy goals, a requirement of the POC, that are established by a therapist, including an occupational therapist, a speech-language pathologist or a physical therapist, or a physician/non-physician practitioner, as applicable. The therapist or physician/non-physician practitioner furnishing the therapy services must not only report the functional information on the therapy claim, but, he/she must track and document the G-codes and modifiers used for this reporting in the beneficiary's medical record of therapy services.

Remittance Advice Messages

Medicare will return a Claim Adjustment Reason Code 246 (This non-payable code is for required reporting only) and a Group Code of CO (Contractual Obligation) assigning financial liability to the provider. In addition, beneficiaries will be informed via Medicare Summary Notice 36.7 that they are not responsible for any charge amount associated with one of these G-codes.

Reference: CR 8005 was issued via two transmittals. The first revises the "Medicare Benefit Policy Manual" and it is available at http://www.cms.gov/Regulations-and-Guidance/Guidance/Transmittals/Downloads/R165BP.pdf on the CMS website. The second transmittal updates the "Medicare Claims Processing Manual" and it is at http://www.cms.gov/Regulations-and-Guidance/Guidance/Transmittals/Downloads/R2622CP.pdf on the CMS website.

Physician Quality Reporting System (PQRS)

The Physician Quality Reporting System (PQRS) was formerly the Physician Quality Reporting Initiative (PQRI). It is a program implemented by Medicare that enables individual eligible professionals (EPs) and group practices to report quality of care information. This assessment tool helps practitioners provide better quality and more timely care.

Individual EPs and group practices can quantify how often they are meeting a particular quality measure by reporting on PQRS. According to the CMS website, "Beginning in 2015, the program will apply a negative payment adjustment to individual EPs and PQRS group practices who did not satisfactorily report data on quality measures for Medicare Part B Physician Fee Schedule (MPFS) covered professional services in 2013. Those who report satisfactorily for the 2015 program year will avoid the 2017 PQRS negative payment adjustment." It is in the best interest of all EPs and group practices to utilize the PQRS for better reimbursement in the future.

Eligible professionals

The CMS website provides a list of eligible professionals who can report on PQRS measures. CMS has deemed professional services paid under or based on the Medicare Physician Fee Schedule to be the only ones who can report on the measures and qualify for PQRS payment adjustments. This includes the following:

- Doctor of Medicine
- Doctor of Osteopathy
- Doctor of Podiatric Medicine
- Doctor of Optometry
- Doctor of Oral Surgery
- Doctor of Dental Medicine
- Doctor of Chiropractic
- Physician Assistant
- Nurse Practitioner
- Clinical Nurse Specialist
- Certified Registered Nurse Anesthetist (and Anesthesiologist Assistant)
- Certified Nurse Midwife
- Clinical Social Worker

- Clinical Psychologist

- Registered Dietician

- Nutrition Professional

- Audiologists

- Advanced Practice Registered Nurse (APRN)

- **Physical Therapist**

- Occupational Therapist

- Qualified Speech-Language Therapist

It is important to note that some professionals are eligible but not able to participate due to their billing practices. CMS indicates this applies to: "Professionals who do not bill Medicare at an individual National Provider Identifier (NPI) level, where the rendering provider's individual NPI is entered on CMS-1500 or CMS-1450 type paper or electronic claims billing, associated with specific line-item services." Also, anyone who uses another fee schedule or method of billing and does not render services under MPFS is not included in PQRS.

2015 Changes to PQRS

According to the APTA website, physical therapists need to keep up-to-date with the specific changes PQRS implements each year. There is now a requirement for private practice physical therapists to report 9 individual measures (or up to 8, if 9 measures do not apply) through claims or registry under the PQRS program. There is also a requirement for at least 1 cross cutting measure, which is a new category. If providers do not heed the requirements, they will incur the 2.0% payment penalty in 2017 (APTA 2015).

The cross cutting measures are as follows:

- Measure 128: Preventive Care and Screening: Body Mass Index (BMI) Screening and Follow-up

- Measure 130: Documentation and Verification of Current Medications in the Medical Record

- Measure 131: Pain Assessment Prior to the Initiation of Patient Therapy and Follow-up

- Measure 182: Functional Outcome Assessment

The measure specifications have changed for many PQRS measures. CMS has announced changes to the medication measure, #130, now requiring reporting of the measure on each visit when 97001, 97002 or 97532 are billed. The low back pain measures, #148-151, and the chronic wound care measure, #245, have been eliminated. Measure #126 for Diabetes Care deleted the numerator code G8406.

The denominator codes G8980, G8983, G8986, G8989, G8992, were added to the FOTO measures, #217-223. If physical therapists plan to participate in PQRS in 2015, they should review the 2015 measures specifications and the qualifying case information, including quality data codes for reporting. APTA claims it has updated its PQRS resources to reflect the 2015 measures changes but encourages providers to review all the measures they are reporting (APTA 2015).

The 2015 list of measure codes has a total of 402 PQRS measures listed and explained in a downloadable spreadsheet via the CMS website. Please refer to this list as needed in practice. Measures Codes - Centers for Medicare & Medicaid Services

Claims-based Reporting

Claims-based submission of data is one reporting method used in the PQRS program. A physical therapist using this method has to submit Quality Data Codes (QDCs) for each PQRS measure on the claim form for each eligible visit. There are only 6 measures available on claims forms in 2015, so all must be completed. The standard to avoid penalty is reporting 9 measures if applicable. Physical therapists need to report on a minimum of 50% of all qualifying Medicare patients in order to meet the claims-based reporting requirements for 2015. The Measure Applicability Validation (MAV) process will be impressed upon any physical therapist reporting via claims. The APTA notes that claims-based reporting is highly discouraged in the future for PQRS (APTA 2015).

The APTA website provides a table summarizing the 2015 claims-based measures. Each of the following measures has to be reported on when billing for PT Evaluation (97001):

- 128 Preventive Care and Screening: Body Mass Index (BMI) Screening and Follow-Up
- 130 Documentation and Verification of Current Medications in the Medical Record
- 131 Pain Assessment Prior to Initiation of Patient Treatment
- 154 Falls: Risk Assessment
- 155 Falls: Plan of Care
- 182 Functional Outcome Assessment

Measure #128 is the only one that does not have to be reported when billing for PT Reevaluation (97002). When billing (97532), measures #130 and #131 must be reported. Refer to the APTA website for the Quality Data Codes associated with each measure (APTA 2015).

Registry Reporting

Another reporting method for PQRS is registry submission. Physical therapists who choose registry submission submit their selected measures through the registry. Feedback from their registry vendor should be received regularly to stay aware of their reporting rate. Reporting rates in 2015 need to be monitored by therapists and maintained at a successful level in order to avoid the 2% penalty in 2017 (APTA 2015).

Once again, the MAV will apply to any therapist not meeting the reporting requirements for 2015 (CMS 2015):

- Reporting at least 9 PQRS measures and 1-3 National Quality Strategy (NQS) domains. (NQS domains include: communication and care coordination; community/population health; efficiency and cost reduction; safety; effective clinical care; person-and caregiver-centered experience and outcomes)

- PQRS reporting on a minimum of 50% of Medicare patients

- Reporting at least 1 cross cutting measure

- At least one patient or procedure in the rate numerator for the measure to be counted as meeting performance.

The MAV is actually a helpful process in avoiding the 2017 penalty of 2%. The alternative to MAV being performed is that MAV will *not* apply, and the 2% penalty will automatically be implemented if any of the following are found (CMS 2015):

- Reporting fewer than 50% Medicare Part B patients

- Not including at least 1 cross cutting measure during a face to face encounter

- No patient or procedure qualifies for the numerator of the performance measure

The APTA website provides this list of 2015 Registry Measures for PQRS. No specific details are given regarding the measures at this time (APTA 2015).

- 126 Diabetes Mellitus: Diabetic Foot and Ankle Care, Peripheral Neuropathy: Neurological Evaluation

- 127 Diabetic Mellitus: Diabetic Foot and Ankle Care, Ulcer Prevention Evaluation of Footwear

- 128 Preventive Care and Screening: Body Mass Index (BMI) Screening and Follow-up*

- 130 Documentation and Verification of Current Medications in the Medical Record*

- 131 Pain Assessment Prior to Initiation of Patient Treatment*

- 154 Falls: Risk Assessment

- 155 Falls: Plan of Care

- 182 Functional Outcome Assessment*

Cross cutting measure

Group Practice Reporting Option (GRPO)

In 2010, the Centers for Medicare & Medicaid Services (CMS) created the group practice reporting option (GPRO) for the PQRS in accordance with the Social Security Act (CMS 2015). Any of the eligible professionals (EPs) such as physical therapists who report in PQRS are automatically registered to report as individuals. When a practice consists of 2 or more PTs, it can register for participation under Group Practice Reporting Option (GPRO). If the practice does not report via registry (as described above), the GPRO option cannot be used. The APTA website states the registration deadline for GPRO is June 30, 2015. The possible benefit of GPRO is the data is analyzed in mass, so a summation of all the therapists' reporting becomes one unified reporting rate for the entire practice (APTA 2015).

Value-Based Modifier

A new program implemented regarding PQRS is the *Value-Based Modifier* in calendar year 2016. Failure to abide by this will result in penalties in the year 2018. The Affordable Care Act mandated CMS to begin applying this Value Modifier under the Medicare Physician Fee Schedule in 2015. The implementation is being phased in, starting with groups of 100 or more eligible professionals (EPs) in 2015 (based on 2013 performance), then groups of physicians with 10 plus EPs (based on 2014 performance), and eventually by 2018, the Value Modifier will apply to Medicare PFS payments for non-physician EPs (physical therapists). This Value Modifier will be aligned with the PQRS to ensure the maximum quality of care is given to beneficiaries of Medicare (CMS 2015).

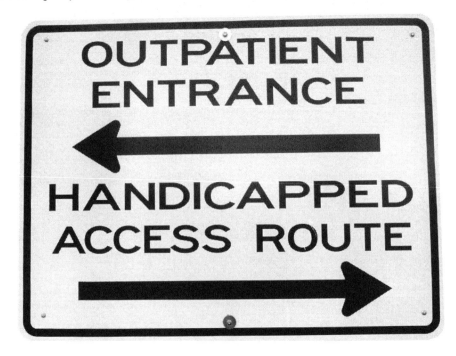

New Medicare Legislation

In the PT in Motion publication on May 5, 2015, the changes accompanying the new Medicare legislation are highlighted. The changes involve the end of the sustainable growth rate (SGR), extending the therapy cap exceptions for 2 more years, changing manual medical review and quality reporting, and offering incentives for participation in alternative payment models. The APTA website further outlines the changes taking place through the MACRA, and the APTA states, "MACRA is laying the groundwork for a significant transformation in how physical therapists (PTs) and other health professionals are paid.

Here are some of the highlights from this article in PT in Motion regarding the future direction for Medicare Part B:

- Manual medical reviews of therapy cap exceptions will not be based solely on dollar amounts as sometime around mid-July, the $3,700 trigger for manual medical review (MMR) will be replaced with a system that links MMR to provider behavior and other factors. CMS will check to see if a provider has an "aberrant" pattern of billing practices, assess the provider's claims denial percentage, check if the provider is newly enrolled, look for what types of medical conditions are being treated, and discern whether the provider is part of a group that includes another provider who has been identified in terms of the those factors. The Merit-Based Incentive Payment System (MIPS) is set to be implemented in the future. Performance will be evaluated according to quality, resource use, meaningful use, and clinical practice improvement. This basically means PQRS, value-based modifiers, and electronic health records meaningful use would be consolidated into this single new quality program.

- CMS will offer 5% bonuses to PTs and health care professionals involved in alternative payment models (APMs) such as accountable care organizations, medical homes, and bundled care systems. In 2026, CMS will stratify annual updates, providing a .75% annual update to health care professionals engaged in APMs, and .25% for those who are not .

- New 1% payment update factor for post-acute care providers.

- Inclusion of physician assistants, nurse practitioners, and nurse clinical specialists as professionals qualified to provide documentation for certain types of durable medical equipment.

- Requirements that Medicare administrative contractors (MACs) provide ongoing outreach, education, training, and technical assistance to providers.

Just in the past few months, the Medicare rules have changed and/or been updated from the start of writing this book to the finish. Keeping up with the most recent news from the CMS and APTA website is essential to know for sure what is applicable here and now for your healthcare practice regarding Medicare Part B.

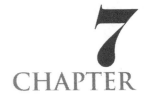

CHAPTER 7

THERAPY CAP, MANUAL MEDICAL REVIEW, & PHYSICIAN FEE SCHEDULE

General Information on the Therapy Cap

The Balanced Budget Act of 1997, P.L. 105-33, Section 4541© set an annual cap for Part B Medicare therapy patients. These limits change annually.

Since the creation of therapy caps, Congress has enacted several moratoria. The Deficit Reduction Act of 2005 directed CMS to develop exceptions to therapy caps for calendar year 2006 and the exceptions have been extended periodically. Exceptions to caps based on the medical necessity of the service are in effect only when Congress deems the exceptions. In 2006, the Exception Processes fell into two categories, Automatic Process Exceptions, and Manual Process Exceptions. As of January 1, 2007, there was no longer a manual process for exceptions. All services that required exceptions to caps were to be processed using the automatic process. The Middle Class Tax Relief and Job Creation Act of 2012 mandated that a manual medical review process for Medicare Part B therapy services that exceed the $3,700 threshold.

All requests for exception are in the form of a KX modifier added to claim lines. The KX modifier is added to claim lines to indicate that the clinician attests that services are medically necessary and justification is documented in the medical record.

2015 Therapy Cap Limitations and Exceptions

On January 1, 2014, the therapy cap exceptions process was extended to March 31, 2014, because Congress passed the Pathway for SGR Reform Act of 2013. Then Congress passed the Protecting

Access to Medicare Act of 2014, which extended the cap exceptions process and manual medical review at $3700 through March 31, 2015. On April 16, 2015, the Medicare Access and CHIP Reauthorization Act of 2015 (MACRA) was enacted. This extended the therapy cap exceptions process through December 31, 2017 and made changes to the manual medical review process. MACRA also extended the application of the therapy cap to outpatient hospitals until January 1, 2018 (APTA 2015).

Therapy caps for 2015 are $1940 for physical therapy and speech therapy combined and $1940 for occupational therapy. Therapy Cap Exceptions Process was to expire April 1, 2015, but the Senate voted 58 to 42 in favor of extending the cap until December 31, 2017 (rather than repeal the cap altogether) (APTA information bulletin April 14, 2015).

For 2015, the $1940 therapy cap with an exceptions process applies to services provided in the following outpatient therapy settings: physical therapists in private practice, physician offices, skilled nursing facilities (Part B), rehabilitation agencies (or ORFs), and comprehensive outpatient rehabilitation facilities (CORFs), critical access hospitals, and outpatient hospital departments. Unlike 2013, the therapy cap now applies when a patient receives outpatient therapy services from a critical access hospital, and those services are subject to extension of the therapy cap exceptions and manual medical review process. If a beneficiary requires therapy services in a critical access hospital beyond the $1940 cap, the CAH needs to submit the claim with a KX modifier, and they will undergo the CMS manual medical review process if services are needed beyond $3700 (APTA 2015).

Fortunately, if a Medicare beneficiary has already exceeded the cap but requires an evaluation (97001) or reevaluation (97002) to determine the need for further therapy, the therapy cap does not apply. These services would be covered for the new or returning patient (APTA 2015).

Questions arise when beneficiaries consider Medicare pays 80% of allowable charges and they pay the remaining 20%. The cap is based on the total allowable charges, combining what Medicare and the beneficiary pay up to $1940 in 2015. Therefore, Medicare will pay 80% of the allowed charges ($1552.00) and the beneficiary will be responsible for the remaining 20% ($388.00).

Medicare Advantage is another plan where the $1940 therapy cap may be applied and require the exceptions process as well. In the past, most Medicare Advantage plans have chosen not to apply a therapy cap. Beneficiaries should always check with their insurance plan regarding payment policies (APTA 2015).

Automatic Exceptions Process

When a beneficiary's condition requires continued skilled therapy that is justified by documentation, an automatic exception to the therapy cap may be applied. Therapy services beyond the $1940 therapy cap require documentation that shows the patient still needs to achieve their prior functional status or maximum expected functional status within a reasonable amount of time. The automatic process for exception can be used for any diagnosis for which providers can justify services exceeding the cap. Unless CMS declares a claim needs to undergo the manual medical review process, a therapist may request an automatic exception (APTA 2015).

In order to submit a request for an automatic exception, the provider must add a KX modifier to the therapy procedure code subject to the therapy cap limits. Codes subject to the therapy cap tracking requirements are listed in a table in the Claims Processing Manual, Chapter 5, Section 20(B), "Applicable Outpatient Rehabilitation Healthcare Common Procedure Coding System (HCPCS) Codes."

A KX modifier should not be added to all Medicare therapy claims. It is only appended to the therapy procedure code when a beneficiary qualifies for a therapy cap exception. By attaching the KX modifier, the provider is attesting that the services billed: 1) Qualified for the cap exception; 2) Required the skills of a therapist and are reasonable and necessary services; and 3) Are justified by appropriate documentation in the medical record (APTA 2015).

Providers do not have to submit specific documentation for automatic process exceptions. The clinician should consult the Medicare Manuals and professional literature to determine if the beneficiary may qualify for the automatic process exception. If the Medicare beneficiaries meet the criteria for an automatic exception, they will automatically be accepted from the therapy cap, and documentation for an exception will not be required. For claims that are selected for manual medical review, documentation justifying the services must be submitted in response to any *Additional Documentation Request* (ADR). (APTA 2015)

Manual Medical Review

Manual Medical Review began October 1, 2012 for Part B Therapy Services. The Middle Class Tax Relief and Job Creation Act of 2012 (MCTRJCA) established a requirement for Manual Medical Review of Part B therapy claims over a $3,700 threshold. Similar to the therapy cap, there is a threshold of $3,700 for OT services and another threshold of $3,700 for PT and SLP services combined. The threshold represents the total allowed charges under Medicare Part B for services furnished by independent practitioners and institutional services under Medicare Part B.

The Manual Medical Review for therapy exceeding the $3,700 threshold requires that providers submit a pre-approval request for exception prior to initiation of the services provided in order to be paid for any additional visits. The provider may request pre-approval of up to 20 treatment days of services per discipline. The FI/MAC will make a decision and inform the provider and beneficiary within 10 business days of receipt of all requested documentation. If the FI/MAC cannot make a decision in 10 days, the therapy will be considered approved. If the request was not approved, the letter communicating the decision must be detailed. If the request was not approved, a provider may submit additional requests and provide additional information for consideration.

The following information is from the APTA website under Frequently Asked Questions regarding manual medical review:

"From January 1, 2014- February 28, 2014 Recovery Audit Contractors (RACs) conducted either prepayment or post-payment review for claims exceeding $3700, depending on the state as follows:

- **Prepayment Review:** Claims submitted in the RAC prepayment review demonstration states will be reviewed on a prepayment basis. These states are Florida, California, Michigan, Texas, New York, Louisiana, Illinois, Pennsylvania, Ohio, North Carolina and Missouri. The MAC will send an ADR to the provider requesting the additional documentation be sent to the RAC. The RAC will conduct prepayment review within 10 business days of receiving the additional documentation and will notify the MAC of the payment decision.

- **Postpayment Review:** In the remaining states, the RACs will conduct immediate postpayment review. The MAC will flag the claims that exceed $3700, request additional documentation and pay the claim. The MAC will send an ADR to the provider requesting that the additional documentation be sent to the RAC. The RAC will conduct post-payment review and will notify the MAC of its decision."

February 28, 2014 the pre- and post-payment manual medical review process changed due to the CMS transition to new recovery audit contracts. Due to the pause in RAC contracts, prepayment reviews stopped, and all claims now undergo post-payment reviews. The 10-day reviewing time frame does not apply to these reviews because of the volume of claims CMS during this transition. The new recovery auditors review the claims in the order that they were paid (APTA 2015).

In July 2015, there will be a new manual medical review process. CMS will consider certain factors to determine which therapy services to review. The APTA website states these factors will include reviewing providers: (1) with patterns of aberrant billing practices compared with their peers; (2) with a high claims denial percentage or who are less compliant with applicable Medicare program requirements; (3) who are newly enrolled; (4) who treat certain types of medical conditions; and (5) who are part of a group that includes another therapy provider identified by the above factors.

The following websites will take you to each Fiscal Intermediaries and Medicare Administrative Contractors (FI/MAC's) manual medical review form to fill out:

Cahaba GBA

http://www.cahabagba.com/documents/2012/09/part-b-pre-authorization-request-form.pdf

CGS

http://www.cgsmedicare.com/Articles/TCE_Request_Form.pdf

First Coast Service Options

http://medicare.fcso.com/Rehabilitation_services/243444.pdf

NGS

http://www.ngsmedicare.com/wps/wcm/connect/0e7308804ca306c786b98e555e90c49f/1319_0912_TherapyServicesPreapprovalForm_V2.pdf?MOD=AJPERES

NHIC

http://www.medicarenhic.com/ne_prov/med_review/J14%20Therapy%20CAP%20Exception%20Cover%20Sheet%20Request%20form.pdf

Noridian Administrative Services

https://www.noridianmedicare.com/partb/coverage/docs/therapy_threshold_pre-authorization_request_coversheet.pdf

Novitas

https://www.novitas-solutions.com/claims/therapy-cap/pdf/ther-cap-a.pdf

Palmetto GBA

http://www.palmettogba.com/Palmetto/Providers.nsf/docsCat/Jurisdiction%2011%20Part%20B~Resources~Forms?open&Expand=1

WPS

http://www.wpsmedicare.com/j5macpartb/forms/_files/therapy-cap-exception-preapproval-request.pdf

Multiple Procedure Payment Reduction (MPPR)

According to the APTA website, under the 2015 Medicare Fee Schedule Calculator section, approximately 44 CPT codes labeled "always therapy services," will incur a 50% reduction of payment to their practice expense value under the multiple procedure payment reduction (MPPR) policy. This applies to physicians and physical therapists in private practice, CORFs, SNFs (Part B), home health (Part B), outpatient hospitals, and rehabilitation agencies. For each code thereafter, the practice expense value will be decreased. As clinicians generally provide several services with CPT codes in a day, the many potential code combinations will determine the total reimbursement (APTA 2015).

Section 4541(a)(2) of the Balanced Budget Act (BBA) (P.L. 105-33) of 1997, which added §1834(k)(5) to the Act, required payment under a prospective payment system (PPS) for outpatient rehabilitation services (except those furnished by or under arrangements with a hospital). Section 4541(c) of the BBA required application of financial limitations to all outpatient rehabilitation services (except those furnished by or under arrangements with a hospital).

2015 Medicare Copays and Deductibles

CMS released information on the copays and deductibles for Medicare Part B services in 2015. The following is the summary found at Federal Register | Medicare Program; Medicare Part B Monthly Actuarial Rates, Premium Rate, and Annual Deductible Beginning January 1, 2015:

"The monthly actuarial rates for 2015 are $209.80 for aged enrollees and $254.80 for disabled enrollees. The standard monthly Part B premium rate for all enrollees for 2015 is $104.90, which is equal to 50 percent of the monthly actuarial rate for aged enrollees or approximately 25 percent of the expected average total cost of Part B coverage for aged enrollees. (The 2014 standard premium rate was $104.90.) The Part B deductible for 2015 is $147.00 for all Part B beneficiaries. If a beneficiary has to pay an income-related monthly adjustment, they may have to pay a total monthly premium of about 35, 50, 65, or 80 percent of the total cost of Part B coverage."

In 2015, the Part B deductible will be $147, staying the same as in 2013, and the Part B copay will remain 20%. Premiums for Part B are based on income, paying $104.90 with individual income less than $85,000 and $335.70 with individual income above 214,000 (CMS 2015).

Outpatient Prospective Payment System (OPPS)

CMS released calendar year 2015 Final Rule for Outpatient Prospective Payment System (OPPS) on October 31, 2014. The changes are those that affect physical therapists in the settings of general acute care hospitals, inpatient rehabilitation facilities, inpatient psychiatric facilities, long-term acute care hospitals, children's hospitals, and cancer hospitals. This list is of changes is taken from the APTA website's summary of the OPPS, last update on 11/12/2014:

- Payment increase of 2.2 percent;

- Revision to the Requirements for Physician Certification of Hospital Inpatient Services

- The implementation of comprehensive APCs to handle payment for the most costly device-dependent services;

- Changes to payment packaging policies for ancillary services;

- The removal of the prosthetic supplies exclusion from payment under the OPPS;

- Changes to the Negative Pressure Wound Therapy APC payment;

- Data collection on services furnished in off-campus provider-based departments;

- Changes to the rural provider and hospital ownership exceptions to physician self-referral law; and

- CMS-Identified overpayments associated with payment data submitted by Medicare Advantage (MA) Organizations and Medicare Part D sponsors.

Medicare Physician Fee Schedule

The Medicare Physician Fee Schedule (MPFS) is not just for physician payment but is also used to pay for Part B therapies in outpatient and nursing facilities. For calendar year 2013, a final rule included a 26.5% reduction to Medicare payment rates for physicians, physical therapists, and other professionals due to the flawed sustainable growth rate (SGR) formula. Congress has enacted legislation preventing the reduction every year since 2003. CMS announced in 2013 that it was "committed to fixing the SGR update methodology and ensuring these payment cuts do not take effect."

After years of physicians, physical therapists, and other health care professionals advocating a repeal of the flawed sustainable growth rate (SGR) formula, Congress passed a bill to repeal it on April 14, 2015. The Medicare Access and CHIP Reauthorization Act of 2015 followed President Obama's April 1, 2014 signing into law the Protecting Access to Medicare Act of 2014, which was one last temporary "fix" to prevent a large payment cut for physicians, physical therapists, and other health care professionals from taking effect. The 2014 law extended the therapy cap exceptions process until March 31, 2015, and then the April 14, 2015 repeal law has further extended the exceptions process to December 31, 2017 (APTA 2015).

Changes in the 2015 Medicare Physician Fee Schedule final rule affect physical therapist practice and payment for 2015. According to the APTA website, the changes that are in effect regarding fee schedule payment rates include the following:

- From January 1-June 30, 2015, there is a slight change from 2014 in the conversion factor for providers. The 2015 conversion factor for the first 6 months is $35.7547 as mandated by legislation. (The 2014 conversion factor was $35.8228.)

- Effective July 1, 2015, there will be a .5% update to the payment rates for the remainder of the year and an extension of the existing 1.0 geographic practice cost index (GPCI) work floor.

Additional Cap Facts for 2015

- If a beneficiary does not qualify for the therapy cap exception, therapy can be continued if the beneficiary chooses to pay out of pocket.

- If continuing therapy beyond the cap and without exception approval, beneficiaries can be billed at a rate decided upon by the provider. Providers are advised not to provide free or deeply discounted rates to avoid violating the anti-kickback statutes.

- How much the beneficiary has accrued toward the therapy cap can be accessed from the ELGA screen inquiries into CWF and the remaining benefit can be accessed through the 270/271 eligibility inquiry and response transaction.

- A provider can use GA/GY/GX codes and bill the secondary insurance plans for reimbursement if the cap exemption ends; however, an ABN should be provided to the beneficiary explaining that services are not covered and submit the claim to Medicare with the modifier for a denial.

- A provider can offer Medicare patients an "aftercare" program at a reduced or flat rate once the cap is met; however, the beneficiary will be financially responsible for these services. The beneficiary should be given an Advanced Beneficiary Notice (ABN).

The APTA advises the following:

"When charging patients out of pocket, it is very important to have a set fee schedule that applies to all patients regardless of their insurer (Medicare or private insurance). Additionally, any discounts offered should also be offered to all patients regardless of their source of insurance coverage and all discount policies should be established in writing. For instance, you may have a policy that offers a 20% discount to patients with income less than a certain dollar amount in a given year or for patients with medical costs that exceed a set limit in a given year."

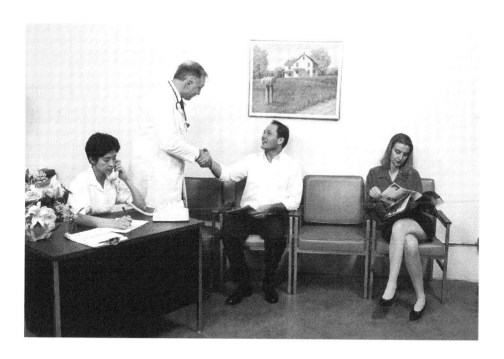

8
CHAPTER

ADMINISTRATIVE MATTERS

Common Billing Errors and How to Avoid Them

Contractors of Medicare receive over two billion claims annually. Not all of these claims can be considered valid because of error in billing or coding methods. Comprehensive Error Rate Testing (CERT) reflects the provider's comprehension with Medicare program payment rules and coverage policies. It also measures the provider's observance of these policies through the Provider Compliance Error Rate. Some denials are caused by wrong billing practices (Part B Virginia Top Claim Denials, 2010).

If Medicare has identified a mistake with the admitting diagnosis, the claim may be denied. To avoid this, the primary/admitting diagnosis code must be valid for the date of service. Billing errors can also occur due to a missing HCPCS code. Another billing error is not indicating the HCPCS code on the HCPCS file and a HCPCS code for a line item is invalid for the date of services on the claim. Before including revenue codes, its accuracy must be confirmed. CPT/HCPCS codes must be reviewed. Also check if a revenue code requires a HCPCS code. And do not forget to check the code's validity. Verify the dates of service on the claim. Make sure the revenue code billed is correctly.

A copy of the patient's Medicare card should be made, and the patient's name and number should match the patient's name and number on the claim exactly. The provider should also confirm the patient's effective date by looking at the patient's Medicare card. Services rendered earlier to the patient's effective date are not eligible for reimbursement. Also, if the patient has terminated his or her Medicare benefits, the services/treatments are not going to be paid. To check a patient's eligibility, providers may look them up on the online inquiry system. Using nicknames on Medicare cards is another ground for denial of claims. If the suffix Jr. or Sr. is included in the patient's name, it should be listed. Once the suffix is not included and it is applicable to the patient, denials can occur. The claim can also be denied because payment for the service has been already given within the valid time period. The service could not be paid with other services on the same day.

Modifiers are used to identify details on a claim and to modify payment of a procedure. Modifiers also help in identifying if a procedure is covered by a claim, and to make sure that reported services are appropriate for Medicare reimbursement. Specific procedure codes must be contained within a Medicare claim, and these codes must match the appropriate procedure that was delivered to the patient. Since codes are updated time to time, it would be better to be updated with CPT codes. A HCPCS manual would also help in choosing the correct procedure code. Providers lose about five percent of their gross revenues because of billing errors and inconsistencies (CPT, 2004).

It would be ideal to have coders and billers, and even registration receptionists, who already have experience, or who have an education related to this healthcare practice. The main reason for billing and coding inconsistencies is human error. Coders and billers must also go through continuous training and be updated with new coding and billing policies (Dunn, 2009).

To help the staff to do their job more effectively and efficiently, billing software systems should be integrated. The right software would help the staff edit and identify mistakes before services are billed. Some software also offers features carrier-specific edits and can flag inconsistencies and make automated corrections. The employee should double check the findings of the software and make necessary edits. As with the staff's knowledge, these billing software systems should always be updated with the correct definitions in case there are new changes in the rules or policies of coding and billing. Another benefit of automation is that it makes the categorization of denials easier.

Although not ideal for all providers, a big organization may benefit from the services of either a data analyst or a computer programmer. In case of an overwhelming number of claims denials, data analysts can make trend reports to cite what has gone wrong and the most common reason for the denial of claims. Programmers could help make or improve existing billing systems.

Automation of billing and documentation complements manual auditing and documentation. The system catches missing charges and sends a daily report on concerned department to resolve relevant issues.

Coordination of Benefits

Nowadays, it is not uncommon for people to have several plans from different insurance providers that are in effect when they undergo treatment or outpatient physical therapy. These plans, normally provided by private companies are active and on top of their Medicare health insurance plans. In situations like these, Medicare plans have the possibility of being covered by another health care plan, making it only a secondary health insurance policy. This means that prior to the billing or even commencement of physical therapy, billers and therapists both need to obtain from their patients all necessary information regarding their health care insurance. In doing so, determining beneficiaries of Medicare is also a must; instead of the usual practice of assuming that Medicare is the primary insurance plan in place.

Coordination of benefits and processing claims based on these must be a key responsibility by billers and practitioners since there is a growing trend of people who are covered by Medicare but opt to use other health insurance plans. These individuals are usually those who are working, even after the age of 65 and are availing the health care insurance plans provided by their respective companies.

In the MSP or the Medicare Secondary Payer and its guidelines, one of the roles being appointed to the physical therapist revolves around coordination of benefits from the health insurance providers of their patients. This role includes the collection of fees and ensuring which insurance plans the patient has covers the services provided by the physical therapist. It should be remembered either by the billers or physical therapists that the Social Security Act requires them to bill insurance service providers first before Medicare for services rendered if Medicare is not the primary payer listed on their plans.

Medicare Payments First

In understanding when Medicare makes payments first for outpatient services provided by the physical therapist, one of the important things is to know what primary payers are. In a general sense, primary payers are companies or insurance providers that take the responsibility of paying for claims made on behalf of customers availing a specific insurance plan they provide. Normally, companies enroll their employees under a group health plan (GHP) for their health insurance needs. This GHP is the one that takes responsibility for being the primary payer for employees when claims are made. Medicare, on the other hand, is considered to be the primary payer for the health services availed by an individual if that person is not covered by any other insurance yet. This is the most general set-up between Medicare and other health care insurance plans (CMS: Medicare Part B Updates, 2014).

To make sure that the payer status of Medicare and other health care insurance providers is properly ascertained, the billers or physical therapists need to collect information about these from the patients or from their employers. All this information is normally collected and kept within what is called a COBC or Coordination of Benefits Contractor. This system is also responsible not only for keeping and storing insurance benefits information but also for sharing the information among all concerned agencies and parties. Physical therapists and billers can also access this information by placing a call to the COBC (CMS, 2013).

Medicare Payments in Event that the Primary Payer Denies Payment Claims

Regardless of the coverage plans availed by patients, there are instances wherein payments are denied for the services rendered. There are a variety of reasons why this happens, but most of them revolve on the technical aspects of billing and payment claims. When such event happens, both the patients and the physical therapists are faced with a conundrum on how to collect the payments. In the past, patients either foot the bill out of their own pockets, or the facility tries to find ways how to collect the payments for services already rendered. In an effort to put a solution to all these and help both parties affected, CMS has made statements that in certain instances, Medicare may consider making payments when the primary payer refuses to do so. This is possible when the services being billed for are covered under a Medicare plan and all necessary requirements for payment claims have been filed accordingly (APTA: Medicare as Secondary Payer, 2011).

It is important that first and foremost, they determine if Medicare is nominated as either primary or secondary payer. In situations where Medicare is nominated as the secondary payer and the primary payer denies making payments, the billers or physical therapists would need to submit the payment claims first to the GHP. The GHP would then ascertain if the claims for which they are being billed are covered by the plan availed by a patient. If the patient's treatment is not part of the benefits and coverage plans, the GHP would need to furnish the biller and therapist a document stating why payment claims have been denied. Reasons can either be because the services being billed for is not part of the plan availed by the patient or simply because the health insurance in general does not cover the service of that type. This document that the GHP issued will be the one that will be presented to Medicare when payments are being claimed (Regulations Regarding Individuals That Qualify For Medicare and Medicaid: Who Qualifies as a "Dual Eligible?, 2010).

Since the document issued by the GHP stating reason for payment denial is important, it is essential for either billers or physical therapists to make sure that the document is complete before they submit to Medicare. Medicare would use this document to determine if payment is going to be released or the claim is to be denied. The determination of payment process is considerably long and quite technical but in the end, if and when Medicare decided to make payments for claims filed, this will be termed as conditional primary payment.

Claiming for Payments when Patients' GHP is Fully Consumed

It is a known fact that most health care insurance plans have caps or limits as to their coverage inclusions. When a patients' health care insurance coverage cap gets depleted, claiming for payments may be coursed through Medicare as a secondary payer. Documents need to be submitted to support the necessity of the claim. In this case, there should be a document indicating all available payment coverage under an existing GHP has been exhausted and the patient is filing for Medicare payment as secondary payer (CMS, 2013).

Medicare secondary payment coverage can also be availed if the GHP of a patient has made payment as a primary payer but reimburses the physical therapist for an amount less than what is actually billed. The balance from that bill can be charged to Medicare as a secondary payer and the physical therapist can expect that if the documents submitted satisfy the guidelines set by Medicare, payment for services rendered can eventually be released. Another thing to consider is that Medicare would facilitate release of payment for claims according to a set table of rates that is approved by them. Normally, the secondary payment benefits of Medicare that falls under this scheme are:

a. The amount that is actually charged by the physical therapist after deducting the charges that were paid by the GHP.

b. The amount of delivered services that Medicare agrees to pay when these services are not originally covered by a GHP. Currently, this amount is capped at $1940.

Plan of Care Document and Medicare

The Plan of Care or POC is one of the essential documents to be included when filing for payment claims under Medicare or any other health insurance plans. When claiming under Medicare coverage, the plan of care that is submitted together with payment claims documents needs to be signed by a physician even if it is originally drafted by a physical therapist. This should be done during the first 30 days of treatment. In the case of treatment that extends more than 90 days, or long-term care for patients, POCs need to be re-certified after every 90 days while the patient is receiving treatment.

Submitting the POC is necessary when reimbursements are claimed for Medicare secondary payer benefits, so this document would need to be signed and certified by a licensed and affiliated physician.

Standard Document Requirements for Claiming Medicare Payments as Secondary Benefits

Claiming payments from Medicare, even if it is through secondary benefit option does not mean that document standards are changed. It is important that the biller complies with the standard required documents in order for payment claims to be processed and reimbursement to be released. This is observed both in primary and secondary payment options in Medicare plans.

The first thing that needs to be considered is the PQRS quality codes. Medicare Part B requires physical therapists to report measures done on their patients either individually or in groups. The use of quality codes would be very helpful in claiming for payments in Medicare Part B or from GHPs when using a sample group. This sample groups' information is to be submitted to the CMS. However, when claims are being made as secondary payment from Medicare and the patients' GHP covers the services being billed for, the biller and the physical therapist should not make a report using the quality codes listed in the PQRS.

Therapy Caps for Medicare Claims on Secondary Payment Scheme

One of the most common questions physical therapists ask when making payment claims under Medicare as secondary payer is about therapy caps and how modifiers can be used when a patient's claims go over the standard $1940 cap. The simplest answer to this is that when Medicare sets a standard rate, it enforces this, and it is followed. At the moment, the standard therapy cap rate is set at $1940. However, there are instances considered as exceptions where Medicare may pay more than the set rate cap if the physical therapist can give justification to the amount in excess of it. This means that apart from the standard documents that need to be submitted to establish the medical necessity of an outpatient therapy done on a patient, a KX modifier code would need to be used when making payment claims.

Medicare Audits on Payment Claims

Most of the time, it is very easy to treat Medicare as just another health insurance plan and a means to collect payments for services rendered by a physical therapist. Billers and therapists alike often oversee the fact that Medicare makes use of Federal funds to pay for those covered by it. However, there is a difference in terms of auditing depending on how Medicare is used and availed. When Medicare is used as a primary payer, their audit is not that highlighted since the claims are made based on the coverage that is listed on the policy or plan availed by a patient. But when Medicare is used as a secondary payer, the chance of audit is increased. Several audits are usually undertaken to check the health care provider who makes claims from Medicare as secondary payment. These audits are usually carried out by Medicare authorized agencies such as the ZPIC (or the Zone Program Integrity Contractors), MAC (the Medicare Administrative Contractor), RAC (Recovery Audit Contractor) and the QIO (or the Quality Improvement Organizations).

Among all these identified auditors, the RAC is considered to be the strictest since it is responsible for auditing practitioners based on payment claims and how they bill Medicare for it. Part of the responsibilities of the RAC is to identify if there are instances where Medicare made either overpayment or underpayment on the claims made when it is billed as a secondary payer. It also makes sure that there are no gaps between the payments made by GHPs and Medicare for therapies done to a patient. Although the manner in which RAC carries out its audits are strict in nature, physical therapists can avoid problems with it by ensuring that they have established rightful information regarding the payment schemes for their outpatients and enforce a proper procedure for collecting these information form their patients prior to making claims. This can be done during the time of admission when the medical necessity for physical therapy is being established or during the time that outpatient services are afforded to their patients.

Denials, Audits and Appeals

In 2006, the CMS drafted a document containing the final provision on how funds were to be recouped from practitioners and providers who were found to have been overpaid for their services to patients covered by Medicare. In the said document, which was published on September 2009 in the Federal Register, it indicated how to settle cases of overpayment and how to make appeals regarding the decision. Those who were found not to have been overpaid could even claim interest for the wrongful identification of being overpaid. This final rule also contained the legal basis used by Medicare on recouping excess payments as per the Medicare Modernization Act of 2003. This law has impacted how Medicare recovers overpayments. Before 2003, the CMS was authorized to collect from providers who were determined to be overpaid and to pay for interest when, after an appeal, the provider was found not to have overcharged. It was a complicated and tedious matter that left both billers and therapists dumbfounded on its merits (Medicare Program; Limitation on Recoupment of Provider and Supplier Overpayments Summary of Final Rule, 2009).

As per the definition, Medicare uses the term recoupment to denote the manner of recovering overpayments. The process involves a reduction in the amount being covered by the health plan and applying the withheld amount to compensate for the previous overpayment. This implies that the law does not authorize that CMS cannot recoup from practitioners who were making an appeal about overpayments. Normally, such appeals are coursed through Qualified Independent Contractors, or QICs, which would then start the process of reconsiderations from the second level of the appeal. This means that after a request is filed with the QICs, the CMS should stop any activities regarding recoupment. This is known as the stage of redetermination and has to be filed within 41 days by the provider. However, the said timeline is not the one to be considered when the practitioner or provider intends to make appeals since the time allotted for filing for redetermination is 120 days, while 180 days is used as a timeline for reconsideration. This means that the provider or therapist may still file over the 41 or 60-day period that is used by the CMS to stop recoupment, but they should not expect recoupment activities to stop after the 41 or 60-day time frame. CMS can take steps to start the recoupment process as soon as the QIC declares the appeal of the provider as invalid. This, however, is not a deterrent for the provider to continue the appeals process beyond the level of the QIC; but, any recouped amount may only be reimbursed if the appeal was found to be valid.

The Medicare Modernization Act of 2008 also affects how interests are paid when the appeals made by providers and practitioners are found to be valid and recouped amounts are returned. The total amount returned to providers may be whole or partial, depending on the result of the appeals process and the level in which the decision has been made. The judicial and administrative levels are considered to be third and fourth levels of appeals. If Medicare needs to reimburse the amount recouped from providers, the Federal Court, Appeals Council or an Administrative Law Judge (ALJ) may dictate how much interest needs to be paid to the provider. Normally, the interest is computed based on when the decision of overpayment was made and its recoupment up to the time reimbursement and interest is given.

The final rule based on the MMA, however, has made no changes on the rule that the CMS puts interests on the charges when they are found to be overpaid and may charge providers and practitioners. Also, it is the CMS's role to pay the provider for overpayment recoupment dues and its associated interests within 30 days after the reversal is made. The interest rate by which Medicare adds to the repayment is based on the comparison between the private consumer's value and the current funds rate value. The higher rate between the two is used to determine the amount of interest to be paid. Payment is expected to be done within the first 30 days from the decision.

Coverage Issues

Like other health care insurance payers, coverage issues are also commonly faced by physical therapists in billing and claiming payments for their services for patients with Medicare Part B coverage. These issues are discussed below in detail (CMS: Medicare Coverage Database, 2014; APTA, 2013).

LCDs or Local Coverage Determination

The Local Coverage Determination (LCD) is a document that Medicare issues, through its contractors, which contains services or procedures that are accepted as necessary, reasonable and therefore billable under Medicare. The LCD was formerly known as the Local Medical Review Policy. In this document there are three primary types of LCDs which therapists should be familiar with in making billing and payment claims. In December of 2003, contractors of Medicare were asked to transition into LCDs from the Local Medical Review Policies that they have been using. One of the differences is with the use of LCDs, there is a need for the establishment of the medical necessity for the procedures and their reasonable values (APTA, 2013).

1. Final LCDs. The final LCDs are also known as active coverage and are used in referring to the Physical Medicine and Rehabilitation component of Medicare. Most Medicare contractors use this for coverage determination. In the final LCD, a specific coverage area should be matched with an effective date. LCDs in this category make use of a detailed description of the services that are under its coverage, an appropriate documentation requirement and the correct information about the ICD 10-CM codes. These codes may be used to express support or lack thereof of the medical need for the services duly provided by the therapist.

2. Draft LCDs. There are instances in which Local Coverage Determination (LCDs) are usually revised to include recently updated information. The revisions of the LCDs that are considered to be draft are no longer requiring billers and contactors to provide an approximate time frame when comments or notices can be made. These items should be provided to concerned parties in cases of revisions of existing LCDs in an effort to revise a current LCD for increased restrictiveness and when an existing LCD is revised for the purposes of correction. When situations like these occur, it is the contractor's duty to post the involved LCD draft and wait for 45 days or more of comment period before incorporating these comments in the final LCD within the next 6 weeks (the prescribed minimum notice period).

In the entire duration of the comment period for the draft LCD, comments and recommendations may be solicited by contractors from a diverse group of people, organizations and other concerned party through the use of survey. These concerned parties include specialty groups and their associations, health care providers and their groups who may be affected with the LCDs, other contractors hired by Medicare, and the general public. The responses given by these groups are collected, summarized, and posted for at least 180 days on a verified contractor website.

3. Retired LCDs. These are LCDs that were previously used, deleted and required by Medicare for its contractors to archive in the event they are needed later for cases in which a final LCD is not available and some of these retired LCDs may be applicable for claiming under a topic of coverage. One of the most important impacts of these LCDs in terms of billing and payment claims is that it serves as guidance in ensuring that correct payment claims are submitted. An advantage in using the LCDs is that it facilitates outlining of how the contractor will conduct a review of the payment claims submitted and ensures that these comply with the requirements set by Medicare. Below are some of the issues that justify the use of LCDs:

1. To help determine what services are under the coverage of Medicare and which ones can be reimbursed to the practitioner.

2. To guide in coding for services being billed. LCDs allow for description of relationships between codes and how to facilitate billing for services.

3. To allow for a partial completion of the requirements for documentation. The LCDs, by nature, describe key information that is part of the medical records of the patients being treated. This key information allows billers and physical therapists to justify the coverage for services where payments are being claimed.

4. To serve as a guideline for the proper utilization of codes; thereby setting standards that would be followed by Medicare and its other contractors.

5. To be used when ICD-10-CM codes do not recognize the combination of CPT and ICD-10 codes for billing and payment claims. When such incident happens, Medicare denies payment and the therapist do not get reimbursed for the services provided to the patient.

Provider-Supplier Enrollment

Medicare computerized the enrollment of practitioners claiming for Medicare in 2008. This computerized provider enrollment is called the PECOS or Provider Enrollment, Chain and Ownership System. This online enrollment process enabled physical therapists a more convenient way of enrolling themselves into the database and updating their information within the comforts of their own offices anytime. The CMS established Internet-based PECOS as an alternative to the CMS-855 paper enrollment. This simplified process has the aim to reduce the total time spent in applying and entering practitioner information in the database, minimize the use of paper-based forms and increase compliance in enrolling with the system for more efficient payment claims submission to Medicare. Internet-based PECOS allows physicians, non-physician practitioners, and provider/supplier organizations to enroll, make changes to their Medicare enrollment, view their enrollment information on file with Medicare, submit a change of ownership, or check on status of a Medicare enrollment application via the Internet. (APTA: PECOS, 2011; CMS, 2013; CMS 2015).

There are several advantages of Internet-based PECOS. PECOS is faster than paper-based enrollment, with 45 day processing time in most cases, vs. 60 days for paper. This is a tailored application process, so only relevant information to the individual provider is supplied. The PECOS gives the provider/supplier more control over enrollment information such as reassignments. This system is easy to check and update information for accuracy. Lastly, PECOS requires less staff time and lower administrative costs to complete and submit Medicare enrollment (CMS 2015)

Physical therapists, as per PECOS, are considered to be suppliers of care. This is also true with physicians and other health care professionals. Facilities and health care agencies are considered to be the providers of care. Physicians and non-physician practitioners may access Internet-based PECOS by using the User IDs and passwords established when application was made on-line to the National Plan and Provider Enumeration System (NPPES) for their National Provider Identifiers (NPIs). Securing the NPI (National Provider Identifier), can be accomplished within 20-30 minutes and is free of charge. This NPI is used by Medicare to identify all professionals instead of the previously recognized billing numbers (CMS 2015).

PECOS enrollment is a beneficial move in the practice of outpatient physical therapy billing and payment claims since it allows for the real time checking of the status of payment claims. However, it is worth noting that practitioners who have been enrolled with Medicare before the year 2003 and do not have updated information since the time of enrollment may have difficulties accessing the PECOS. To be able to enroll in this, practitioners are asked to furnish paper-based application to facilitate access to PECOS in the future. When access information is granted, CMS Form 588 and 460 may be needed to be filled out to authorize Medicare to carry out automatic fund transfers.

In enrolling in the PECOS, therapists should remember that only those who are into PTPP settings are required to register in the 8551 applications to be entitled for receiving payments made by Medicare for the services they provided (APTA: PECOS, 2011). Further detailed information on Internet-based PECOS can be found at Internet-based PECOS - Centers for Medicare & Medicaid Services.

Supervision: Use of Students, Aides and PTAs

Health care facilities have varied staffing patterns in place in caring for their patients. Some facilities are used as training institutions for students of the allied medical professions, while some are employing the services of aides and assistants to ensure safe, effective and efficient patient care within the facility. Physical therapists caring for their patients across varied health care settings may be tasked to supervise, assist in training or even employ the assistance of the abovementioned groups of people as they care for their patients. Ideally, this would not be a cause of concern in terms of care provision, but there may be instances where the billers or physical therapists are claiming payments for their patients' care under Medicare Part B and may result in a complication in claiming for payments.

To clarify the confusion regarding the involvement of students, physical therapy aides and assistants, especially when billing and claiming for payments under Medicare Part B, the CMS issued a memorandum to clarify matters on payments and billing concerns when the physical therapists are supervising any of the three groups of individuals.

Supervision of Students

Physical therapy undergraduate students, during the entire course of their baccalaureate degree are involved in both theoretical and clinical care concepts. This means that after lectures and discussions are given to them in their classes, there is a need to make these concepts come alive through actual care of patients, both in the inpatient and outpatient settings. It is worth knowing for physical therapists whether the participation of the students on supervision is billable under Medicare Part B (APTA; Use of Students Under Medicare Part B, 2014).

Probably considered the trailblazers into the questioning of how involvement of students can affect billing, the American Speech Language and Hearing Association or ASHA made a similar query during 2001 on the matter of billing for the services provided by physical therapy students. This query was given a response by the CMS on November of the same year. In this response the CMS stated that in order for the therapists to bill and get paid for the services they rendered their patients, they have to have valid evidence that they are providing care for their patients while acting and observing practice within the scope that their licensure allows them to act on. A year after the ASHA made its position known, another organization, the AOTA, made the same query on what policies are in place for payments on the services rendered by students to patients under the coverage of Medicare Part B. This was answered by the CMS on January 2002 and was done by the CMS not in the effort to make another guideline, but rather to elucidate on the matter.

On April 11, 2011, memorandum AB 01-56 was issued by the CMS to clarify matter on how physical therapy students provide outpatient care for patients claiming benefits under Medicare Part B. Most of the contents of this memorandum revolve on answering some of the most frequently asked questions regarding the matter of payment claims. In this memorandum, the CMS made its stand on the ruling that services rendered by physical therapy students may not be billed under Medicare Part B, even if these are carried out under the supervision of a licensed physical therapist. This answer stems from the fact that Medicare only makes payments for the services that are provided by physicians and other licensed practitioners such as physical therapists given authority by their respective states to practice their professions (APTA 2015).

To make the matter simpler, the CMS gravitated on the fact that physical therapy students, regardless of their level of current education, do not meet the minimum requirements to be considered as practitioners as defined by the CMS statutes. This was met by more questioning from physical therapists, stating that even if students provided the actual therapy, they are present and are supervising. The CMS, on the other hand, stood firm in its directive, stating that only the actual care provided by the licensed therapist will be billed and paid under Medicare Part B. It also clarified that the physical therapists can bill for payments of their services to their patients if they are the ones who provided the treatment even if there are students present in the room (APTA 2015).

In recapitulating the important points on the stand of the CMS in billing and payment claims made for Medicare Part B coverage, the following are enumerated:

1. The physical therapist or qualified practitioner making the billing and payment claims should be one who is recognized by the beneficiary of Medicare Part B. He or she should be the professional who is responsible in each session with the patients or when care is being provided.

2. The therapist who is referred to as the qualified practitioner need to be inside the room during the entire time the session is ongoing. If a physical therapy student is involved in providing care, the qualified physical therapist should be present as he directs how the service is to be provided. He has to make sure that he is the one making skilled judgment while taking responsibility for the assessment and all other components of treatment.

3. 3. The qualified physical therapist should be putting his attention on the patient of the student he is guiding as care is being provided and not directing his attention in another patient or task within the same time period. This is to ensure that safe and effective care is given to the patients.

4. 4. In terms of providing services to patients and billing for their therapies, the qualified practitioner should take it upon himself to sign all documentation related to billing and payment claims for Medicare Part B. He cannot delegate this task to a student since payments for Medicare is based on the services provided by a qualified therapist and not on the students' care, no matter what their skill level.

Acceptable Billing Practices

The American Physical Therapy Association has made recommendations about how billing and payment claims are to be made when both the physical therapist and the student engages in the care of a patient covered by Medicare Part B. This is based on a series of information emanating from the MedPAC and the CMS. Both of these organizations agree on the fact that there is a possibility for the physical therapist to bill and claim for payments when the student and therapist jointly render the services. The following factors are suggested by the APTA to be considered when determining whether or not a patient is to be billed under Medicare Part B.

1. Professional judgment should be employed by the physical therapist in determining when services can be billable under Medicare Part B coverage.

2. There is a need for the physical therapist to be able to properly distinguish the difference between a students' ability to care for patients and the capacity of the physical therapist to bill Medicare for the care rendered by students on their patients. There may be certain states or territories in which care provided by student to patients are allowed, although this does not mean that these services can be billed.

3. Medicare will only pay and consider billing for the services provided by physical therapists to their patients themselves. The degree or level of involvement the physical therapist have in the provision of services to patients is one of the most important things to consider when making the decision to bill Medicare or not. One of the key factors to consider when making this decision is to make sure that there is active involvement and engagement in provision of services to patients being billed. This is supported by the second statement on the important points regarding the stand of the CMS in billing for Medicare Part B when student physical therapists are involved in care provision.

4. The physical therapist should make a conscious decision whether or not he or she would bill the patient more or the same when a student is involved in care provision. The rule of thumb in this situation is that regardless of the degree of involvement a student has in the care of patients, the physical therapist should not bill them more than the usual rate he sets for similar services. The presence of a student physical therapist while providing care for patients should not be an excuse for the qualified practitioner to think of financial benefits in enriching these students' clinical experiences.

When supervision of students are entrusted to qualified physical therapists, they should be conscious about their ability to comply with the rules and guidelines set forth by Medicare, especially when it comes to billing and making payment claims. Allowing a physical therapy student to take part in actual care provision does not entitle them to collect payments since this is part of their learning experience. One of the thrusts of the APTA is on advocacy to ensure physical therapy students who are in the clinical training are going to benefit more out of this stage in their education to mold them and allow them to be good practitioners capable of providing cost-efficient, safe and effective care for their patients.

Physical Therapy Assistants

Similar to other professions, physical therapy may have different categories of qualified practitioners depending on the duties and responsibilities associated with their licenses. Most States recognize physical therapists as licensed providers of care, and physical therapy assistants as performing a supportive function to the duties and responsibilities of the physical therapist. In most States, practice acts dictate that supervision is a responsibility of the licensed physical therapist over the functions of the physical therapy assistants. Most of the time, the regulations set about by state boards are stricter than those set by Medicare and Medicaid (APTA: Use of Physical Therapy Assistants Under Medicare, 2014).

In considering safe practice and compliance, the presence of a physical therapist is needed when the physical therapy assistant is delegated to perform certain tasks or activities. The elements in which the concept of presence varies from one state to another, but the main thing is that supervision, regardless if it is direct or general, is required of the physical therapist to comply with the requirements set forth both by the State and Medicare for billing and payment claims.

There are several forms of outpatient settings and facilities in which the services of a physical therapy assistant are employed in the delivery of care. Depending on the type of setting or facility, Medicare requirements may vary for billing and payment claims processing.

a.   CRAs or Certified Rehabilitation Agencies. These institutions are required by Medicare to have dedicated qualified personnel who are responsible for providing the initial direction of how care is going to be provided to the patients. Also, part of the job of the qualified personnel is observation of the performance of the physical therapy assistant while doing his tasks and periodically assessing the said performance based on set standards. Medicare requires that CRAs have PTAs that meet the qualifications set for assistant level practitioner, and if the staffs are not yet able to comply with this requirement, then a physical therapist must be within the premises of the facility in any given time.

b.   CORFs (Comprehensive Outpatient Rehabilitation Facility). These facilities are designed to provide over all rehabilitative care for individuals on an outpatient basis. Because of the nature of the services that these facilities offer, Medicare requires that the services offered and provided in this setting are done by qualified practitioners when billing and payment claims are made. However, in instances where care is provided by a physical therapy assistant, a qualified practitioner should be present during care provision while providing care instructions to the assistant. The supervision to be performed by the physical therapist include, but is not limited to guidance on the techniques of providing patient care, safe and effective management of services and teaching these assistants to be responsible for their actions. Furthermore, because comprehensive lines of services are offered in these facilities, there should be a separate person responsible for each service the facility offers.

c. HHA (Home Health Agencies). For these facilities, Medicare payment claims require that services be performed while observing proper safety precautions and under the direct supervision of a skilled general therapist. This means that as an assistant is tasked to care for a patient, the qualified physical therapist is to give him or her initial directions on the service to be rendered while ensuring that it is safely and effectively performed. The main difference in the guidelines for HHA as compared with other facilities is that there is no need for the qualified individual to be always on the premises as care is being provided.

d. Inpatient Hospital Services. These settings would require the presence of active supervision of a physical therapist on the actions of the assistant. There is also the need for the physical therapist to determine the capacity of the assistant to perform services safely and effectively. One confusing concept in caring for patients in inpatient settings is that there is no definite limitation on the tasks that an assistant can perform and delineate on how much supervision is required of the qualified physical therapist and on what manner is this to be provided. In most cases, the assistant is required to refer to his or her immediate supervisor (who in this case is the physical therapist) when questions arise regarding the functions he or she needs to perform.

e. Outpatient Hospital Services. For outpatient services, an assistant with the supervision of a qualified physical therapist should effectively and safely perform physical therapy. The rest of the considerations for assistants being supervised by physical therapist on providing services in inpatient hospital setting also applied to outpatient services.

f. Physician's Office. When billing Medicare for payment claims for services provided by a physical therapy assistant in doctor's offices, there is a need for direct supervision to occur while services are being rendered. The person required to supervise assistants in performing their functions is a physical therapist with an enrollment in Medicare as a provider. This means that a doctor, regardless of the services he has supervised the PTA to do, cannot possibly bill Medicare for his own actions. This means that the corresponding provider number of the physical therapist is to be used for claims processing.

g. Skilled Nursing Facility. When physical therapy assistants are providing services to their patients in skilled nursing facilities, Medicare requires that these services be provided while a supervising physical therapist directly monitors performance of their tasks. However, despite the need for direct supervision, Medicare does not stipulate if there is a need for the ongoing presence of the said supervisor as the task is being performed.

CMS: Medicare Coverage Database

The Centers for Medicare and Medicaid Services has elected the CMS: Medicare Coverage Database (or MCD) website to be used by health care providers, private contractors and other stakeholders to access information regarding billing, payment claims and matters regarding Medicare and Medicaid coverage and services. The website also allows practitioners to search related information they need to ensure billing, payment claims, and other documentation guidelines are followed. In this website, updates and other related information regarding CMS, ICD updates and legislation affecting Medicare and Medicaid beneficiaries and how services for them may be billed and reimbursed are listed.

In most specific terms, the MCD houses most information regarding the National Coverage Determinations (NCDs), as well as LCDs (or Local Coverage Determinations). Apart from these, physical therapists and billers can take advantage of the information listed in numerous articles, and proposed NCD documents to improve and better coordinate billing and payment claims. Coding documents and related analyses are also contained in the site, as well as information from the NCA (National Coverage Analyses), MEDCAC (Medicare Evidence Development and Coverage Advisory Committee) and CALS (Coding Analyses for Labs).

Durable Medical Equipment, Prosthetic, Orthotic and Supplies (DMEPOS)

Another area of concern for Medicare Part B billing and payment claims is the use of DMEPOS used in outpatient therapies. DMEPOS, or Durable Medical Equipment, Prosthesis and Supplies are defined by Medicare as those equipment which are designed to be able to take the rigors of repeated usage, are used for medical reasons and therefore only useful to people with injuries or illnesses that affects their functional capacities and that these supplies are also appropriate to be used inside homes. DMEPOS include things such as wheelchairs, bedside commodes, crutches and braces and even specialized hospital beds. Supplies on the other hand, include items that are consumable and disposable such as gauze pads, bandages, catheters and pads, and gloves. These items are basically not built to last or designed for single use only.

For therapists billing Medicare for DMEPOS as part of the care given to patients, it is necessary to prove why such equipment is used and the purpose of its inclusion in the care plan (e.g., a patient with musculoskeletal weakness given crutches to improve mobility). It is also important to show Medicare that the billed equipment will be used in the home of the patient so payments can be made. This includes equipment that is rented, if purchase is not feasible for both coverage inclusions and patient needs. Furthermore, prior to the procurement of the DMEPOS, it is important to secure a valid physician's prescription for it and a duly signed Certificate of Medical Necessity for each particular piece of equipment being billed.

Prosthesis and orthotic devices are also covered as part of DMEPOS under Medicare Part B as long as they fit into the definition provided by Medicare. This definition specifies billable devices are prosthetic body parts required to be used by the patient because of a change in health status and functional capacity. These may include braces, arm and leg prosthesis, artificial eyes and their respective replacements when necessary. Orthotic devices may have limitations in their use, such as braces that are used in a specific part of the body and are implemented independent from other treatments or equipment given to patients.

Medicare only covers orthotic devices that are rigid or semi-rigid in nature and are primarily employed to support a weakened or deformed part of the body as a result of a valid medical condition. It may also be used to facilitate motion and function on an affected part of the body. On its guidelines, Medicare includes coverage for orthotic devices that are prefabricated or custom made for safe and effective use of the beneficiaries. When including prosthetics for billing, it is worth knowing that Medicare would not release payment for the use of prosthetic and orthotic devices for purposes other than rehabilitative such as prevention or palliation. It may also not be billed if prosthetics and orthotics were prescribed as part of a research study. In addition to these restrictions, prosthesis and the accessories needed for their safe and effective use are also covered by Medicare Part B and therefore may be billed.

One of the documents being used to support the guidelines set by Medicare about the coverage for DMEPOS is found on section 427 of BIPA of the United States Social Security Act. In this document, it is mentioned that there will be no payments given for billing prosthesis or orthotic device unless the device is prescribed by a qualified practitioner. In the same document, qualified practitioners are health care professionals such as physical therapists, physicians, or occupational therapists. The definition of the term "qualified practitioner" is also expanded to include certified orthotists and prosthetists.

In terms of considering what orthotics sometimes mean, physical therapists become confused about the nature and the inclusion of shoe inserts into the DMEPOS. Ideally, shoe inserts are not covered even if they are used to treat patients with foot drop or to prevent complications in diabetic patients, but there are instances when they can be billed as long as there are valid documents to support the claims.

Claims for DMEPOS are usually submitted to four carriers that were identified by the CMS to process payments and reimbursement for this equipment. These carriers include HealthNow, which is based in New York, Administar Federal, Palmeto GBA and Cigna Healthcare. Collectively, they are called the DMERC or the Durable Medical Equipment Regional Carriers. These carriers are divided as such to cover certain geographic areas in the country to ensure efficient and faster payment claims and reimbursement.

- DMERC A is managed by HealthNow and includes 9 states. These are Connecticut, Delaware, Maine, Massachusetts, New York, New Hampshire, New Jersey, Rhode Islands and Vermont.

- DMERC B is under the management of Administar Federal and has 10 states in the region. These states are District of Columbia, Illinois, Indiana, Maryland, Minnesota, Ohio, Virginia, West Virginia and Wisconsin.

- DMERC C is under the management of Palmetto Government Benefits Administration and includes Alabama, Arizona, Colorado, Florida, Georgia, Kentucky, Louisiana, Mississippi, New Mexico, North Carolina, South Carolina, Tennessee, and Texas. It even includes US Territories such as Puerto Rico and the Virgin Islands.

- DMERC D is managed by Cigna and the region has 17 states and 3 United States Territories. These are Arkansas, Arizona, California, Hawaii, Idaho, Iowa, Kansas, Missouri, Montana, Nevada, North Dakota, Oregon, South Dakota, Utah, Washington and Wyoming. The territories are Guam, American Mariana Islands and Samoa.

Medicare Advantage

Practitioners, billers and even patients most commonly know Medicare Advantage as Medicare Part C. This feature of Medicare allows private companies and insurance providers to enter in a contract with the Federal government to make the benefits of Medicare available to their beneficiaries. These plans were previously known as Medicare + Choice and were later changed to what we now know as Medicare Advantage. This allows the beneficiary to have the option of choosing Medicare coverage plans on top of another health plan. This allows them to avail of services paid for by Medicare but have the benefits of Medicare made available to them through their respective private health insurance plans, or HMOs (http://www.apta.org/Payment/Medicare/Advantage).

Medicare Advantage's main design is to serve as an alternative to the fee-for-service scheme of payment for claims which gained popularity during the 1970s. There are several programs that Medicare Advantage has under its coverage. These are Health Maintenance Organizations and Private Provider Organizations (or collectively known as coordinated care plans), medical savings account plans (MSA) and the private fee-for-service (PFFS) plans.

The acceptance of practitioners and billers in the Medicare Advantage plan facilitated its evolution as a response to the changes impacted upon it by different guidelines, rules and requirements enacted by the Congress throughout the years. Primarily, Medicare Advantage plans cover almost all the same services as that of the regular Medicare plan. In the regular Medicare plan, Part A is known to be responsible for covering inpatient and other hospitalization benefits while Part B is covering outpatient services. But beneficiaries who have Medicare Advantage plans can have parts A and B benefits plus other coverage such as dental treatments, vision-related appointments with physicians and treatments and even services that tend to focus more on the preventive aspect. Medicare Advantage plans can also be used to cover the medication expenses for its beneficiaries, especially among those needing long-term therapy.

Similar to most health care insurance plans, Medicare Advantage also has therapy caps, and there may be instances in which patients may have out-of-pocket spending that is set every year. The CMS is the agency that has authority over these caps, but it is clear that plan holders of the Medicare Advantage have higher therapy caps than those with Medicare A and B only. Furthermore, Medicare Advantage plans also follow the LCD for payments and billing guidelines. This means that all services prescribed in the original Medicare plan must be covered, and statues set by the NCD and LCDs are also considered in Medicare Advantage. This is a unique feature for Medicare Advantage plan because, while it is required by the CMS to cover all those things included in Parts A and B, Medicare Advantage cannot give a patient or beneficiary lower than what is actually given in Medicare as detailed by the LCDs and NCDs.

One thing therapists and billers would have to bear in mind when using Medicare Advantage to claim payments for services rendered is that it has a difference as compared with Medicare Part A and Part B. Coverage information in Medicare Advantage is similar to what private health care insurance companies offer, so there is a need for either the billers or physical therapists to conduct a process to verify benefits under which the patient may be covered. This may be done prior to providing actual treatment so problems with payment claims are minimized. Furthermore, there is also a need for the billers and therapists to know which specific type of Medicare Advantage plan the patient has and how it works for the practitioners and the patients. These different Medicare Advantage plans are:

1. Coordinated Care Plans. These plans are basically dependent on other health insurance providers (usually referred to as a network) to deliver benefit packages as approved by the CMS. The coordination would allow these plans to exert control over how services are utilized by their beneficiaries through certain mechanisms. Examples of these are referrals in which physicians would act as gatekeepers in checking the quality of care provided as compared to the cost being billed. If the claim for services is seen by these gatekeepers as being cost-effective, incentives are usually provided to encourage maintenance of the cost-effectiveness and high quality of care.

   a. Health Maintenance Organizations or HMOs. One of the most common types of coordinated care plan under Medicare Advantage, HMOs are characterized by linkages with contracted service providers. This means that the beneficiary or patient would need to avail of the services needed from those providers who are part of the network to claim benefits. In most cases, there are accredited providers registered with these HMOs, but services rendered by other practitioners may be paid if these are not offered within members of the network, the patient has chosen out-of-network option, or if the care provided falls within what is considered as emergency.

   b. PPOs or Preferred Provider Organizations. Similar to the HMOs, PPOs also operate by relying on a network of care providers that agrees to deliver the care to their beneficiaries within the bounds of agreed reimbursement amounts. An advantage, however, of PPOs is that patients may receive services outside the networks of accredited care providers since PPOs are required to pay for all the benefits under the plan availed by the patient, whether they be provided within or outside the network.

2. Special Needs Plan or NSP. As the name implies, Special Needs Plans are intended for those patients who have specialized care needs as compared with other patients. Special care needs include chronic or debilitating conditions, confinement in nursing homes and other institutional type of care. Some of those who are under SNPs are also dually eligible for Medicare and Medicaid benefits.

3. PFFS or Private Fee-For-Service Plans. These plans operate on paying for claims via a fee-for-service scheme. However, it is the company that deems if such claims are payable under the health insurance plan in place and if there is such a contract as to the rate to be reimbursed. Despite this, one positive thing for beneficiaries regarding fee-for-service plans is that they are not limited to getting care from a network or accredited providers. Billers and practitioners can submit payment requests and can expect to be paid for services billed as long as the proper documentary requirements are submitted and providers conform to the payment scheme offered by the PFFs.

However, because of the unclear lines as to what the coverage of PFFs is and how the process of deeming rightful services and reimbursable treatments occurs, the process changed in 2011. This change has brought about the implementation of a system that is similar to the process employed by those billing and collecting payments under Original Medicare plans. This is based on the MIPPA or the Patients and Providers Act of 2008 which obliges the PFFS to have an accessible network of providers of care that belongs within their area of operations and that they have reasonable reimbursement systems. This includes both individual plan holders and company-sponsored plans for their employees.

Physical therapists need to understand that it is for their own good to know if the patients to be treated have PFFS plans that belong to a multiple-network Medicare Advantage plan within the area. If the patient to be treated does not belong to such, then the therapist would be deemed as part of that particular network. This means that if the therapist does not want to be identified within that network, he or she cannot treat the patient.

4. MSA or Medical Savings Account Plans. The Medical Savings Account plans are health care coverage plans where MSAs are combined with deductible health plans to cover for their beneficiaries' care needs. The MSA is where Medicare makes annual deposits intended for the payments and reimbursements for therapies availed by their beneficiaries. In these plans, the beneficiary is required to make payments to meet an annual deductible coverage, which can be used to pay for the services availed.

Medicare Claims Audits

Billers and physical therapists alike would admit that one of the most challenging aspects they watch out for in billing and making payment claims is facing claims audits. This is because claims audit are usually carried out by Medicare, Medicaid or other health care insurance companies to assess if there have been instances when they are overcharged by one practitioner for services rendered for their beneficiaries. Most of the time, independent contractors hired by Medicare for the purpose mentioned above carry out claims audits.

The RACs or Recovery Audit Contractors are tasked to assess not only claims made for Medicare Part B, but also audits on Part A coverage. Most settings in which assessments are made include clinics, hospitals, private physical therapy practices, home health settings, and other health care related facilities.

Audits are not only made to check for appropriateness of billing as compared with the patients' care needs, they are also carried out to ensure equipment used and availed during the care of patients are correctly billed as well as other parties who were hired to contribute to the total care of the patient.

At the onset of summer 2009, the CMS started implementing audits to ensure that overpayment and underpayment does not happen for those claiming for Medicare benefits. The implementation of this program caused some confusion at first, prompting the APTA to come up with a guide that was posted on their website to practice good billing to avoid problems with the claims audit, the RCA and of course, receiving payments for the services that is rightfully given to patients.

The following steps are recommended by the American Physical Therapy Association to make compliance with the CMS guidelines for claims audit simple.

1. Be familiar with the process related to audits and appeals. Knowing how the process works is an advantage. Usually, when such instances arise, there is a series of five steps included in the process for making appeals on audit results. Normally, appeals occur because there have been findings where the billers or therapists need to return a certain amount of money to Medicare because they have been found to bill more than what Medicare finds rightful to pay for. This appeal may be done within 30 days from when it was found.

According to CMS and the APTA, physical therapists and billers can avoid such occurrences through furnishing all needed documents when making claims for services rendered for Medicare beneficiaries. These are needed to prove to the payers and the auditors that there is indeed a medical need for the provision of such services to patients. It is also important to know which guidelines are to be followed for filing claims to determine the coverage criteria for beneficiaries of health insurance plans.

2. The need to know improper payments and how they were found as such is important to avoid the mistake having the same matter found on payment claims made for services of the physical therapists. Observe for the presence of errors when making claims and ensuring that such claims are rightfully carried out. This means that there is a need for stakeholders to know what guidelines are to be followed and how best to comply with such requirements, avoiding things that may be interpreted as fraud and watching out for errors in billing.

3. Avoid having low audit findings and reports by having internal auditing on practice. Doing an internal audit even before Medicare sends one ensures that problems identified are remedied, thereby reducing specific areas of practice auditors may find to be noncompliant. Another good thing about this, especially when done on a continuous basis, is that trainings and staff development programs are implemented to improve performance and to achieve better results when the practice is being audited. And lastly, when internal audits are in place there is increased competency to foresee future problems and address them even before they become apparent.

4. Having knowledge about RAC and its designated regions can greatly help establish effective and efficient billing and payment claims, as well as reducing negative audit results. The country

was divided by the CMS into four different regions under one RAC regional office that is responsible for conducting audits in their specific areas. Because of the intricacies and variations of practice guidelines in each region, these RACs are required to have a system in place that will enable providers to conduct tracking on the auditing process that is currently taking place. This system would include knowing the status of appeals for audits that were negative, and the necessary information that needs to be prepared for audits.

Another advantage of the establishment of a regional RAC website is the presence of support where therapists can communicate with various members of the health care workforce about matters pertaining to the activities and related matters regarding the RAC. There is an email directory and update system where therapists can subscribe to receive periodic email newsletters letting them know of the various activities of the RACs in their respective regions.

5. There is a need to be familiar with the different terminologies employed by contractors. This action is essential in ensuring that appropriate fees are paid by Medicare to the physical therapist for services rendered. Knowing the similarities and differences between the most common terms used by contractors for audits would mean that therapists have greater success of submitting needed documents for payment processing and that the claims audit has a higher probability of yielding favorable results. Example, knowing the difference between automated and complex review would help greatly in knowing which review is done to determine if and when there are overpayments and underpayments. To put it more simply, contractors use automated review when there is a need to review data or information sets regarding claims. A complex review is usually implemented when the patients' records are the ones that need to be reviewed.

6. Always be ready if there is a need to provide a response for a request forwarded by the RAC. Probably one of the most stressful things to experience is the receipt of a correspondence from the RAC in the mail. Sometimes, the fear of knowing what is written in the letter is compelling enough for some to ignore it, causing bigger problems in the long term. No matter what the reasons for some wanting to ignore the correspondence, the best course of action is always responding to whatever is written on it. Not all letters from the RAC deal with letting therapists know there have been claims audit findings of overpayment. One of the possible reasons for the correspondence is letting the stakeholders know there are contractors coming to conduct an audit. The RAC are composed of contractors from different organizations, and it will be easier to communicate to practitioners about these matters if the correspondence originates from the RAC.

Health Care Reform

The Health Care Reform, also commonly known as the Affordable Care Act was implemented as a law after it was signed in March of 2010. The main purpose of this law was to enhance the quality of health care provided for patients and to increase the manner by which health insurance plans are availed and afforded by the masses. Also, with the enactment of ACA, the Federal government wished to lower the number of people without health care insurance to cover for their health care needs. Since it has been made into a law, more and more people are using the provisions of the health care reform to secure for themselves health insurance plans. More and more patients who avail outpatient physical therapy pay their health care providers using this plan.

Under the EHB clause, patients with Medicare and Medicaid plans are expected to be availed of the following benefits starting the year 2014:

    a. Patients availing of ambulatory health care services;

    b. Emergency health care services;

    c. Hospital confinement;

    d. Care during pregnancy and early newborn periods;

    e. Treatments for conditions within the domain of mental health;

    f. Services that are rehabilitative and restorative in nature;

    g. Wellness interventions and treatments that are preventive in nature; and

    h. Care for pediatric patients as well as care for the eyes and oral health.

The inclusion of the coverage to rehabilitative services and even use of devices on the essential benefits lists of the ACA is most concerning. Since the health care reform supports the nature of services offered by physical therapists, billers could rest assured they could collect payments for services rendered by physical therapists to their patients. Probably more good news physical therapists can consider in providing outpatient service for patients under the ACA is that most health plans would be including physical therapy and other similar rehabilitative services in their plan coverage. This would be mandatory and sanctioned by the ACA. However, because of the possible financial repercussions of this rule, limits may be imposed upon the number of visits a therapist may bill for a patient, dollar price caps and other restrictions similar to most private insurance plans.

In making sure they are not underpaid for the services they provide their patients while following the ACA guidelines, steps should be taken in educating other stakeholders into the value of providing rehabilitative care. Furthermore, they should also emphasize facts that availing this may result in eventual savings for health care costs not only for patients but also for parties providing health care insurance to them.

Refinements in payment plans are also included in the ACA to make sure that payments are correlated with the quality of care provided to patients. Various programs are being employed towards this end such as the PQRS program. This program is one of the most widely used payment programs apart from the typical electronic health record system used in most facilities. Under such payment software programs, services provided by therapists and the coding and billing mechanisms are pegged against most recent trends and issues in reimbursement and payments.

Payment Reforms Under Practice Administration

In an effort to increase the efficiency of billing and claiming payments from patients, insurance providers and other parties on the services provided by physical therapists, the APTA has made steps in proposing reforms on how payments are to be made. The current trend for collecting payments for services rendered is the *fee-for-service* scheme, where a patient gets billed for each procedure performed on him. This scheme, while leaning towards increasing profits for the physical therapist is not as efficient in the long run. By turning the payment system into a per-session-payment scheme, the APTA plans to carry out this reform in hopes of not only ensuring billing and payments are done efficiently, but that services are provided with the highest possible quality. With the new payment system in place, the physical therapists' clinical judgment will be improved and further promoted to increase the integrity of the decisions that they dispense.

Documentation

One of the most vital aspects in provision of care from the phase of assessment until evaluation and follow-up is documentation of care provided and other matters that has a direct influence upon it. Documentation not only affects the quality of care the physical therapist provides for his patients, it also affects how billing is done and payments are filed for claims and eventually received.

Medicare has adopted a documentation system that physical therapists can use to support their claims for payment when billing outpatient therapy under Medicare Part B. This system is known as the CERT (Comprehensive Error Rate Testing) and is used to make a composite description of the most common errors committed related to billing for outpatient therapy services.

One of the reasons for the development and adoption of the CERT is the need for the CMS to come up with a program that can produce the error rates for the Medicare Fee-For-Service for the entire country. This data is needed to be submitted as part of complying with the Improper Information Act. The CERT chooses a sample from the FFS claims filed with Medicare and examines these records against the claims protocols. Also, attached medical records from health care providers are reviewed as part of this to ensure billers and practitioners have complied with guidelines related to Medicare coverage, billing rules and coding systems.

The CMS has taken steps to accurately assess and measure how processing contractors for Medicare claims perform. Calculating the error rates related to provider compliance and the national FFS paid claims by Medicare allows the CMS also to gain insight into the mater while measuring performance of concerned contractors.

In order to accurately measure the performance of the Medicare claims processing contractors and to gain insight into the causes of errors, CMS calculates both a national Medicare FFS paid claims error rate and a provider compliance error rate. The results of the reviews are published in an annual report and semi-annual updates disseminated through accredited organizations such as the APTA.

Another goal by which the CMS has established CERTS is to ensure that the trust funds held by Medicare are protected and improper payment processes are eliminated. By the start of the use of CERT, the CMS has identified the most common issues related outpatient physical therapy services and how they are billed. The following are problems identified by the CERT in terms of documentation and how it impacts billing and making payments claims:

1. Some therapists have been found to submit documents with care or treatment plans that are either incomplete or altogether missing.

2. Documents submitted sometimes have missing signatures for concerned physicians and therapists. In some instances, dates of treatment and submission were also missing.

3. Therapists and billers also overlook the fact that the total treatment time for procedures and other care modalities need to be included in the documentation.

4. Certification and recertification documents are also found to be missing in some claims.

Documenting Outpatient Physical Therapy Services that Have CERT Findings

CERT findings about outpatient physical therapy care filed for claims would require billers and therapists to directly implement inclusion of a written plan of care or treatment plan in making claims for payments. These specific treatment plans should be made prior to the onset of treatment, except in some special cases. This means that therapists and other practitioners can confidently make claims because therapy plans are established.

It is important to remember therapy plans are only considered to be established when a physician, an NPP, an occupational therapist, physical therapist or speech language pathologist is the one who created it. Although these plans may be dictated and encoded by other staff, the practitioners must make treatment plans.

CERT minimum requirements for treatment plans to be submitted are the following:

1. Statement about the diagnosis/diagnoses of the patient

2. Treatment goals (especially long term ones)

3. Each specific type of therapy (PT, OT or SLP) should be identified based on the interventions carried out and modality observed. This is done to verify proper coding procedures and to support billing.

4. The number of sessions given as part of the treatment plan expressed in daily counts.

5. Length of each session

6. Number of sessions given in a week

In submitting the treatment plan, the practitioner who made it should attach his signature on the document, including any revisions made in the said plan as soon as it was made. If such changes are made, there is a need for a physician or an NPP to certify this. The general idea of this is to ensure that care plans implemented and undertaken in treatment of patients can contribute greatly to safe, effective and efficient care while aiming for the best possible outcomes.

Initial Certification of Treatment Plans

Certifications for the treatment or care plans being implemented are mostly attained through the attestation of an NPP or a physician. They can carry out such certifications regardless of the presence of an order if the document to be certified meets all the necessary requirements during the entire time the plan is in force, a 90 day period, or whichever among the two time frames is shorter. These initial treatment plans should contain the necessary assessment made by the practitioner that necessitates the need for a care plan to be valid. **Moreover**, there is a 30-day period where the NPP or the physician should certify either in writing or verbally from the onset of treatment. However, protocols dictate that if such verbal orders were given about the certification, the document would need to be properly signed within 14 days from the verbal certification.

The Process of Recertification

Recertification is required when the previously submitted treatment plan needs either to be modified or continued as per the patients' condition. The process requires that practitioners observe recertification when there are significant modifications to the plan of care. Ideally, this should be done at least within the 90-day period from the onset of treatment. However, there are instances where recertification may be delayed. The reasons for such delays would be determined by the CMS as either valid or invalid depending on the submitted supporting documents. Additionally, when the patients' treatment plans last for less than 90 days, the recertification needs to be done right away if it is indeed necessary.

Billing Procedures and Associated Modality Units

It is also worth noting when using HCPCS, some codes would specify the need to include how many minutes are allotted per treatment and how long the treatment actually lasted. Services that are performed in 8 minutes or less are not eligible for billing, unless its repeated performance totals to a minimum of 15 minutes per day. This would mean the total time devoted to the treatment of the patient, whether using timed or untimed codes, should be documented.

Ensuring Documents are Error Free on CERT

The CERT program is designed to pay specific attention to detect document errors for claims submissions. To ensure that the medical records submitted comply with CERT and errors are minimized, they should contain:

1. A complete plan of care. This means that apart from the date when the plan was made, it should also contain the signature of the practitioner.

2. Indicate or attach a document if the original plan of care was modified. This should also include an explanation about how modifications were made and why it was made in the first place.

3. Have appropriate certification (or recertification, when necessary).

4. Ensure that the total time spent for treatment is documented both in the timed code portion and ensure that these are all reflected in the record of the patient.

HIPAA Policies

One of the most important ethical rules in medical service is confidentiality of patient information. Medical practitioners in all fields are bound by the rules of their profession to maintain confidentiality regarding the personal information and medical records of any patient who engages their services. Whether you are a cardiologist or chiropractor, the rule applies to you. HIPAA of 1996 created the wide-ranging federal regulations that governed the privacy of individual-protected health information. HIPAA classifies wide categories of health information while establishing confidentiality standards. Stiff penalties are administered by the HIPAA in cases of breached confidentiality. The policy of confidentiality must therefore be adhered to with absolute compliance. This includes both you and the people under your employment working with you at your health facility.

HIPAA was ratified in order to guarantee the privacy and confidential management of medical information for all patients in the United States. Its major policies that support this standard of confidentiality apply to all U.S. medical service providers. It is the job of the HIPAA Compliance Officer to make sure that medical practitioners adhere to certain requirements. The Compliance Officers have access to all information related to compliance activities, such as patient records, billing records, and research data.

Hence, in adherence with HIPAA rules and regulations, the employees at your health facility must all undergo what are called HIPAA training sessions. The law that penalizes breached confidentiality in the medical profession also affects everyone who collects employer health benefits, which means that a training session on the basics and importance of the HIPAA should be part of the employee orientation. You can hold your own HIPAA training sessions provided that you have a reliable trainer/ facilitator to perform the discussions. Below are a few simple steps on how to initiate HIPAA training sessions for your clinic employees.

Step 1. Provide your employees with a handy compilation of summary information regarding HIPAA topics such as the HIPAA Privacy Rule. However, be sure that a HIPAA regulatory specialist or legal counsel takes a look at your binder of HIPAA information to certify its overall accuracy and approve its dissemination. Remember to include any of your company's policies or procedures regarding protected health information.

Step 2. Designate the specific date, time, and venue for your employees to assemble for the training session. A session should last at least two hours so there is plenty of time for your employees to ask relevant questions.

Step 3. During the training session, give a brief introduction about HIPAA, including its history and the latest status of the law. Explain the most important terms in the HIPAA, such as "protected health information." Give strong emphasis on the legal consequences and sanctions of illegal disclosure of such information.

Step 4. Next, elaborate on your company's established policies and procedures in direct connection with HIPAA. Among these is the exchange of information involving the company and any third-party vendors of employee services such as medical-insurance agencies or labor unions.

Step 5. Employees must be encouraged to ask questions during the training sessions. If an answer to a question remains unclear, the question must be discussed later on when a sufficient answer is found.

Step 6. Lastly, distribute a survey form to the participating employees to help improve future HIPAA training sessions. Have your employees sign a statement acknowledging their active participation in the training session, which is to be included in their permanent employee file.

The HIPAA has standardized disciplinary procedures for violations. The following selection of HIPAA-related violations and their corresponding penalties is an excerpt from the UC Davis Health System website (Year):

"Penalties Under HIPAA 42USC1320d-5 General penalty for failure to comply with requirements and standards:

(a) General penalty

(1) In general except as provided in subsection (b), the Secretary shall impose on any person who violates a provision of this part a penalty of not more than $100 for each such violation, except that the total amount imposed on the person for all violations of an identical requirement or prohibition during a calendar year may not exceed $25,000.

* * *

42USC1320d-6 Wrongful disclosure of individually identifiable health information

(a) Offense

A person who knowingly and in violation of this part

(1) Uses or causes to be used a unique health identifier; (2) obtains individually identifiable health information relating to an individual; or (3) discloses individually identifiable health information to another person, shall be punished as provided in subsection (b).

(b) Penalties

A person described in subsection (a) shall-

(1) Be fined not more than $50,000, imprisoned not more than 1 year, or both; (2) if the offense is committed under false pretenses, be fined not more than $100,000, imprisoned not more than 5 years, or both; and (3) if the offense is committed with intent to sell, transfer, or use individually identifiable health information for commercial advantage, personal gain, or malicious harm, be fined not more than $250,000, imprisoned not more than 10 years, or both."

As part of your practice's compliance with HIPAA regulations, you are obligated to provide a "Notice of Privacy Practices," a "Business Associates Agreement," and an "Authorization to

Disclose Protected Health Information" form (Magmutual, 2009).

HIPAA makes it compulsory that all the people from whom you collect medical information must be given a "Notice of Privacy Practices" so that they are aware of their rights to confidentiality and privacy. The following pages are sample forms for "Notice of Privacy Practices" and "Authorization to Disclose Protected Health Information."

By now you must understand the significance of following HIPAA rules and regulations. They provide a safeguard for the trust that patients give their attending physician or healthcare provider and protect the integrity of the medical profession as a whole.

Sample HIPAA Notice of Privacy Practices Statement:

Notice of Information Practices and Privacy Statement for Imaginary Health Services Nonprofit

(Your Physical Address and Complete Contact Information)

How We Collect Information About You: Imaginary Health Services Nonprofit. (IHSN) and its employees and volunteers collect data through a variety of means including, but not necessarily limited to, letters, phone calls, emails, voice mails, and from the submission of applications that is either required by law or necessary to process applications or other requests for assistance through our organization.

What We Do Not Do With Your Information: Information about your financial situation and medical conditions and care that you provide to us in writing, via email, on the phone (including information left on voicemails), contained in or attached to applications, or directly or indirectly given to us, is held in strictest confidence.

We do not give out, exchange, barter, rent, sell, lend, or disseminate any information about applicants or clients who apply for or actually receive our services that is considered patient confidential, is restricted by law, or has been specifically restricted by a patient/client in a signed HIPAA consent form.

How We Do Use Your Information: Information is only used as is reasonably necessary to process your application or to provide you with health or counseling services that may require communication between IHSN and healthcare providers, medical product or service providers, pharmacies, insurance companies, and other providers necessary to do the following: verify your medical information is accurate; determine the type of medical supplies or any healthcare services you need including, but not limited to; or to obtain or purchase any type of medical supplies, devices, medications, insurance.

If you apply or attempt to apply to receive assistance through us and provide information with the intent or purpose of fraud or that results in either an actual crime of fraud for any reason including willful or un-willful acts of negligence, whether intended or not, or in any way demonstrates or indicates attempted fraud, your non-medical information can be given to legal authorities including police, investigators, courts, and/or attorneys or other legal professionals, as well as any other information as permitted by law.

Information We Do Not Collect: We do not use cookies on our website to collect data from our site visitors. We do not collect information about site visitors except for one hit counter on the main index page (www.yourwebpage.org) that simply records the number of visitors and no other data. We do use some affiliate programs that may or may not capture traffic date through our site. To avoid potential data capture that you visited a website, simply do not click on any of our outside affiliate links.

Limited Right to Use Non-Identifying Personal Information from Biographies, Letters, Notes, and Other Sources: Any pictures, stories, letters, biographies, correspondence, or thank-you notes sent to us become the exclusive property of IHSN. We reserve the right to use non-identifying information about our clients (those who receive services or goods from or through us) for fundraising and promotional purposes that are directly related to our mission.

Clients will not be compensated for use of this information and no identifying information (photos, addresses, phone numbers, contact information, last names, or uniquely identifiable names) will be used without client's express advance permission.

You may specifically request that NO information be used whatsoever for promotional purposes, but you must identify any requested restrictions in writing. We respect your right to privacy and assure you no identifying information or photos that you send to us will ever be publicly used without your direct or indirect consent.

(Wolfe, 2009).

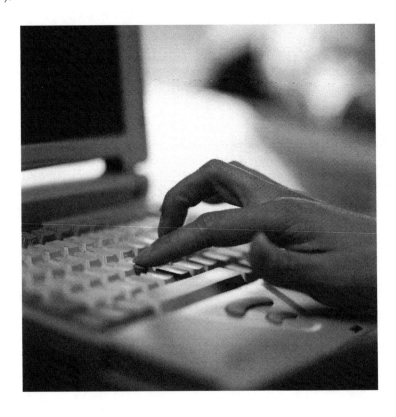

Sample HIPAA Authorization to Disclose Protected Health Information:

(Note: "You" refers to the person(s) to whom this Authorization is directed. "I," "me" or "my" refers to the Patient.)

AUTHORIZATION FOR DISCLOSURE OF PROTECTED HEALTH INFORMATION

To the following person(s) or class of persons:

Any and all physicians, healthcare providers, healthcare facilities, or healthcare entities that provide or have provided healthcare services to the patient named below.

Patient Name: _____

Date of Birth: _____

Address: _____

AUTHORIZATION

You are hereby authorized to disclose my Protected Health Information, whether oral, written, or electronic healthcare information pertaining to my complete medical record, including, but not limited to, HIV and AIDS confidential information.

You are hereby authorized to disclose my Protected Health Information specifically pertaining to my mental health, including but not limited to: psychiatric and psychological information, drug, and alcohol abuse treatment information.

You are hereby authorized to disclose such Protected Health Information to any physician, healthcare provider or healthcare facility that has provided healthcare services to me. Additionally, you are hereby authorized to disclose such Protected Health Information to any attorney at law representing such physician, healthcare provider or healthcare facility.

Discussions Related to My Care. You are hereby authorized to discuss my care and treatment with any attorney or representative of an insurance provider if I assert a claim against another physician, healthcare provider, healthcare facility, or healthcare entity.

This authorization expires three (3) years after the date of execution shown below.

PATIENT'S RIGHTS

I understand I do not have to sign this authorization to receive healthcare benefits (treatment, payment or enrollment) from the person(s) to whom this authorization is directed. I may revoke this authorization in writing at any time. If I do so, it would not affect any actions already taken by someone in reliance on this authorization. I may not be able to revoke this authorization if its purpose was to obtain insurance coverage. If I wish to revoke this authorization, I shall do so by sending a letter to the person(s) to whom this authorization is directed. Once the healthcare provider discloses health information, any person or organization that receives it may re-disclose it. Patient privacy laws may no longer protect that information. I must sign an authorization form to take part in a research study, or to receive health care when the purpose is to create health information for a third party.

_____   _____

Patient or Legally Authorized Individual Signature Date

_____

Printed Name (If Signed on Behalf of Patient)

Relationship (Parent, Legal Guardian, etc.): _____

Reference: Magmutual, 2009.

PURCHASING CLINICAL EQUIPMENT

A health facility is only as good as the quality of both its service and its clinical equipment. In order for your patients to stay loyal, you must show them first-rate equipment that is clean and safe to use. A client may only be satisfied with your services if you offer them the kind of treatment they deserve using first-rate equipment. They will tell their friends, family, and acquaintances how impressed they were with the clinical equipment at your facility. You should purchase this equipment at reasonable prices without sacrificing quality.

Clinical equipment can be divided into four categories—Testing Equipment (i.e., X-ray machine, equipment for range of motion and manual muscle, sphygmomanometer); Procedural Equipment (i.e., treatment tables); Exercise Equipment (i.e. mirrors, weights, treadmill; must be simple, focused, and automated); and Equipment for Modality (Halley, 2008).

Have a checklist of clinical equipment and clinical furniture you need to purchase. Determine what is absolutely necessary. In other words, purchasing medical equipment while your facility is still new will require prioritization. Also, determine what equipment will need to be replenished monthly or quarterly. Depending on your profession, you can choose from the following list:

Name of Equipment

14 × 17 Full Speed Blue Film	Pulse oximeter
8 × 10 Green Sensitive Film	Reflex hammer
Blue Fast Detail Film	Sacral blocks
Boxes of gloves	Sphygmomanometer
Boxes of paper	Standard Weight Vest kilt Apron
Cold packs	Stethoscope
CPR mannequin	TENS
Defibrillator	Theraband (red, green, blue, black)
Educational posters	Thumper
Emergency light	Traction table
Exam gowns	Transport 2-Channel Electrotherapy
Freezer	Transport with 19 Diode Cluster Applicator
Goniometric apparatus	Travel cards
Headrest paper	Treatment table
Hot pack handling tongs	Tuning fork
Hot packs	Ultrasound
Hydrocollator	Ultrasound gel/lotion
ID printer	Weighing scale
Inclinometer	X-ray caliper
Iontophoresis delivery device	X-ray film developer
Laser	X-ray film fixer
Lead shield	X-ray film storage bin
Literature rack	X-ray ID cards
Magazine rack	X-ray illuminator
Opthalmoscope	X-ray machine (requires installation and inspection)
Otoscope	X-ray mailer
Oxygen tanks	X-ray marker
Pinwheel	

You can search on the Internet for various online suppliers of clinical equipment. The nearer their offline store location is to your facility, the cheaper the transportation fees are. Although you may purchase certain items for bargain prices on eBay, be cautious and do extensive research on the eBay seller you are buying from. Set aside a budget for your medical equipment. Make the most out of your purchases. While it is good to be a thrifty buyer, do not sacrifice good quality in order to save a few dollars. As was discussed before, your medical equipment will reflect the kind of services you can provide, and impressing your clientele will require standard, quality medical equipment. So select only the best that you can offer to your clients. You can find really good buys at dotmed.com or craigslist.org.

The Facility

When looking for the right location for your practice, it is important to consider the building itself. You cannot hope to persuade clientele to become regular patients if they see that your building is decrepit, disorganized in design and arrangement, or has an unhygienic or shabby ambiance. The facility itself must be designed and furnished in such a way that the overall effect is conducive to healing and recovery. To do so requires careful planning of the architecture and arrangement of clinical equipment and office furniture.

When evaluating a building for your facility, you may have to do some remodeling but you are indeed lucky if the place needs little or no modifications in its design. Things to look for when choosing the right structure include abundant natural lighting, great window placement, good ventilation, spacious and open patient areas, hygienic conditions, good state of utilities (i.e., water and electricity supply), and a capacious and inviting waiting/reception area (Halley, 2008). Make it your goal to have a facility that one can truly regard as a "healing environment" for your patients. Think of having a health facility in a building that is both functional and attractive. A building should look good on the outside and should make people feel good when they walk in.

The facility should have separate areas for the therapy of the patients (private treatment rooms for evaluation, hydrotherapy pool, and therapy gymnasium), the records and files room, the waiting/reception area, your main office, the bathrooms and private area for staff. Other things to consider include storage space, line of sight design for exercises, lighting, electrical outlets, computer workstations, floor drains, use of a hydrocollator tank, and where to get your facility's supply of linens (Halley, 2008). Decorating your facility should be the least of your concerns since you still have to prioritize the purchase and arrangement of the facility's clinical equipment, office supplies and furniture. Proper arrangement is key in helping your facility win the confidence of your patients.

Since your facility is a health service provider, you must follow several rules and regulations that are necessary for Medicare facility compliance. These include:

- Appropriate parking space for the handicapped

- Bathrooms for both males and females must have grab bars installed

- Clearly marked points of entry and exit

- Doors must have an opening of at least 32 inches and must open at 90 degrees

- Floor must be carpeted with a maximum

- thickness of one-half inch

- Ramps

- The front desk must be at least 36 inches

- in height and length

For a health facility that has enough space for a practitioner who is just starting out, a space ranging approximately from 1,500–2,000 sq. ft. can be quite sufficient.

New Patient Area

Patients must have a separate waiting area where they can wait comfortably and fill out all necessary forms. You may provide a small part of the receptionist's counter specially marked for the new patients so that they will not be confused as to where they should start first (Halley, 2008). This way, the forms for new patients can be placed easily within reach while returning patients are free to move more quickly when completing other forms.

The area should be well-organized for the coming and going of patients who have arrived for their appointments. The clients must have ample space to move about and have enough comfortable seats to sit on while waiting, completing forms, or watching patient educational videos.

Patient Care Area

In its Standard for Health Care Facilities (NFPA, 1999), NFPA defines a patient care area as "any portion of a health care facility wherein patients are intended to be examined or treated." Quiet, beautiful, natural, easy, and soothing would be the adjectives that should come to mind when designing the patient care area. Things you should consider include color selection & coordination, concept design, fixture planning, cabinet design, specific materials and finishes, textile & fabric selection, equipment selections, furniture and upholstery, accessorizing, window, wall, flooring treatments, lighting layout and selection.

Point of Sale Area

Have a product display section as well as product inventory area that can be securely locked up when left unattended. The fact that your facility's products are being displayed allows customers to browse through them and see if they would like to purchase any of them. Having a product display stand or glass case is one way to promote the products that are for sale (Halley, 2008). Another part of increasing your cash flow is your point of sale (POS) system. A POS involves having a POS computer, a cash drawer, a receipt printer, and reliable POS software. These make POS procedures easier to perform, thus making the entry of cash more efficient. Your POS system software must also be up-to-date so that you will have an easier time managing your cash flow.

Billing Area

When automating regular operations, the billing station is where your competent staff handles the daily billing and the management of fee slips. The employee in charge of billing will use references for ICD-9/10 (International Statistical Classification of Diseases and Related Health Problems) codes and CPT (Current Procedural Terminology) so these must on hand for easy referral (Halley, 2008). Daily operational procedures must be improved to ensure swift, secure, and precise performance of tasks.

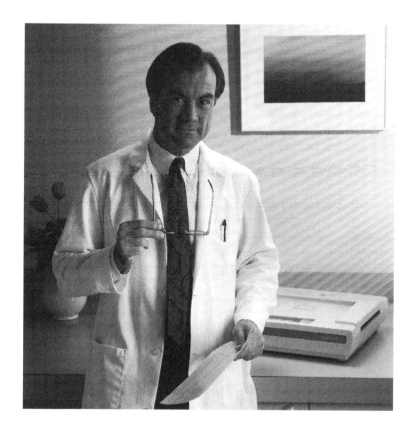

————— *Starting your Own Practice from Scratch* —————

Office and Furniture Supplies

Your facility will not be complete without your office and furniture supplies. They are your next priority after the building and clinical equipment. Buy them at select stores where you can take advantage of discounts by buying in bulk. Purchase items only if they are necessary and if they can bring value. Investing money in frivolous items at this point is not an option, so stick to your budget.

Office supplies include appointment books and cards, patient folders and charts, alphabetizing stickers, business checks, mailing labels, staplers, staple wire, adhesive tape, reams of paper, paper clips, pens, a literature rack, and scissors. They can also include customized items such as brochures, business cards, letterheads, envelopes, and postcards. Check out your local Staples or Quill for office supplies. As for other necessary office items, be sure to buy trash bags, toilet seat dispensers, toilet seat covers, disinfecting wipes, rolls of toilet paper, and paper towels.

Aside from a front desk, waiting room chairs and filing cabinets, you should also consider purchasing LCD television sets for the waiting room and evaluation rooms, wall mounts for these television sets, one coat/hanger rack, an all-in-one printer, one computer, a telephone, and a sound system.

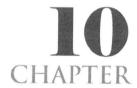

10
CHAPTER

MARKETING PLAN

Regardless of how many years you are in any particular business, constantly updating your marketing plan is key to achieving and maintaining success. Marketing is highly significant in terms of building meaningful customer relationships and spreading product or service awareness. A company that does not have an effective marketing strategy risks not gaining any new customers as well as losing their current loyal customers. This leads to revenue loss and absence of company growth. Marketing facilitates so many benefits for business that it is a booming industry on its own.

A marketing plan outlines the precise actions you intend to execute to capture the interest of prospective clientele in your community. The goal is to ultimately convince these clients to buy the services you offer. Your marketing plan must clearly illustrate how you will implement your marketing strategy. "True Marketing" entails defining who you are, knowing what you are good at and what it is you can offer. Finally, brainstorm all the possible and effective marketing actions you will be willing to take. This can help you narrow down your choices and think of specific parameters and details for each marketing action you will list in your marketing plan. True marketing lets you see things practically since you will have to think about your weaknesses and strengths and how to use these to your advantage (Halley, 2008).

Below is a list of actions divided into several categories that you must incorporate into your marketing plan:

Internal Marketing Actions	External Marketing Actions
Order business cards for ready use	Attend and sponsor public awareness seminars
Have a family and friends voucher	Have a referral pad
Order "Thank You" postcards for ready use	Have your health facility's name and contact details placed in the local Yellow Pages
Publish a newsletter	Place a brief yet effective ad or article in the local newspapers
Order caps, t-shirts, and other promotional material as freebies for returning clients and good employees	Local mailers to community – product/service specials
Make use of online promotion via a website	In your website, include Staff Profile, an introduction to your facility, updated lists of programs, services, specialized equipment, and testimonials
Gather patient testimonials	Have your website make use of tracking tools to count the number of visitors
Gather MD testimonials	Hold public speaking engagements such as lectures and workshops in the community and even in your office
	Hold free health screenings for scoliosis, blood pressure, etc.
	Build alliances with attorneys, dentists, podiatrists, health food store owners, spas, nursing homes, dance schools, yoga teachers, etc.
	For your professional acquaintances that you have alliances with, hold lunch and dinner meetings for collaboration discussions

To help you have a better idea of time regarding marketing certain activities, you may use the suggestions below:

Time Orientation	Action
Daily	Check brochures / cards available in the lobby Send thank you postcards
Monthly	Flyers Referral pads
Quarterly	Publish ads/articles in local newspapers Direct mailer
Semi-annually	Collect recommendation letters from best referring people
Seasonally	Send Christmas postcards during Christmas

Part of building a good relationship with your clientele is making them feel special and letting them know how thankful you are for their choice of health facility or their continued patronage. Sending thank-you cards to show your appreciation is a good idea. This marketing tactic is more effective if you also include three business cards (so that they may readily refer you to a friend or family member) and a survey (to evaluate your facility's overall performance and give useful suggestions for improvement) (Halley, 2008).

There are hundreds of other ways to promote lasting relations with your customers, and all you have to do is look for them and decide which will best suit your business. Last but not the least, remember that people like to feel valued, and you must consider this first when devising your marketing plan. Check out paloalto.com for Marketing Plan Pro, software that will help you design a marketing plan.

Creating a Website for Added Promotion and Public Accessibility

Very frequently, we make the mistake of believing that in order for a marketing technique to be truly effective, we have to shell out hundreds and even thousands of dollars. This misconception has caused many business establishments to lose thousands of dollars each year. You can actually promote your health facility for so much less with even more successful results. One such cost-effective marketing technique is to create an official website for your online promotion.

With rapidly expanding Internet access in households, marketing businesses have taken advantage of this medium. People now turn to the Internet to purchase many of their needs, regardless of whether it is a simple product or a specific service, which is why even offline businesses choose to promote themselves on the Web. Shopping online is now the norm, and there is no sign in any way that the trend is going away any time soon. It is logical, therefore, to ride the wave of online promotion to make more people aware of your health facility's services.

For those of you who already have extensive knowledge of computers and the Internet, this is an excellent way to forge new alliances and attract potential customers. And for those who have limited experience with computers and surfing the Web, you can engage the professional services of reliable web designers who can design you a website according to your particular specifications.

The demand for physical therapy, occupational therapy, and chiropractic care does not fade given the number of people who suffer from all sorts of injuries and disabilities each year. However, for your location, there will most likely be dozens of other medical practitioners in those fields already. How can one medical professional possibly stand out from the rest? Simply by having clients look to you for service.

That's what a website can do for you. Creating and maintaining a promotional website provides many benefits. Online users typing in a search on Google for "Occupational Therapist in Chicago" will receive innumerable directory listings, names, contact numbers, and site addresses. There are even those directory listings that go as far as posting the latest reviews coming from previous patients along with their personal ratings of the health facilities.

Having a website would allow you to "introduce" yourself better to your potential clients. Information about your educational and professional background and a little bit about your personal life would provide prospective clients with a feel of their would-be health professional. What you say about yourself on your website can help make them feel less apprehensive about engaging your services, especially if you address them with a warm, accommodating tone.

Websites can facilitate better improvements for your practice, thanks to feedback systems. Through a feedback application on your site, clientele would be able to directly make suggestions and maybe even add constructive criticism regarding your health facility and its services (Tresellers, 2009). Having a website also helps prospective customers make better choices about treatment. A lot of people are reluctant to see a therapist, but when they have singled out one they seem to like or are comfortable with; this is one more opportunity for you to start a long-term business relationship with them.

In addition to the other benefits, creating your own website for the clinic would make it possible for you to attract patients in search of a specific technique or an alumnus of a specific school. Building alliances with attorneys, dentists, podiatrists, health food storeowners, spa owners, nursing home staff, dance schoolteachers, and yoga teachers, can also readily be achieved via an online presence.

To design your website, seek the advice of master web designers and set your focus on four things: content, visual appearance, functionality, and visibility (Tresellers, 2009). If you wish to coordinate with a designer, then you may collaborate with him or her on all four aspects to get the exact tenor that you want your site to have.

Content refers to the information posted on the website. This needs to be carefully written and strategically formatted to help your website become visible online. Regularly update your content, making sure it contains no grammatical or typographical errors, and check the tone of your sales pitch to make sure it does not end up sounding like a hard sell. Relevant content and targeted keywords will rank your website higher in search engine results (Tresellers, 2009). Aim to be on the main page of the results listings by using search engine optimization. That is the kind of visibility that you need in order to catch potential clients' attention.

Regarding functionality and appearance choose a design that is visually attractive and interesting, yet easy to load. Color combinations should be pleasant to the eye. Pictures can also be engaging points of interest. Images and videos may look good, but refrain from using those that take too long to load. Impatient site visitors might switch to another website if you make them wait too long. Make the site functional by having an easy navigational interface (http://blog.traffic-resellers.net/?p=61). This means that you have to make things uncomplicated for your user-clients to move around the website. Let them be free to browse your site's webpages without any kind of hassle.

In terms of visibility, you can make your website rise in search index position by implementing what are known as Search Engine Optimization (SEO) techniques. The higher your ranking in a particular search engine results page, the greater the chances are that a customer will click through to your website and thus learn about your health facility (Tresellers, 2009). If you are unfamiliar with SEO methods, it is recommended that you do a little research on your own and then hire an SEO company to help you out. Cost-effective SEO methods and online promotional techniques include Article Marketing, Video Marketing, social bookmarking, blogging, social networking websites, etc. You can also advertise online by utilizing Google Adwords and Yahoo Marketing Solutions. You can set a daily spending limit of $2.00 per day!

One of the biggest internet phenomena in recent years has been the rise of daily deal sites such as Groupon or Living Social. These sites offer discounts, generally of between 40 and 60 per cent, for products and services available in specific cities around the world. These deals are expensive for merchants. Groupon takes about half the revenue that the vouchers generate. But although merchants may make a short-term loss during the deal, the potential benefit is of long term growth due to the repeat business from new customers. John Byers and Georgia Zervas from Boston University and Michael Mitzenmacher from Harvard University studied over 16,000 Groupon deals in 20 US cities between January and July this year. They monitored each deal every ten minutes or so to determine how sales varied over time and also counted the number of Facebook likes that each deal generated. At the same time, they collected Yelp reviews--some 56,000 of them for 2,332 merchants who ran 2,496 deals--examining how merchant reputations changed before and after a Groupon deal. They found that a Groupon deal seems to have an adverse impact on reputation as measured by Yelp ratings.

The real test, of course, is the long-term revenue that the deals generate for merchants and this study provides no data on that. So ultimately, only the merchants themselves can know how successful these deals really are (arxiv.org/abs/1109.1530). These sites are expensive to the starting clinician. Therefore, if you are starting your practice from scratch, I do not recommend using this model.

Pre-Open Advertising

We have already discussed certain advertising methods to help you build your identity as well as those that are ideal components of a marketing plan. To differentiate what is called pre-opening advertising from the promotional tactics that were outlined in the previous chapters, pre-opening advertising is an intensive set of promotional methods that are specifically chosen and systematically scheduled for implementation before the opening date of a new business establishment (Halley, 2008). The main goal of pre-opening advertising is to ensure that by the time your business doors open, you have generated awareness and support for your new establishment.

The primary goal of advertising with regards to building brand is to help build and maintain a positive relationship shared by your health facility and others involved with your business, namely your clientele, investors, distributors, media, and your employees. Pre-opening advertising guarantees that when the opening date of your practice finally arrives, you can rest assured that you have done everything possible to reach out to your targeted customers as well as all alliances (doctors, lawyers, dentists, health clubs, and yoga instructors, to name a few).

Before your practice opens its doors for business, you must have already scheduled your pre-opening advertising tactics. Your target audience is divided into two—your potential customers and your referral sources. As with preparing any organized plan, you have to focus and write lists of actions to be done and people to reach out to before integrating everything into one comprehensive document. Below is a sample list that you can use to understand who your target population is for your pre-opening advertising. (With your referral sources, you can immediately start listing the names of the alliances you wish to solicit support from.)

Customers

a. Target city or area_____

b. Target age_____

c. Target gender_____

d. Other:_____

      Referral sources

a. Target city(s)_____

b. Specialties_____

c. Other:

      Name: XXXXX XXXXX
      Specialty:
      Residential Address:
      Clinic Address:
      Contact details: (E-mail address, landline number, mobile phone number, fax, etc.)

      Name: XXXXXX XXXXX
      Specialty:
      Residential Address:
      Clinic Address:
      Contact details: (E-mail address, landline number, mobile phone number, fax, etc.)

Here is a simple checklist for you to determine if you have prepared and then successfully implemented the feasible pre-opening advertising tools available to you. It will also serve as a list of suggestions for the possible marketing actions you can implement. Check the pre-opening advertising methods you have planned and performed.

Prepared	Schedule of Implementation	Completed	Date Accomplished	Pre-opening Advertising Tool
				Invitations for Open House
				Invitations for free workshop/ seminar
				Free giveaways (t-shirts, coffee mugs, caps, etc.)
				Local newspaper article/s (for best results, provide them with your resume, a copy of your license, a facility brochure, and your business card)
Prepared	Schedule of Implementation	Completed	Date Accomplished	Pre-opening Advertising Tool
				Local newspaper ad/s
				Newsletter (Online)
				Postcard for a product promo related to your service
				Postcard communicating your services
				Poster/s
				Flyers/Postcards to be left with local merchants
				Fax: All MDs and other possible referral services
				Put your name and business in the local Yellow Pages
				Radio announcements

To assist you in setting a good timeframe for your activities for your pre-opening advertising campaign, here is an ideal timeline indicating the right time to implement each advertising method.

1 year prior to opening date	6 Months prior to opening date	3 Months prior to opening date	1 Month prior to opening date	Week 4,3,2 prior to opening date	Week 1 prior to opening date
Yellow page ad					
Mailing list					
Newsletter	Newsletter	Newsletter	Newsletter		
Service postcard	Service postcard	Service postcard	Service postcard	Service postcard	
1 year prior to opening date	**6 Months prior to opening date**	**3 Months prior to opening date**	**1 Month prior to opening date**	**Week 4,3,2 prior to opening date**	**Week 1 prior to opening date**
	Newspaper	Newspaper	Newspaper	Newspaper	Newspaper
	Giveaways	Giveaways	Giveaways	Giveaways	Giveaways
		Referral Program	Referral Program	Referral Program	Referral Program
			Radio ads	Radio ads	
			Invitations	Invitations	

When speaking to your target audience, adopt a tone that speaks from the heart (i.e., "Be free from pain for life!"). Doing so will give them more of a connection to you than cold, extremely business-like lines would. Also, it is important that in all your ads not to communicate more than two niche services since things can get very confusing (Halley, 2008). Concentrate on a maximum of two niche services and you will have less complicated concerns to deal with when addressing your pre-opening advertising audience.

Setting Up Your Online Appointment Scheduler

An online appointment scheduler software can help your health facility. What this particular computer software basically does is allow your customers to securely book their own appointments online. The beauty of this lies in the fact that your clients, especially the returning ones, need not trouble themselves with the hassle of going to your clinic just to set up an appointment. They can easily check the available appointment slots of the health facility and pick their desired date and time for consultation and/ or treatment, all within the safety and comfort of their home. Plus your clients may also pay you immediately online via your PayPal account, credit card, or other payment form available through the vendor.

Since more and more people are opting for Internet access, you will find transacting business online as advantageous. Computerization of schedules of appointments is definitely a business essential more than ever (Halley, 2008).

You do not have to look far to obtain this useful software since it can easily be purchased via the Internet. Many companies are selling their version of an online appointment scheduler, each one having different special features, product packages, and terms of use. But plainly speaking, with an online appointment scheduler as part of your site, a "Schedule Now" button should appear on your homepage, which is what a prospective client clicks for an appointment. A "booking page" designed to match the rest of your site will be displayed where the client can log in and book an appointment. Both you and that client will then receive a notification by e-mail, and the client's appointment will appear on your online calendar.

After a client finishes his/her appointment with you, do not forget to set the next schedule for evaluation, re-evaluation, and presentation of a report of findings, if necessary. This saves you and your client the trouble of talking over the phone to settle that schedule.

Moreover, this type of software is highly customizable so that it can easily be modified to fit any scheduling requirement. There are also numerous features available to make everything even easier, such as:

- Limitless online bookings
- Confirmations that are automated
- Phone appointments (bookings made over the phone can be accepted while automatic
- Updates will be made on the available slots on your website)
- Automatic creation of a client database for every customer who books an appointment online
- Automatic suggestions for alternate appointments when a client wants a slot that is already booked

Usually online appointment scheduler software marketers will allow customers like you to enjoy a 30-day free trial period. Simply download their trial version software at their official website. Monthly fees for the software range between $5.00 to $160.00. Be a wise buyer and compare prices and features first before making a purchase.

Have a set of policies regarding several important issues concerning appointments booked online. Have a "No Show" policy for clients who fail to appear on the scheduled date and time, a cancellation or reschedule policy, as well as a "Recommended Late" policy. Whether or not you will implement some kind of penalty for clients who do not follow the appointment rules will be up to you.   There are 2 top online appointment schedulers that are currently in the market.

Schedulicity

Since it launched in 2010, 15,000-plus subscribers have booked more than 10 million appointments through Schedulicity across the United States and Canada, making it the largest service. Schedulicity is also the most robust, with strong customer-relationship management tools and customizable deals and promotional tools. Schedulicity provides a ScheduleNow button for your website or Facebook page. A client who wants to schedule an appointment clicks the button and then, with the aid of a pop-up, walks through choosing a service and provider and picking a time from among your open spots--all without leaving the browser or having to install anything. After creating an account with Schedulicity, clients gain access to a personalized scheduling page with one-click rebooking, appointment reminders, and links to cancel or reschedule appointments. Schedulicity won't track is money. Clients can't use the service to pay in advance for services, and you can't use it to keep track of deposits that you may require clients to pay in order to hold a time slot. This limitation isn't a big deal if your policy is for clients to pay at the time that they receive your service, but if you require a deposit to secure a time, you'll have to track that separately.

Schedulicity lets you send mass email messages to your clients based on various templates, including industry-specific artwork, newsletters, seasonal promotions, and invitations to book or connect online. You can also invite Facebook fans and Twitter followers to check out your online listing and book online. The price is $19 per month for a single user and $39 per month for 2 to 20 users.

Appointy

Appointy stands out from the crowd by covering basic online booking at no cost. Higher tiers of service that include more-advanced features are available at rates ranging from $10 to $40 per month. Appointy launched in 2007 and now supports more than 21,000 customers in 78 countries. In 2011, 1 million users booked more than 3 million appointments through Appointy. Setting business hours in Appointy is easier than in any competing service. Appointy lets you accept--or require--prepayment through PayPal or Authorize.Net. This feature enables you to require deposits or to accept prepayments without having to store credit-card information. When booking a new appointment, you can select from existing clients or add a new one. You can also create recurring appointments, and Appointy allows clients to set up their own recurring appointments, showing dates available for the selected time slot. Clients can enter coupon codes and choose to pay later, or they can pay up-front with PayPal. Appointy displays your cancellations policy to the client along with the booking confirmation.

Appointy will maintain a basic list of your clients and their contact information, but it doesn't provide a way to import your current list. Customers can submit reviews and you can choose whether the reviews will display their name or appear anonymously. The basic plan is free, $10 per month for Plus plan (adds Google Calendar linking); $20 per month for Pro plan (adds customizations, analysis, prepayments, and recurring bookings); $40 per month for Business plan (adds separate staff logins).

Here are other companies:

http://aceplanner.com	http://www.clickbook.net
http://checkappointments.com/index.html	http://www.effexis.com/achieve/planner.htm
http://essentialpim.com	http://www.genbook.com
http://flashappointments.com	http://www.myintervals.com
http://personaltaskmaster.com	http://www.mylifeorganized.net
http://www.appointment-plus.com	http://www.simplifythis.com/index.htm
http://www.appointmentquest.com	http://www.taskline.com/default.asp
http://www.bookfresh.com	https://www.chaossoftware.com/secure/purchase.asp

Getting Referral Sources

You will need good sources of referrals to have a steady line of referrals coming to your health facility's doorstep. Orthopedists, neurologists, physicians, other chiropractors, physical therapists, occupational therapists, high school sports coaches, massage therapists, the people at the local rotary club, contacts at the Social Service at nearby hospitals, personal injury attorneys, medical directors of health maintenance organizations (HMO), and so on, are good sources of referrals (Halley, 2008).

Winning over the support of these potential sources of patient referrals requires courtesy, sincerity, tact, and diplomacy. You cannot just barge in on them and ask them to start sending referrals your way. You cannot just assume that they will all say yes to your request, either. Bear in mind that these people for the most part do not even know you (although it is a good idea to start with people whom you know or who are acquaintances). Be courteous at all times and refrain from badgering them incessantly if they say no or do not send a reply to your request. Pestering them during their free time is also a big mistake, unless they explicitly ask that you meet them during non-working hours. Before anything else, you must have the person's complete contact address and number.

The first most suitable step would be to send a well-composed letter which is direct and devoid of unnecessary chit-chat or hollow flattery (Halley, 2008). Nothing turns off people more than a person who is asking for a favor and yet takes a long time to state things simply. It is simply irritating when there are too many flowery words, so compose a letter that is neat, coherent, humble, and sensible (Halley, 2008). Remember to include a company brochure and newsletter to help the person learn more about what you do, what services you offer, and what your facility stands for.

Next, follow up the letter with a phone call. Call at a suitable hour when you think the timing is most right. Be polite, regardless if you speak with the front desk receptionist of the person you are calling. State your purpose and ask if you could schedule appointment.

Once the other party has agreed to see you, pay the person a visit. While conversing with them, do not be pushy and let them finish everything that they have to say. When it is your turn to speak, thank them for lending you their precious time before telling them all about you and your new facility. Tell them directly why you are unique as a healthcare service provider and enumerate your most interesting programs and services, without sounding too overconfident or presumptuous. Bring referral pads and newsletters to leave behind. However, do not offer these until you feel the timing is right to offer them to the person or wait until they ask for the items.

Send a thank-you card to those who have agreed to be one of your referral sources. Have it done using a customized letterhead, envelope, and postcard (Halley, 2008). For the enclosed gift, it is recommended that you to give a useful promotional item that your prospect is likely to keep around that have your contact information on it (e.g., business card magnets, promotional pens, coffee mugs and drink ware).

In general, almost all industries today have their own respective trade associations in every state or region. A trade association, otherwise known as an industry trade group, is generally composed of businesses all belonging to one specific kind of industry whose main objective for organizing themselves is to initiate public relations programs and collaborations between themselves for the mutual benefit of all the members. Trade associations are typically non-profit organizations and are for the most part funded by the regular contributions of all the members.

These business associations offer numerous benefits for their members which is the main reason why you should join one. Your connections with your profession's trade organization will reward you in more ways than one but you must also be aware of the responsibilities that go along with your membership.

Join Trade Associations

Members of trade associations not only get an opportunity to interact with one another to boost their industry's overall public image, but they also get the chance to organize themselves and lobby on legislation issues that can potentially affect their particular industry. If a certain legislation is in the best interest of a certain line of trade, that industry's trade association can help in promoting it. Likewise, if there is legislation that can have possible adverse effects on the industry, the trade association's members can collectively voice their sentiments against it.

Trade associations serve as forums to further disseminate relevant information to the general public regarding a particular industry and its functions. Such forums also allow the public to become more educated on the chief services and products that are currently being offered by the industry as well as the latest developments in the field. Educating the public through easily understandable facts and figures can help generate their interest and raise awareness about a particular product or service the trade association is promoting.

To a certain extent, a trade association provides protection for the integrity of a given industry. It generally sets standards that each member must adhere to in order to be regarded in good standing. Members who refuse to comply with the said standards set by their trade organization face being excluded from the association as well as losing a large amount of credibility in the consumer public's eyes. This paves the way for the individual members to gain better reception for their marketing efforts.

By joining, you are given opportunities to attend conferences sponsored by your trade association. Conferences are organized to help better the overall function of the industry through the provision of relevant information that each conference attendee can take in and relay at the company home base. Most trade associations sponsor at least one industry conference or seminar-workshop per year. Through this, a trade organization can offer valuable resources for its members to help them acquire additional skills as well as increase their education. Try to learn if the association you plan to join offers educational literature, relevant magazines, mentoring, and accreditation programs that are aimed for the professional development of its members.

Networking is another advantage to joining a trade organization. You can make valuable business contacts as well as search for potential job opportunities. You can also obtain a competitive edge from trade associations since they can provide you with the most up-to-date industry news and technology. Lastly, a great number of trade and professional associations that are influentially powerful and have sound integrity can acquire special discounts and pricing for their members. These professional discounts can apply to business insurance, expensive conferences, and other services related to your profession.

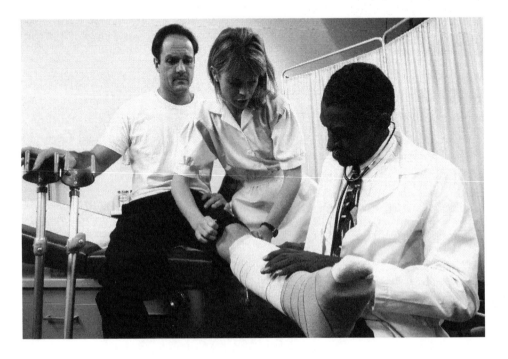

—— *Starting your Own Practice from Scratch* ——

Before joining a particular trade association, you have to take time to learn about your options and research each potentially deserving association (Halley, 2008). It pays to ask around and do your research. The following are suggestions on finding and joining the right trade association.

Research and come up with a list of registered associations for your industry. The best method to do this would be to go online and use a search engine. Type in the words "trade association" or "professional organization" and your line of industry (physical therapy, occupational therapy, or chiropractic care) for your query and click submit. An index of possible associations will then be given to you. Try Google's Business Directory, which has an "Associations" category that lists them by industry.

Choose the association that best suits your needs and has the most benefits. At this point, it would be wise to ask those in your field who are more experienced about which associations are better than others. Your colleagues can give you some pointers on what they already know about trade associations in your field. There are international trade associations that have local chapters, so do not exclude them when searching for the best organization.

Weigh the costs versus benefits. As a member, you are obligated to pay membership fees periodically. You are then entitled to avail of the association's benefits. Trade associations vary in terms of member privileges and advantages, so it is up to you evaluate which association will give you the most value for your monetary contribution to the group.

Joining a trade association need not be a tiresome task or unproductive endeavor. You can gain so much from your membership that you actually cannot afford to let the opportunity just pass you by. Be wise in your choice of association and you will soon see just how much you stand to gain by joining.

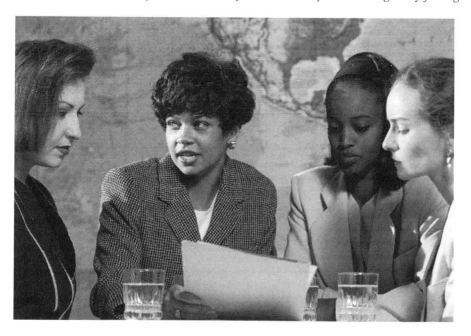

—— *Starting your Own Practice from Scratch* ——

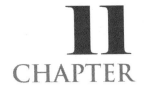

CHAPTER

KEEPING TRACK

In any business, money is the primary lifeblood that sustains all activity in the establishment. Regardless of how you look at it, a business needs money to run. People go into business generally for the sake of earning substantial profit from the money they invested as business capital. In order to determine whether a business establishment is earning more than it is spending, one must track productivity as well as the cash flow that occurs daily in the company. For businesspeople who do not record the money that goes in and out of their business, sooner or later they will find out that much of their invested money has "vanished into thin air" since they have no record as to how much money was spent and whether it was compensated by any incoming profit. Such neglect is any businessperson's downfall, which is why early on in the game, one must be prepared to diligently engage in tracking daily productivity and cash flow (Kishel, 2005).

Once in while we forget to list things we spend money on in our simple, daily lives, despite having a restricted budget. However, when it comes to business, listing the company's daily expenses is imperative to monitor the financial status of the company (Kishel, 2005). Spending more than what the facility earns will mark your facility for future failure so have your most trusted employee make an itemized list for every expense (both cash and credit) that your facility incurs every day. Several times a week, go over the list with your employee and ask to see the receipts for every payment made on the list. You must also be sure that the person who will take charge of this duty is reliable, meticulous, and above all, trustworthy. Double-check the list when possible, using the receipts or by phoning the establishment.

Daily expenses can be divided into two major categories—those that are fixed and those that are variable. Fixed expenses are those that remain constant, are paid every month, and do not fluctuate even if time passes by. Examples include rent, telephone, Internet connection, insurance, subscription fees, and taxes.

In contrast, variable costs are those that change depending on your consumption of a product or service and are much more unpredictable compared to fixed expenses. Examples include car rental fees, hotel room fees, and plane ticket fares.

Below are some common business expenses that your facility will need to pay on a more or less regular basis:

- Accounting/bookkeeping, and financial consulting fees
- Advertising expenses
- Automobile expenses (only the percent that is used for business)
- Bank service charges and fees
- Books and periodicals
- Business/trade conventions
- Business gifts
- Business meals
- Computer, printer, and software
- Consultant fees
- Credit card processing fees
- Depreciation and amortization
- Dues for professional and trade associations
- Education expenses for maintaining or improving required skills
- Email, Internet access, and web hosting services
- Fax machine
- Insurance expense
- Lease
- Legal and attorney fees
- License fees and taxes
- Office furniture and equipment
- Office supplies
- Online services used for the business
- Printing and duplication
- Rent Utilities
- Self-employment taxes
- Start-up expenses (amortized over 60 months)
- State and local business taxes
- Preparation of business tax return
- Telephone expense (only for a separate business line)
- Travel expenses

To keep track of your incoming cash flow, keep a separate list for the income you earn each day. This goes along the lines of the cash payments that your patients pay, reimbursements, product sales, etc.

To track daily productivity, record the number of hours that you and each employee on your payroll work each day, collecting incident reports, chart reviews, as well as tracking how many patients come in daily. Client turnovers data are very important and they include both old and new clients who visit your health facility. To specifically gauge customer satisfaction, you can send the patient satisfaction survey forms to your clientele through the mail or by e-mail. Record the data from the completed survey forms when the clientele send them back to you. Take note of their answers, criticisms, and suggestions.

Keeping track of your clinic's overall productivity enables you to measure the progress and efficiency of your health facility. You can use the data that you gathered to make improvements in your workforce so that you can provide maximum "output" at the end of each week. Let the data help you find your weaknesses and then act accordingly. If you are spending too much on a non-essential item, cut down on that cost. If your clientele report in the survey that they find the waiting room stuffy, do something about the air-conditioning or ventilation, and so on. Treat the process of tracking productivity not as a chore, but as a safeguard to your business.

Employees

Hiring employees is an integral part of owning a healthcare establishment since medical practitioners definitely cannot work on their own without the help of reliable staff. The tasks involved in operating your establishment are too many for a single person. You will need people to accommodate incoming patients at the front desk, handle the forms that need to be completed, arrange the patient medical files and important documents, assist you while you treat patients, manage the health facility's website, handle appointment schedules (especially when clients cancel), receive telephone calls, etc. Having dependable, loyal employees should be one of your priorities if you want your practice to operate smoothly and efficiently. Even though you have to go through the trouble of getting insurance, additional paperwork and taxes, hiring employees should not be put off. Employees are, without doubt, valuable assets that will greatly contribute to the success of your medical facility (Podmoroff, 2005).

The hiring process starts first and foremost with writing job descriptions. Develop a clear understanding of the employee position that you wish to fill. A job description can be defined as a concise enumeration and explanation of the requirements, duties, and responsibilities of the person who will hold the position in question. Once you have developed a satisfactory job description, you must then define the academic and experiential qualifications that the employee must have in order to qualify for the position. Next, study the salary range of people in similar job situations so that you can decide on the earnings the position will be entitled to (Podmoroff, 2005).

The second step would then be to recruit possible candidates. Since you already have a clear job description, you will be able to communicate to jobseekers exactly what you are looking for. Your objective at this stage is to attract a good number of highly qualified individuals as job applicants (Podmoroff, 2005). You can recruit employees by placing ads on online job sites, running print advertisements via local newspapers or professional journals, and engaging executive search firms. If you are in search for a physical/occupational therapist and cannot find one, consider sponsoring a foreign-trained physical/occupational therapist for an H1-B visa (working visa). This is a lengthier process, but at least you are guaranteed that you will have an employee for three years (which can be extended another three years). See PTSponsor.com for details.

Here is a list of things you should include when announcing a job vacancy:

A brief description of your health facility, its objectives, and its goals

The job description (name of position, duties and responsibilities, qualifications)

Salary and benefits (specify salary range/starting salary)

Starting date and deadline of application

The requirement of non-personal references

Your health facility's name and address

Your health facility's website address

After posting notices of the vacant job position, applicants will then respond. The third step is to screen candidates, which should be done before any interviews are done. Screening the initial applicants helps ensure that you do not have to waste time interviewing people who actually do not have the proper qualifications to apply for the job (Podmoroff, 2005). In order to screen your potential employees, you can simply review their resumes and conduct brief phone interviews. It is also wise to conduct background checks for any record of criminal history, drug use, bad credit, etc.

Now that you have narrowed down your list of applicants, move on to step four, which is the more intensive portion of the hiring process. Here you hold interviews and do more in-depth background checks by following up on references. Schedule the interviews at convenient times and be sure not to ask invasive or offensive questions. Reference checks should be done meticulously since they may simply be lies or exaggerations. Never settle for just any applicant for the position. Choose one who is above average. Selecting the best candidate from many qualified ones may be difficult, but sooner or later you will have to decide.

After you have finally chosen your new employee, you must now process legal paperwork. Remember to apply for an Employer Identification Number (EIN), obtain worker's compensation insurance, handle your employees' social security tax payments, etc. You will also need to have the following forms: offer of employment, W-4 Form, I-9 Form, employee rules of conduct agreement, terms of employment, time card, time off request form, probation policy sheet, specific job description, plus operations and employee manuals (Podmoroff, 2005; State Office of Risk Management, 2009). Companies such as ADP, Paychex, Surepayroll, and Paycycle can help you with most of the tasks listed.

Part of having employees is the responsibility of having to train, motivate, and pay your hired people. A training manual is a must, so do not assume that everything can just be discussed by word of mouth

Sample Letter Making a Bona Fide Offer of Employment:

(Certified Mail Return Receipt #)

(Date)

(Employee name)

(Address 1)

(Address 2)

Re: Offer of Employment

Dear (Employee name):

After reviewing the information provided by _____ , we are offering you the following temporary work assignment.

This assignment is within your capabilities as described by your doctor on the attached Work Status Report (DWC-73). You will only be assigned tasks consistent with your physical abilities, skills and knowledge. If any training is required to do this assignment, it will be provided.

Position title: _____
—

Description of physical requirements of this position: _____

Location: _____

Duration of assignment: From: (_____) To: (_____)

Work Hours: From: (_____) To: (_____)

Wages: _____(Hour, Week, Month)

Department: _____

Supervisor: _____

This job offer will remain open for seven (7) calendar days from your receipt of this letter. If you do not respond within seven (7) calendar days, we will presume you have refused this offer. Refusing this offer may impact your income benefits.

We look forward to your return. If you have any questions, please do not hesitate to contact me (include phone number or email address).

Sincerely,

(Signature)

　　　(Typed name and title)

　　　EMPLOYEE:

_____ I have read and understand the requirements of the position and accept the position.

_____ I have read and understand the requirements of the position but do NOT accept the position.

_____   _____

Employee's Signature   Date Signed

　　　(State Office of Risk Management, 2009).

alone. If it's not written, the training manual does not exist. Training your employees should include orientations through verbal explanation and demonstration of the training manual.

Employee performance is highly affected by how you motivate them in the workplace. Aside from the employee's monthly salary, a reward system may be another way to motivate them (Kishel, 2005). Show appreciation for a job well done with little tokens of gratitude. Recognizing talent and effort can really make your employees feel valued and appreciated. The more they feel that way, the more they will be motivated to do their jobs well. When paying your employees, use the payroll method that can easily be organized via computer software.

Feedback on employee performance is an essential part of improving your customer service, so do not forget to evaluate your staff's performance on a routine basis (Kishel, 2005). Check up on who is slacking off, arriving late too many times, lying habitually, etc. If worse comes to worst, remove the delinquent employee from your workforce. (State Office of Risk Management, 2009).

Start-Up Expenses

With any medical practice start-up, it is essential to carefully approximate all the initial expenses that one will incur. This is important to help you determine the total amount of money you should prepare for the entire process of setting up your clinic as well as keep costs within their allocated budget (Kishel,

2005). Your start-up capital should be more than your start-up expenses, so if you keep within the limits of your list of start-up expenditures, then you have fewer chances of spending beyond what you can actually afford. A list of start-up overhead is also needed to help you remember which tasks are prerequisites to other tasks, which is very important since mixing up your priorities out of sequence can possibly cause significant delays in the opening of your medical practice.

The list can serve as a checklist for you to see just how much money is actually spent. That way, it will be easier to monitor the progress of your health practice in relation to the status of your entire fund after every purchase or payment. You should also bear in mind that some overhead costs for start-up are only paid once while others are paid periodically so that you can adjust your preliminary estimates.

There are two basic types of start-up expenses to help you in finalizing your initial overhead estimates: the fixed costs and the variable costs. Fixed costs are those that remain constant and do not fluctuate regardless of you selling one or more unit of your service or products. Examples of fixed costs include:

- Professional Fees—Refers to service fees incurred for engaging an accountant, solicitor, lawyer, or other expert professional

- Insurance

- Finance—Refers to any loans or finance including interest payments and arrangement fees

  - Variable costs are expenses that increase each time you sell one or more unit of your service or products. They can also be defined as costs that fluctuate periodically depending on how much of a product or service you use (Kishel, 2005). Here are some examples of variable costs:

- Premises Costs—Includes construction cost of premises, rental fee, and utilities like telephone, electricity, and water

- Staffing and Employment—Refers to money spent in advertising and recruiting for employees, including their training

- Sales and marketing—Includes costs of the initial launch and promotion of your health facility, its products and services (i.e., website creation, flyers, promotional giveaways, etc.)

To help you get an idea on how to go about making your list of initial overhead, here are some examples of start-up expense list.

Start-up Costs	Actual	Budgeted
Legal		
Stationery etc.		
Brochures		
Consultants		
Insurance		
Rent		
Licensing		
Research and Development		
Computers and Software		
Print Advertising and Report Production		
Office Furniture		
Clinical Equipment		
Total Start-up Expenses		
Start-up Assets Cash Required		

Samples of One-Time and Monthly Start-Up Expenses Checklists:

One-Time Start-Up Costs

Start-up Costs

Clinical Equipment	$X.XX
Office furniture	$X.XX
Computer hardware and software	$X.XX
Setup, installation and consulting fees	$X.XX
Business cards and stationery	$X.XX
Decorating and remodeling	$X.XX
Fixtures, counters, equipment and Installation	$X.XX
Starting inventory	$X.XX
Deposits with public utilities	$X.XX
Legal and other professional fees	$X.XX
Business licenses and permits	$X.XX
Advertising and promotion for opening	$X.XX
Signage	$X.XX
Rent and security deposit (often equals 3 months rent)	$X.XX
Operating Cash	$X.XX
Other	$X.XX
Subtotal	$X.XX

Monthly Expenses

    Start-up Costs

Salary of owner-manager (amount you need to pay yourself)	**$X.XX**
All other salaries, wages, and commissions	**$X.XX**
Payroll taxes or self-employment tax	**$X.XX**
Rent	**$X.XX**
Equipment lease payments	**$X.XX**
Advertising (print, broadcast and Internet)	**$X.XX**
Supplies (inks, toners, labels, paper goods, etc.)	**$X.XX**
Telephone	**$X.XX**
Utilities	**$X.XX**
Internet connection	**$X.XX**
Website hosting and maintenance	**$X.XX**
General business insurance	**$X.XX**
Business vehicle insurance	**$X.XX**
Health insurance	**$X.XX**
Interest and principal on loans and credit cards	**$X.XX**
Inventory	**$X.XX**
Legal and other professional fees	**$X.XX**
Franchise fee	**$X.XX**
Miscellaneous	**$X.XX**
Subtotal	**$X.XX**

Estimate the number of months needed to find customers and get established.

Monthly expense for X months	**$X.XX**
One time start-up expense	**$X.XX**
	_____
Total Start-up Expenses	**$X.XX**

Your Accounting System

Your health facility must have a reliable accounting system, payroll system, and means of credit card processing. These will all need the help of computer software. In this day and age, the best option is for you to choose software that can easily be backed up by the Internet. Also, your accounting system needs different people to handle its various areas of responsibility and duties. Assign specific employees to handle task areas such as:

Overall responsibility for the accounting system

Management of the computer system

Accounts receivable

Accounts payable

Order entry

Cost accounting

Monthly reporting

Inventory control

Payroll (even if you use an outside payroll service, someone must be in control and responsible)

Internal accounting control

Fixed assets

A business checking account is also a necessary part of creating an efficient accounting system; so opening one with a reliable bank should be done as soon as possible (Kishel, 2005). Opening a business checking account requires that you first assess your business establishment's needs as well as determine which bank you want to do business with. A business checking account will help you manage your business operations or make account information more accessible to your financial managers. Next, gather and organize all the necessary information needed to open a business checking account, which can possibly require your business employment identification number, your previous year's business

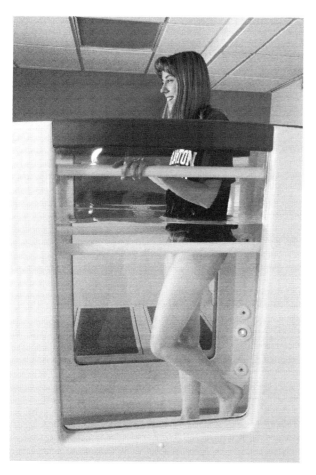

tax forms, social security number, and any preceding bank statements (Kishel, 2005). If you are going to apply for a business checking account online, log on to your chosen bank's official website. Be sure to follow the instructions on their website. Contact the bank's online customer service department around two business days subsequent to opening your account. Verify whether the account was properly opened and if everything is properly set up. Many banks offer online business checking accounts and all you have to do is search the words "open a business checking account" on any of the major search engines to receive a list of such banks. Determine which bank will suit your business needs.

Quickbooks is one of the most highly recommended software systems when it comes to preparation of basic financial statements and reports, entering sales receipts, sales tax tracking and payment, inventory management, purchase order processing, tracking expenses, preparing and sending invoices, check printing, and options for employee payroll and time tracking. It is a line of business accounting software that is marketed by Intuit. Many business establishments make use of Quickbooks because of its proven solutions for business management concerns. You may try it out for yourself and then you will see the difference it will make with your facility's overall accounting system efficiency.

12

CHAPTER

GRAND OPENING

Day Planning

You have been through months of preparation and hard work, months of planning, budgeting, marketing, purchasing, and arranging. Now all is in place, waiting for that one big event—your Grand Opening. But even such a celebration needs preparation in order to have maximum positive effect, especially with your potential clients. In general, a grand opening is considered as a promotional tool for a business to declare to the public that it is fully prepared to serve its clients competently and professionally (Kishel, 2005). It is your way of announcing your health facility's official opening in your new location.

Many grand opening events have a festive atmosphere, which includes food, celebratory signs, music, prizes, giveaways, colorful balloons, and maybe even a fireworks display. However, you still do have to manage your budget wisely, so allocate just the right amount for the affair. Here are some suggestions to help you prepare a successful grand opening event:

Selecting the Date and Time. Avoid holding your grand opening on a major holiday, or on a Saturday or Sunday. The most suitable days of the week to ensure good attendance are Tuesday, Wednesday, and Thursday. Morning grand openings should commence no earlier than 8:00 A.M.

Prizes. Holding a simple contest or a raffle draw is one way of drawing an interested crowd to your opening event. Free items can attract customers especially if these are related in some way to your services and products.

Extra Staff. In any grand opening, the business owner will never be absolutely sure as to the exact number of people who will attend. So it might actually be a good idea to have your complete staff working on that date or maybe even add a few extra people just for the day. Being under-staffed on that day is courting trouble.

Give Back to the Community. You may want to try hosting a charitable cause at your health facility's grand opening by offering to donate to the community a certain sum coming from the earnings from your first few weeks of business. Giving back to the people in the area is a good way of inviting goodwill and trust between you and the local community (Kishel, 2005).

Entertainment. Entertainment for your guests need not be costly. Why not try inviting the local church choir or high school band to help things be livelier at the celebration? It shows that you support the community and is a great way of keeping your guests entertained.

Hold a Ribbon-Cutting Ceremony. This is quite a popular gesture at grand openings and is appropriately symbolic despite its simplicity. Simply buy a ribbon and a few flower arrangements and you are all set to cut the ribbon with a pair of scissors to officially open your health facility.

If you have followed your marketing plan, you have probably drummed up enough publicity for the community to take notice and gather around your health facility for its grand opening. You must also make sure that most of the important people you have invited to the opening can make it. Call them up to ask for their confirmation, but do not hold grudges if they cannot make it to the event. Having an important local government official at your opening event is also a good idea. You should also invite

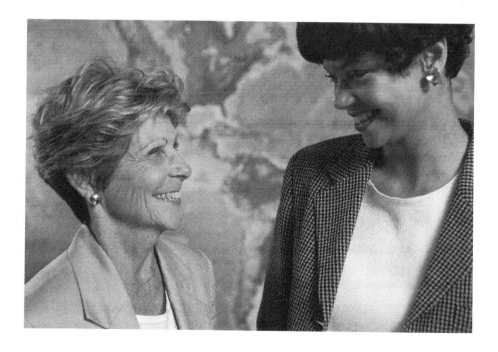

—— Starting your Own Practice from Scratch ——

the local journalists to join you at the special event. The newspapers need to write about your opening in their local business section so remember to hand them invitations.

Be more than punctual on the day of your grand opening. Keep your confidence levels up and be alert always. Mingle with your guests, answer their questions patiently, and say everything with a smile. You have done all that is possible to help make your health facility a success, so face the future with courage and you will have no regrets

Conclusion

The implementation of Medicare Part B is ideally designed to help patients get high quality care in the most cost-efficient way possible. It also intends to help practitioners and independent physical therapists make proper payment claims for the services they render their patients. While it is important that the services required by patients be given promptly when and where they need it and as often as necessary, it is also important that physical therapists are paid and reimbursed accordingly for the services they provide their patients. In the inpatient setting, the problem of documenting care and making payment claims is not as complicated as making claims for outpatient physical therapy. There are considerations to be taken such as knowing codes and how these affect billing, coding and making payment claims.

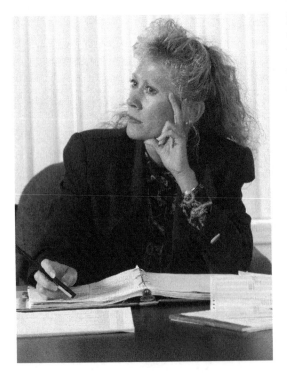

Through the vigilant efforts of the APTA in protecting and advocating the rights of physical therapists, changes in coding and how it affects billing and making payment claims have been undertaken. Physical therapists find themselves to have improvements in terms of receiving payments for the care rendered and that more and more of the services provided to outpatient are being paid and reimbursed by Medicare and other health care insurance companies. With the integration of patient electronic health records into the practice of the profession, information about patients becomes more accessible, and the exchange of information between billers and payers are made faster.

The issue is, however, despite all the advances, underpayment for services being billed are common because codes are not mastered enough or utilized appropriately in relation to a patient's condition or the procedure being performed. There are instances where Medicare has decided a therapist or biller has made a payment claim higher than what is allowed, and processes were enforced to recoup payments. In more unfortunate cases, payment claims are denied, and the physical therapist is not paid what is due. With so many repercussions associated with improper or incomplete knowledge of Medicare Part B and its intricacies, only one solution remains, and that is to better understand Medicare Part B and its provisions so the physical therapist can better focus on providing safe, efficient and effective care for outpatient beneficiaries and not become preoccupied with billing, coding and making payment claims.

References/Resources

2010 ICD-10-CM. Centers for Medicare and Medicaid Services. Accessed October 16, 2014.

2015 ICD-10-CM and GEMs - Centers for Medicare & Medicaid Services. Available at http://www.cms.gov/Medicare/Coding/ICD10/2015-ICD-10-CM-and-GEMs.html. Accessed May 20, 2015.

About Local Coverage Database. APTA, 2013. http://www.apta.org/Payment/Medicare/CoverageIssues/LCD/About/ Accessed October 29, 2014.

Allen, S. (n.d.) Choosing a location for your business: There's more to consider than just cost. Retrieved from http://entrepreneurs.about.com/od/gettingstarted/a/chooselocation.htm.

American Medical Association; American Medical Association (COR); Michelle Abraham; Jay T. Ahlman, Angela J. Boudreau, Judy L. Connelly (30 October 2010). CPT 2011 Professional Edition. American Medical Association Press. ISBN 978-1-60359-217-8. Retrieved 26 May 2011.

American Physical Therapy Association House of Delegates. Support of Electronic Health Records in Physical Therapy. HOD P06-08-13-11. American Physical Therapy Association; 2008. http://www.apta.org/uploadedFiles/APTAorg/About_Us/Policies/HOD/Practice/Support.pdf#search=%22support of electronic%22.

APTA Summary of the Correct Coding Initiative (CCI). Available at http://www.apta.org/Payment/Medicare/CodingBilling/CCI/.

APTA; Use of Students Under Medicare Part B, 2014. Available at https://www.cms.gov/Regulations-and-Guidance/Guidance/Transmittals/downloads/AB0156.pdf

APTA: Expansion of Coverage Under Health Care Reform. http://www.apta.org/ExpansionofCoverage/

APTA: Health Care Reform. http://www.apta.org/HealthCareReform/

APTA: Use of Physical Therapy Assistants Under Medicare, 2014. Available at http://www.cms.gov/Medicare/Billing/TherapyServices/downloads/61004ptartc.pdf

Arxiv.org. (2009). Daily Deals: Prediction, Social Diffusion, and Reputational Ramifications. Retrieved from Billing Scenarios for PTs and OTs. Centers for Medicare and Medicaid. Available at: https://www.cms.gov/Medicare/Billing/TherapyServices/downloads/11_Part_B_Billing_Scenarios_for_PTs_and_OTs.pdf. Accessed October 30, 2014.

Chaudhry B, Wang J, Wu S et al. Systematic review: impact of health information technology on quality, efficiency, and costs of medical care. Ann Intern Med. 2006 May 16;144(10):742-52. Epub 2006 Apr 11. Review. PubMed PMID: 16702590.

Ciolek & Hwang 2008 – Available at https://www.cms.gov/Medicare/Billing/TherapyServices/downloads/2_CY2006OutpatientTherapyUtilizationReport_PDF_Final.pdf Accessed April 20, 2015.

Ciolek & Hwang, 2004 – Available at http://www.cms.gov/Medicare/Billing/TherapyServices/downloads/projectrpt111504.pdf

CMS Publication 100-03, Medicare NCD, Section 30.1

CMS, 2013. http://www.cms.gov/Medicare/Provider-Enrollment-and-Certification/MedicareProviderSupEnroll/indcx.html?redirect=/MedicareProviderSupEnroll/

CMS: Medicare Part B Updates, 2014. Available at https://www.cms.gov/Medicare/Billing/SNFConsolidatedBilling/2014-Part-A-MAC-Update.html

CMS: National Correct Coding Initiative 2014

CMS: National Correct Coding Initiative Edits 2014

Coding and Billing APTA 2014: http://www.apta.org/Payment/CodingBilling/

Coding Intepretations. One-on-One and the Group Code. http://www.apta.org/Payment/Coding/OneonOneGroup/

Coverage Issues Manual, Sections 35-72 and 35-77

Crandell, Deborah JD (2012). Compliance Matters: Selecting an EHR Vendor. PT in Motion. September 2012. Available at http://www.apta.org/PTinMotion/2012/9/ComplianceMatters/. Accessed on October 29, 2014.

Dick RS, Steen EB, Detmer DE (eds). The Computer-based Patient Record: An Essential Technology for Health Care. Washington, DC: National Academies Press; 1991. http://www.nap.edu/openbook.php?isbn=0309055326.

Dunn, Abe. Does Competition Among Medicare Advantage Plans Matter?: An Empirical Analysis of the Effects of Local Competition in a Regulated Environment. 2009. http://www.justice.gov/atr/public/eag/248399.pdf.

Elias, S. (2007). *Trademark: Legal care for your business and product name* (8th ed). Berkeley, CA: Nolo. Costhelper. (Year). Chiropractor cost. Retrieved from http://www.costhelper.com/cost/health/chiropractor.html.

Falkenstein, L. C. (2000). *Nichecraft: Using Your specialness to focus your business, corner your market and make customers seek you out* (2nd ed.). Portland, OR: Niche Press.

FAQ: 2015 Medicare Therapy Cap. Available at http://www.apta.org/Medicare/TherapyCap/FAQ/2015/. Accessed May 16, 2015.

Federal Register | Medicare Program; Medicare Part B Monthly Actuarial Rates, Premium Rate, and Annual Deductible Beginning January 1, 2015. Available at https://www.federalregister.gov/articles/2014/10/10/2014-24248/medicare-program-medicare-part-b-monthly-actuarial-rates-premium-rate-and-annual-deductible. Accessed May 23, 2015.

Functional Reporting - Centers for Medicare & Medicaid Services. Available at http://www.cms.gov/Medicare/Billing/TherapyServices/Functional-Reporting.html. Accessed May 16, 2015.

Gillikin, J. (n.d.) How to conduct a HIPAA training session for employees. Retrieved from http://www.ehow.com/how_5603080_conduct-hipaa-training-session-employees.html.

Guide to Physical Therapist Practice 3.0. Alexandria, VA: American Physical Therapy Association; 2014. Available at: http://guidetoptpractice.apta.org/. Accessed October 10, 2014.

Halley, M. D., & Jerry, M. J. (2008). *The medical practice start-up guide.* Phoenix, MD: Greenbranch Publishing.

Hobday, G. (n.d.) What type of business organization is best for you?. Retrieved from http://www.myownbusiness.org/s4/.

ICD - ICD-10-CM - International Classification of Diseases, Tenth Revision, Clinical Modification. Available at http://www.cdc.gov/nchs/icd/icd10cm.htm. Accessed May 20, 2015.

ICD-10 - Centers for Medicare & Medicaid Services. Available at http://www.cms.gov/Medicare/Coding/ICD10/index.html. Accessed May 20, 2015.

Ingenix, Inc. Staff. (n.d.) Brush up on CPT/HCPCS modifiers. Retrieved from http://health-information.advanceweb.com/Article/Brush-Up-on-CPTHCPCS-Modifiers.aspx.

Internet-based PECOS - Centers for Medicare & Medicaid Services. Available at http://www.cms.gov/Medicare/Provider-Enrollment-and-Certification/MedicareProviderSupEnroll/InternetbasedPECOS.html. Accessed May 23, 2015.

Kenny, P. (n.d.) Why is business insurance important? Retrieved from http://www.streetdirectory.com/travel_guide/141785/insurance/why_is_business_insurance_important.html.

Kishel, G. F. (2005). *How to start, run, and stay in business: The nuts-and-bolts guide to turning your business dream into a reality* (4th ed.). Hoboken, NJ: Wiley.

Krotz, J. L. (n.d.) How to build a company identity from scratch. Retrieved from http://www.microsoft.com/smallbusiness/resources/marketing/advertising-branding/how-to-build-a-companyidentity-from-scratch.aspx#Howtobuildacompanyidentityfromscratch.

Laura Southard Durham (1 June 2008). Lippincott Williams and Wilkins' Administrative Medical Assisting. Lippincott Williams and Wilkins. pp. 2–. ISBN 978-0-7817-9789-4. Retrieved 26 May 2011.

Magmutual. (Year). HIPAA authorization to disclose protected health information. Retrieved from http://www.magmutual.com/mmic/articles/HIPAA-authorization-sample.pdf.

Manual Medical Review Process for Therapy Claims. Available at http://www.asha.org/Practice/reimbursement/medicare/Manual-Medical-Review-Process-for-Therapy-Claims/. Accessed May 23, 2015.

Maxwell, S., C. Basseggio, and M. Storeygard. 2001. Part B therapy services under Medicare, 1998–2000: Impact of extending fee schedule payments and coverage limits. Washington, DC: Urban Institute.

Mdsr.ecri.org. (2009). Electrical Safety Requirements: Patient Care Areas versus Non-Patient-Care Areas. Retrieved from http://www.mdsr.ecri.org/summary/detail.aspx?doc_id=8286

Measures Codes - Centers for Medicare & Medicaid Services. Available at http://www.cms.gov/Medicare/Quality-Initiatives-Patient-Assessment-Instruments/PQRS/MeasuresCodes.html. Accessed May 23, 2015.

Medicare As Secondary Payer. APTA, 2011. Available at http://www.apta.org/Payment/Medicare/CoordinationofBenefits/SecondaryPayer/FAQ/. Accessed November 4. 2014.

Medicare Coverage Database. Available at http://www.cms.gov/medicare-coverage-database/. Accessed November 8, 2014.

Medicare Part B- Current Updates. March 2014 Edition. Centers for Medicare and Medicaid Services. Available at: http://www.ismanet.org/pdf/membership/32114handouts.pdf. Accessed October 10, 2014.

Medicare Part B- Current Updates. March 2014 Edition. Centers for Medicare and Medicaid Services. Available at: http://www.ismanet.org/pdf/membership/32114handouts.pdf. Accessed October 10, 2014.

Medicare Physician Fee Schedule. Available at http://www.apta.org/Payment/Medicare/CodingBilling/FeeSchedule/. Accessed May 16, 2015.

Medicare Physician Quality Reporting System (PQRS). Available at http://www.apta.org/PQRS/. Accessed May 16, 2015.

Medicare Program; Limitation on Recoupment of Provider and Supplier Overpayments Summary of Final Rule. September 2009. APTA.

Medicare Therapy Cap. Available at http://www.apta.org/Payment/Medicare/CodingBilling/TherapyCap/?navID=10737430585. Accessed May 16, 2015.

Michelle Abraham; Jay T. Ahlman; Angela J. Boudreau; Judy L. Connelly, Desiree D. Evans, Rejina L Glenn (30 October 2010). CPT 2011 Standard Edition. American Medical Association Press. ISBN 978-1-60359-216-1. Retrieved 26 May 2011.

Morebusiness.com. (2007, October 31). Building your company identity: Image branding. Retrieved from http://www.morebusiness.com/building-company-identity.

Murray, J. (n.d.) Fixed expenses. Retrieved from http://www.wisegeek.com/what-are-fixed-expenses.htm.

National Correct Coding Initiative Edits. Centers for Medicare and Medicaid. Available at: http://www.cms.gov/Medicare/Coding/NationalCorrectCodInitEd/index.html?redirect=/nationalcorrectcodinited/. Accessed May 16, 2015.

National Quality Forum. http://www.qualityforum.org/Home.aspx and http://www.qualityforum.org/Setting_Priorities/Partner ship/Measure_Applications_Partnership.aspx

Nichols and Albanese, Implementing ICD-10 Diagnostic Codes. APTA Learning Center Webinar handout. March 27, 2015.

Payment Methodologies: Advantages vs. Disadvantages for Practice. APTA. Available at http://www.apta.org/Payment/PrivateInsurance/PaymentMethodologies/ Accessed October 25, 2014.

PECOS. APTA, 2011. Available at: http://www.apta.org/Payment/Medicare/Enrollment/PECOS/. Accessed November 5, 2014.

Physician Fee Schedule. APTA. Available at: http://www.apta.org/Payment/Medicare/CodingBilling/FeeSchedule/2013/FAQ/

Physician Quality Reporting System - Centers for Medicare & Medicaid Services. Available at http://www.cms.gov/Medicare/Quality-Initiatives-Patient-Assessment-Instruments/PQRS/. Accessed May 23, 2015.

Podmoroff, D. (2005). *How to hire, train, and keep the best employees for your small business.* City: FL: Atlantic Publishing Group.

PQRS Claims-Based Reporting. Available at http://www.apta.org/PQRS/ClaimsBasedReporting/. Accessed May 16, 2015.

Ready for the Post-SGR World? APTA Offers Highlights of New Medicare Law Available at http://www.apta.org/PTinMotion/News/2015/5/5/MACRAHighlights/. Accessed May 24, 2015.

Registry Based Reporting and GPRO. Available at http://www.apta.org/PQRS/RegistryReporting/. Accessed May 16, 2015.

Regulations Regarding Individuals That Qualify For Medicare and Medicaid: Who Qualifies as a "Dual Eligible?". APTA, December 2010.

Sculley, Michael J. (2013). Physical Therapy Billing. http://www.freept.com/PhysicalTherapyBilling/. Accessed October 19, 2014

Sculley, Michael J. (2013). Physical Therapy Billing. http://www.freept.com/PhysicalTherapyBilling/. Accessed October 19, 2014.

Shamus & Stern. Effective Documentation for Physical Therapy Professionals. McGraw-Hill Medical. 2004.

Standards Related to Essential Health Benefits Offered in the State Health Insurance Exchanges: Final Rule Summary. APTA. February 22, 2013

Stanford University Center for Health Policy: Model contractual language for medical necessity. Developed at the workshop, Decreasing Variation in Medical Necessity Decision Making. 1999 Mar 11-13; Sacramento (CA). Available at http://www.chcf.org/~/media/MEDIA%20LIBRARY%20Files/PDF/M/PDF%20medicalnec.pdf.

State Office of Risk Management. (n.d.) Letter making a bona fide offer of employment. Retrieved from http://www.sorm.state.tx.us.

Straube, D. M. (n.d.) HCPCS codes: Frequently asked questions. Retrieved from http://www.nls.org/av/FAQ%27s%20HCPCS.pdf.

Therapy Services - Centers for Medicare & Medicaid Services. Available at https://www.cms.gov/Medicare/Billing/TherapyServices/index.html?redirect=/TherapyServices. Accessed May 16, 2015.

Tracy, B. (n.d.) Analyzing your competition. Retrieved from http://www.briantracy.com/blog/sales-success/analyzing-your-competition/

Tresellers.com. (2009, December 24) Three crucial steps on website promotion. Retrieved from http://blog.traffic-resellers.net/?p=61.

UC Davis Health System. (n.d.) Penalties under HIPAA. Retrieved from http://www.ucdmc.ucdavis.edu/compliance/guidance/privacy/penalties.html.

Use of Physical Therapy Aides Under Medicare. APTA, 2013. http://www.apta.org/Payment/Medicare/Supervision/UseofAides/Accessed May 23, 2015.

Van Der Hope, E. V (2008). *Mastering niche marketing: A definitive guide to profiting from ideas in a competitive market.* Los Angeles, CA: Globalnet Publishing.

Ward, S. (n.d.) Do you have the business insurance you need? Part 1: Contents and property insurance. Retrieved from http://sbinfocanada.about.com/cs/insurance/a/insurancetypes.htm.

Ward, S. (n.d.) Starting a business: Choosing a business name. Retrieved from http://sbinfocanada.about.com.

Wojciechowski , Michele (2009). Third-party Payers: Strategies for Private Practice PTs. Available at http://www.apta.org/PTinMotion/2009/4/Feature/ThirdPartyPayers/. Accessed October 20, 2014.

Wolfe, L. (2009). HIPAA law requires you to give a privacy practices statement to all patients, sample HIPAA notice of privacy practices statement. Retrieved from http://womeninbusiness.about.com/od/insuranceandlegalissues/a/hipaa-privstate.htm.

Wolfe, L. (2009). HIPAA notice of privacy practices statement. Retrieved from http://womeninbusiness.about.com/od/insuranceandlegalissues/a/hipaa-privstate.htm.

Appendix A

Coding Algorithm

Medical Diagnoses: V57.89

Treatment Diagnoses: V54.81, V43.64, V15.88, 719.7

V57.89	Care involving other specified rehabilitation procedure	Z51.89	Encounter for other specified aftercare
V54.81	Aftercare following joint replacement	Z47.1	Aftercare following joint replacement surgery
V43.64	Hip joint replacement	Z96.649	Presence of unspecified artificial hip joint
V15.88	History of fall	Z91.81	History of falling
719.7	Difficulty in walking	R26.2	Difficulty in walking, not elsewhere classified

Assigning diagnoses for cases with six or more:

If you have more than five diagnoses, then you will need to place additional diagnoses on the medical diagnoses line. In cases of more than five diagnoses, assign diagnoses in order of importance based on the algorithm with the first few diagnoses identified on the medical diagnoses line and then the remainder of the diagnoses will be place on the treatment diagnoses line.

Example:

Medical Diagnoses: V57.89, V54.81, V43.64

V57.89	Care involving other specified rehabili-tation procedure	Z51.89	Encounter for other specified aftercare
V54.81	Aftercare following joint replacement	Z47.1	Aftercare following joint replacement surgery
V43.64	Hip joint replacement	Z96.649	Presence of unspecified artificial hip joint

Treatment Diagnoses: V15.88, 719.7, 719.45, 728.87

V15.88	History of fall	Z91.81	History of falling
719.7	Difficulty in walking	R26.2	Difficulty in walking, not elsewhere classified
719.45	Pain in joint, pelvic region and thigh	M25.559	Pain in unspecified hip
728.87	Muscle weakness (generalized)	M62.81	Muscle weakness (generalized)

Algorithm Step 1:

Encounter Type (Use for Part A and NGS Part B only)

V57.89	Care involving other specified rehabili-tation procedure	Z51.89	Encounter for other specified aftercare
V57.1	Care involving other physical therapy	Z51.89	Encounter for other specified aftercare
V57.21	Encounter for occupational therapy	Z51.89	Encounter for other specified aftercare
V57.3	Care involving speech-language therapy	Z51.89	Encounter for other specified aftercare

Algorithm Step 2: Aftercare /Late Effects

Aftercare for healing Traumatic Fractures (V54.1X). Excludes: fractures repaired with a joint (total or hemi) replacement (see V54.81) and late effect of healed traumatic fractures (see 905.0-905.5):

V54.11	Aftercare for healing traumatic fracture of upper arm	S42.309D	Unspecified fracture of shaft of humerus, unspecified arm, subsequent encounter for fracture with routine healing
V54.12	Aftercare for healing traumatic fracture of lower arm	S52.009D	Unspecified fracture of upper end of unspecified ulna, subsequent encounter for closed fracture with routine healing
V54.13	Aftercare for healing traumatic fracture of hip	S32.309D	Unspecified fracture of unspecified ilium, subsequent encounter for fracture with routine healing

(Continued)

V54.15	Aftercare for healing traumatic fracture of upper leg	S72.23XD	Displaced subtrochanteric fracture of unspecified femur, subsequent encounter for closed fracture with routine healing
V54.16	Aftercare for healing traumatic fracture of lower leg	S82.009D	Unspecified fracture of unspecified patella, subsequent encounter for closed fracture with routine healing
V54.17	Aftercare for healing traumatic fracture of vertebrae	S12.130D	Unspecified traumatic displaced spondylolisthesis of second cervical vertebra, subsequent encounter for fracture with routine healing
V54.19	Aftercare for healing traumatic fracture of other bone	S02.113D	Unspecified occipital condyle fracture, subsequent encounter for fracture with routine healing

Aftercare for healing Pathologic Fractures (V54.2X). Excludes fractures repaired with a joint (total or hemi) replacement (see V54.81):

V54.81	Aftercare following joint replacement	Z47.1	Aftercare following joint replacement surgery
V54.21	Aftercare for healing pathologic fracture of upper arm	M84.421D	Pathological fracture, right humerus, subsequent encounter for fracture with routine healing
V54.22	Aftercare for healing pathologic fracture of lower arm	M84.431D	Pathological fracture, right ulna, subsequent encounter for fracture with routine healing
V54.23	Aftercare for healing pathologic fracture of hip	M84.459D	Pathological fracture, hip, unspecified, subsequent encounter for fracture with routine healing
V54.25	Aftercare for healing pathologic fracture of upper leg	M84.453D	Pathological fracture, unspecified femur, subsequent encounter for fracture with routine healing
V54.26	Aftercare for healing pathologic fracture of lower leg	M84.469D	Pathological fracture, unspecified tibia and fibula, subsequent encounter for fracture with routine healing
V54.27	Aftercare for healing pathologic fracture of vertebrae	M84.40XD	Pathological fracture, unspecified site, subsequent encounter for fracture with routine healing
V54.29	Aftercare for healing pathologic fracture of other bone	M84.48XD	Pathological fracture, other site, subsequent encounter for fracture with routine healing

Late effect of fracture (905.X): Excludes: aftercare for a healing traumatic fracture (V54.1X), aftercare for a healing pathologic fracture (V54.2X), and late effect of pathologic fracture. Use when late effect related to a healed traumatic fracture is reason for referral or complexity impacting treatment:

905.0	Late effect of fracture of skull and face bones	S02.8XXS	Fractures of other specified skull and facial bones, sequela
905.1	Late effect of fracture of spine and trunk without mention of spinal cord lesion	S22.009S	Unspecified fracture of unspecified thoracic vertebra, sequela
905.2	Late effect of fracture of upper extremities	S42.209S	Unspecified fracture of upper end of unspecified humerus, sequela
905.3	Late effect of fracture of neck of femur	S72.009S	Fracture of unspecified part of neck of unspecified femur, sequela
905.4	Late effect of fracture of lower extremities	S82.009S	Unspecified fracture of unspecified patella, sequela
905.5	Late effect of fracture of multiple and unspecified bones	M84.40XS	Pathological fracture, unspecified site, sequela

Aftercare for joint replacements (V54.81 and V43.6X): This applies for elective joint replacements and joint replacements after a fracture. Requires two codes. First code V54.81, then code the site.

V54.81	Aftercare following joint replacement	Z47.1	Aftercare following joint replacement surgery
V43.61	Shoulder joint replacement	Z96.619	Presence of unspecified artificial shoulder joint
V43.62	Elbow joint replacement	Z96.629	Presence of unspecified artificial elbow joint
V43.63	Wrist joint replacement	Z96.639	Presence of unspecified artificial wrist joint
V43.64	Hip joint replacement	Z96.649	Presence of unspecified artificial hip joint
V43.65	Knee joint replacement	Z96.659	Presence of unspecified artificial knee joint
V43.66	Ankle joint replacement	Z96.669	Presence of unspecified artificial ankle joint
V54.89	Other orthopedic aftercare	Z47.89	Encounter for other orthopedic aftercare

Late effects of musculoskeletal and connective tissue injuries:

Aftercare for amputation (V54.89 and V49.6X or V49.7X): Requires two codes. First code V54.89, then code the site. Excludes: late effect for healed amputation (see 905.9):

905.6	Late effect of dislocation	S03.0XXS	Dislocation of jaw, sequela
905.7	Late effect of sprain and strain without mention of tendon injury	S83.90XS	Sprain of unspecified site of unspecified
905.8	Late effect of tendon injury	M67.90	Unspecified disorder of synovium and tendon, unspecified site
V54.89	Other orthopedic aftercare	Z47.89	Encounter for other orthopedic aftercare

Code first: Aftercare for orthopedic, other

Code second: Site upper extremity/lower extremity

V49.61	Thumb amputation status	Z89.019	Acquired absence of unspecified thumb
V49.62	Other finger(s) amputation status	Z89.029	Acquired absence of unspecified finger(s)
V49.63	Hand amputation status	Z89.119	Acquired absence of unspecified hand
V49.64	Wrist amputation status	Z89.129	Acquired absence of unspecified wrist
V49.65	Below elbow amputation status	Z89.219	Acquired absence of unspecified upper limb below elbow
V49.66	Above elbow amputation status	Z89.229	Acquired absence of unspecified upper limb above elbow
V49.67	Shoulder amputation status	Z89.239	Acquired absence of unspecified shoulder
V49.71	Great toe amputation status	Z89.419	Acquired absence of unspecified great toe
V49.72	Other toe(s) amputation status	Z89.429	Acquired absence of other toe(s), unspecified side
V49.73	Foot amputation status	Z89.439	Acquired absence of unspecified foot
V49.74	Ankle amputation status	Z89.449	Acquired absence of unspecified ankle
V49.75	Below knee amputation status	Z89.519	Acquired absence of unspecified leg below knee
V49.76	Above knee amputation status	Z89.619	Acquired absence of unspecified leg above knee
V49.77	Hip amputation status	Z89.629	Acquired absence of unspecified hip joint

Late effect of amputation (905.9): Use when late effect related to an old amputation is reason for referral or complexity impacting treatment:

905.9	Late effect of traumatic amputation	S48.919S	Complete traumatic amputation of unspecified shoulder and upper arm, level unspecified, sequela

Excludes: late amputation stump complication (997.60-997.69)

V58.42	Aftercare following surgery for neoplasm	Z48.3	Aftercare following surgery for neoplasm
V58.43	Aftercare following surgery for injury and trauma	Z48.89	
V54.10	Aftercare for healing traumatic fracture of arm, unspecified	S52.90XD	Unspecified fracture of unspecified forearm, subsequent encounter for closed fracture with routine healing
V54.11	Aftercare for healing traumatic fracture of upper arm	S42.116D	Nondisplaced fracture of body of scapula, unspecified shoulder, subsequent encounter for fracture with routine healing
V54.12	Aftercare for healing traumatic fracture of lower arm	S52.009E	Unspecified fracture of upper end of unspecified ulna, subsequent encounter for closed fracture with routine healing
V54.13	Aftercare for healing traumatic fracture of hip	S32.309D	Unspecified fracture of unspecified ilium, subsequent encounter for fracture with routine healing
V54.14	Aftercare for healing traumatic fracture of leg, unspecified	S82.90XD	Unspecified fracture of unspecified lower leg, subsequent encounter for closed fracture with routine healing
V54.15	Aftercare for healing traumatic fracture of upper leg	S72.23XD	Displaced subtrochanteric fracture of unspecified femur, subsequent encounter for closed fracture with routine healing
V54.16	Aftercare for healing traumatic fracture of lower leg	S82.009D	Unspecified fracture of unspecified patella, subsequent encounter for closed fracture with routine healing
V54.17	Aftercare for healing traumatic fracture of vertebrae	S12.001D	Unspecified nondisplaced fracture of first cervical vertebra, subsequent encounter for fracture with routine healing
V54.19	Aftercare for healing traumatic fracture of other bone	S32.19XD	Other fracture of sacrum, subsequent encounter for fracture with routine healing
V58.44	Aftercare following organ transplant	Z48.298	Encounter for aftercare following other organ transplant
V42.0	Kidney replaced by transplant	Z94.0	Kidney transplant status
V42.1	Heart replaced by transplant	Z94.1	Heart transplant status
V42.2	Heart valve replaced by transplant	Z95.3	Presence of xenogenic heart valve

(Continued)

V42.3	Skin replaced by transplant	Z94.5	Skin transplant status
V42.4	Bone replaced by transplant	Z94.6	Bone transplant status
V42.5	Cornea replaced by transplant	Z94.7	Corneal transplant status
V42.6	Lung replaced by transplant	Z94.2	Lung transplant status
V42.7	Liver replaced by transplant	Z94.4	Liver transplant status
V42.9	Unspecified organ or tissue replaced by transplant	Z94.9	Transplanted organ and tissue status, unspecified
V42.81	Bone marrow replaced by transplant	Z94.81	Bone marrow transplant status
V42.82	Peripheral stem cells replaced by transplant	Z94.84	Stem cells transplant status
V42.83	Pancreas replaced by transplant	Z94.83	Pancreas transplant status
V42.84	Organ or tissue replaced by transplant, intestines	Z94.82	Intestine transplant status
V42.89	Other specified organ or tissue replaced by transplant	Z94.89	Other transplanted organ and tissue status
V58.71	Aftercare following surgery of the sense organs, NEC	Z48.810	Encounter for surgical aftercare following surgery on the sense organs
V58.72	Aftercare following surgery of the nervous system, NEC	Z48.811	Encounter for surgical aftercare following surgery on the nervous system
V58.73	Aftercare following surgery of the circulatory system, NEC	Z48.812	Encounter for surgical aftercare following surgery on the circulatory system
V58.74	Aftercare following surgery of the respiratory system, NEC	Z48.813	Encounter for surgical aftercare following surgery on the respiratory system
V58.75	Aftercare following surgery of the teeth, oral cavity and digestive system, NEC	Z48.814	Encounter for surgical aftercare following surgery on the teeth or oral cavity
V58.76	Aftercare following surgery of the genitourinary system, NEC	Z48.816	Encounter for surgical aftercare following surgery on the genitourinary system
V58.77	Aftercare following surgery of the skin and subcutaneous tissue, NEC	Z48.817	Encounter for surgical aftercare following surgery on the skin and subcutaneous tissue
V58.78	Aftercare following surgery of the musculoskeletal system, NEC	Z48.89	Encounter for other specified surgical aftercare

Acquired absence of organ (V45.7X)

V45.71	Acquired absence of breast and nipple	Z90.10	Acquired absence of unspecified breast and nipple
V45.72	Acquired absence of intestine (large) (small)	Z90.49	Acquired absence of other specified parts of digestive tract
V45.73	Acquired absence of kidney	Z90.5	Acquired absence of kidney

(Continued)

V45.74	Acquired absence of organ, other parts of urinary tract	Z90.6	Acquired absence of other parts of urinary tract
V45.75	Acquired absence of organ, stomach	Z90.3	Acquired absence of stomach [part of]
V45.76	Acquired absence of organ, lung	Z90.2	Acquired absence of lung [part of]
V45.77	Acquired absence of organ, genital organs	Z90.79	Acquired absence of other genital organ(s)
V45.78	Acquired absence of organ, eye	Z90.01	Acquired absence of eye

Late Effects of Cerebrovascular Disease (438.0-438.9): This category is to be used to indicate conditions in 430-437 as the cause of the late effects. The "late effects" include conditions specified as such, or as sequelae, which may occur at any time after the onset of the causal condition.

438.0	Late effects of cerebrovascular disease, cognitive deficits	I69.91	Cognitive deficits following unspecified cerebrovascular disease
438.11	Late effects of cerebrovascular disease, aphasia	I69.920	Aphasia following unspecified cerebrovascular disease
438.12	Late effects of cerebrovascular disease, dysphasia	I69.921	Dysphasia following unspecified cerebrovascular disease
438.13	Late effects of cerebrovascular disease, dysarthria	I69.922	Dysarthria following unspecified cerebrovascular disease
438.14	Late effects of cerebrovascular disease, fluency disorder	I69.923	Fluency disorder following unspecified cerebrovascular disease
438.21	Late effects of cerebrovascular disease, hemiplegia affecting dominant side	I69.951	Hemiplegia and hemiparesis following unspecified cerebrovascular disease affecting right dominant side
438.32	Late effects of cerebrovascular disease, monoplegia of upper limb affecting non-dominant side	I69.933	Monoplegia of upper limb following unspecified cerebrovascular disease affecting right non-dominant side
438.7	Late effects of cerebrovascular disease, disturbances of vision	I69.998	Other sequelae following unspecified cerebrovascular disease
438.81	Other late effects of cerebrovascular disease, apraxia	I69.990	Apraxia following unspecified cerebrovascular disease
438.82	Other late effects of cerebrovascular disease, dysphagia	I69.991	Dysphagia following unspecified cerebrovascular disease
438.83	Other late effects of cerebrovascular disease, facial weakness	I69.992	Facial weakness following unspecified cerebrovascular disease
438.84	Other late effects of cerebrovascular disease, ataxia	I69.993	Ataxia following unspecified cerebrovascular disease
438.85	Other late effects of cerebrovascular disease, vertigo	I69.998	Other sequelae following unspecified cerebrovascular disease
438.89	Other late effects of cerebrovascular disease	I69.898	Other sequelae of other cerebrovascular disease

Late effects of injuries (906.X) to skin/subcutaneous tissue:

906.0	Late effect of open wound of head, neck, and trunk	S01.90XS	Unspecified open wound of unspecified part of head, sequela
906.1	Late effect of open wound of extremities without mention of tendon injury	S41.009S	Unspecified open wound of unspecified shoulder, sequela
906.2	Late effect of superficial injury	S00.90XS	Unspecified superficial injury of unspecified part of head, sequela
906.3	Late effect of contusion	S20.20XS	Contusion of thorax, unspecified, sequela
906.4	Late effect of crushing	S07.9XXS	Crushing injury of head, part unspecified, sequela

Late effect of injuries to the nervous system (907.X):

907.0	Late effect of intracranial injury without mention of skull fracture	S06.9X9S	Unspecified intracranial injury with loss of consciousness of unspecified duration, sequela
907.1	Late effect of injury to cranial nerve	S04.9XXS	Injury of unspecified cranial nerve, sequela
907.2	Late effect of spinal cord injury	S14.109S	Unspecified injury at unspecified level of cervical spinal cord, sequela
907.3	Late effect of injury to nerve root(s), spinal plexus(es), and other nerves of trunk	S34.9XXS	Injury of nerve root of lumbar spine, sequela
907.4	Late effect of injury to peripheral nerve of shoulder girdle and upper limb	S44.90XS	Injury of unspecified nerve at shoulder and upper arm level, unspecified arm, sequela
907.5	Late effect of injury to peripheral nerve of pelvic girdle and lower limb	S74.90XS	Injury of unspecified nerve at hip and thigh level, unspecified leg, sequela

Late effect of burns (906.X): First code the residual condition such as contracture or scar and then the appropriate late effect code:

906.5	Late effect of burn of eye, face, head, and neck	T20.00XS	Burn of unspecified degree of head, face, and neck, unspecified site, sequela
906.6	Late effect of burn of wrist and hand	T23.009S	Burn of unspecified degree of unspecified hand, unspecified site, sequela
906.7	Late effect of burn of other extremities	T22.00XS	Burn of unspecified degree of shoulder and upper limb, except wrist and hand, unspecified site, sequela
906.8	Late effect of burns of other specified sites	T21.00XS	Burn of unspecified degree of trunk, unspecified site, sequela

Late effect of other and unspecified injuries (908.x):

908.0	Late effect of internal injury to chest	S27.9XXS	Injury of unspecified intrathoracic organ, sequela
908.1	Late effect of internal injury to intra-abdominal organs	S36.90XS	Unspecified injury of unspecified intra-abdominal organ, sequela
908.2	Late effect of internal injury to other internal organs	S37.90XS	Unspecified injury of unspecified urinary and pelvic organ, sequela
908.3	Late effect of injury to blood vessel of head, neck, and extremities	S09.0XXS	Injury of blood vessels of head, not elsewhere classified, sequela
908.4	Late effect of injury to blood vessel of thorax, abdomen, and pelvis	S25.90XS	Unspecified injury of unspecified blood vessel of thorax, sequela
908.5	Late effect of foreign body in orifice	T15.90XS	Foreign body on external eye, part unspecified, unspecified eye, sequela
908.6	Late effect of certain complications of trauma	T79.9XXS	Unspecified early complication of trauma, sequela
908.9	Late effect of unspecified injury	S16.9XXS	Unspecified injury of muscle, fascia and tendon at neck level, sequela

Algorithm Step 3: Pressure Ulcer/Non Pressure Ulcer

Pressure Ulcer (707.0X and 707.2X): Requires two codes. First code site. Second code stage.

Code first: Site

707.01	Pressure ulcer, elbow	L89.009	Pressure ulcer of unspecified elbow, unspecified stage
707.02	Pressure ulcer, upper back	L89.119	Pressure ulcer of right upper back, unspecified stage
707.03	Pressure ulcer, lower back	L89.139	Pressure ulcer of right lower back, unspecified stage
707.04	Pressure ulcer, hip	L89.209	Pressure ulcer of unspecified hip, unspecified stage
707.05	Pressure ulcer, buttock	L89.309	Pressure ulcer of unspecified buttock, unspecified stage
707.06	Pressure ulcer, ankle	L89.509	Pressure ulcer of unspecified ankle, unspecified stage
707.07	Pressure ulcer, heel	L89.609	Pressure ulcer of unspecified heel, unspecified stage
707.09	Pressure ulcer, other site	L89.899	Pressure ulcer of other site, unspecified stage

Code second: Stage

707.23	Pressure ulcer, stage III	N/A	Not Available
707.24	Pressure ulcer, stage IV	N/A	Not Available

Algorithm Step 3: Non Pressure Ulcer

Ulcer of lower limbs, except pressure ulcer (707.1X):

Includes: ulcer, chronic, of lower limb.

Code, if applicable, any causal condition first: atherosclerosis of the extremities with ulceration (440.23), chronic venous hypertension with ulcer (459.31),

440.23	Atherosclerosis of native arteries of the extremities with ulceration	I70.25	Atherosclerosis of native arteries of other extremities with ulceration
459.31	Chronic venous hypertension with ulcer	I87.319	Chronic venous hypertension (idiopathic) with ulcer of unspecified lower extremity
459.33	Chronic venous hypertension with ulcer and inflammation	I87.339	Chronic venous hypertension (idiopathic) with ulcer and inflammation of unspecified lower extremity
249.80	Secondary diabetes mellitus with other specified manifestations, not stated as uncontrolled, or unspecified	E08.618	Diabetes mellitus due to underlying condition with other diabetic arthropathy
249.81	Secondary diabetes mellitus with other specified manifestations, uncontrolled	E08.69	Diabetes mellitus due to underlying condition with other specified complication
250.80	Diabetes with other specified manifestations, type II or unspecified type, not stated as uncontrolled	E11.618	Type 2 diabetes mellitus with other diabetic arthropathy
250.81	Diabetes with other specified manifestations, type I [juvenile type], not stated as uncontrolled	E10.618	Type 1 diabetes mellitus with other diabetic arthropathy
250.82	Diabetes with other specified manifestations, type II or unspecified type, uncontrolled	E11.69	Type 2 diabetes mellitus with other specified complication with: E11.65 Type 2 diabetes mellitus with hyperglycemia
250.83	Diabetes with other specified manifestations, type I [juvenile type], uncontrolled	E10.69	Type 1 diabetes mellitus with other specified complication with: E10.65 Type 1 diabetes mellitus with hyperglycemia
459.11	Postphlebetic syndrome with ulcer	I87.019	Post thrombotic syndrome with ulcer of unspecified lower extremity
459.13	Postphlebetic syndrome with ulcer and inflammation	I87.039	Post thrombotic syndrome with ulcer and inflammation of unspecified lower extremity

Then, code location.

707.10	Ulcer of lower limb, un-specified	L97.909	Non-pressure chronic ulcer of unspecified part of unspecified lower leg with unspecified severity
707.11	Ulcer of thigh	L97.109	Non-pressure chronic ulcer of unspecified thigh with unspecified severity
707.12	Ulcer of calf	L97.209	Non-pressure chronic ulcer of unspecified calf with unspecified severity
707.13	Ulcer of ankle	L97.309	Non-pressure chronic ulcer of unspecified ankle with unspecified severity
707.14	Ulcer of heel and midfoot	L97.409	Non-pressure chronic ulcer of unspecified heel and midfoot with unspecified severity
707.15	Ulcer of other part of foot	L97.509	Non-pressure chronic ulcer of other part of unspecified foot with unspecified severity
707.19	Ulcer of other part of lower limb	L97.809	Non-pressure chronic ulcer of other part of unspecified lower leg with unspecified severity

Speech Codes- Dysphagia and Other

787.21	Dysphagia, oral phase	R13.11	Dysphagia, oral phase
787.22	Dysphagia, oropharyngeal phase	R13.12	Dysphagia, oropharyngeal phase
787.23	Dysphagia, pharyngeal phase	R13.13	Dysphagia, pharyngeal phase
787.24	Dysphagia, pharyngoesophageal phase	R13.14	Dysphagia, pharyngoesophageal phase
787.29	Other dysphagia	R13.19	Other dysphagia
780.93	Memory loss	R41.2	Retrograde amnesia
784.3	Aphasia	R47.01	Aphasia
784.41	Aphonia	R49.1	Aphonia
784.42	Dysphonia	R49.0	Dysphonia
784.51	Dysarthria	R47.1	Dysarthria and anarthria
784.52	Fluency disorder in conditions classified elsewhere	R47.82	Fluency disorder in conditions classified elsewhere
784.60	Symbolic dysfunction, unspecified	R48.9	Unspecified symbolic dysfunctions
784.61	Alexia and dyslexia	R48.0	Dyslexia and alexia
784.69	Other symbolic dysfunction	R48.8	Other symbolic dysfunctions
314.00	Attention deficit disorder without mention of hyperactivity	F90.9	Attention-deficit hyperactivity disorder, unspecified type
314.01	Attention deficit disorder with hyperactivity	F90.1	Attention-deficit hyperactivity disorder, predominantly hyperactive type
780.93	Memory loss	R41.2	Retrograde amnesia
331.83	Mild cognitive impairment, so stated	G31.84	Mild cognitive impairment, so stated

(Continued)

437.7	Transient global amnesia	G45.4	Transient global amnesia
781.8	Neurologic neglect syndrome	R41.4	Neurologic neglect syndrome
799.51	Attention or concentration deficit	R41.840	Attention and concentration deficit
799.52	Cognitive communication deficit	R41.841	Cognitive communication deficit
799.53	Visuospatial deficit	R41.842	Visuospatial deficit
799.54	Psychomotor deficit	R41.843	Psychomotor deficit
799.55	Frontal lobe and executive function deficit	R41.844	Frontal lobe and executive function deficit
799.59	Other signs and symptoms involving cognition	R41.89	Other symptoms and signs involving cognitive functions and awareness

Musculoskeletal/Nervous System

V13.51	Personal history of pathologic fracture	Z87.311	Personal history of (healed) other pathological fracture
V13.52	Personal history of stress fracture	Z87.312	Personal history of (healed) stress fracture
V15.51	Personal history of traumatic fracture	Z87.81	Personal history of (healed) traumatic fracture
V15.52	Personal history of traumatic brain injury	Z87.820	Personal history of traumatic brain injury

**If providing care for late effect of TBI, assign appropriate code

907.0	Late effect of intracranial injury without mention of skull fracture	S06.9X9S	Unspecified intracranial injury with loss of consciousness of unspecified duration, sequela

**If providing care for late effect of nontraumatic brain hemorrhage, apply appropriate 438.XX code
Cannot be coded as primary diagnosis

V15.88	History of fall	Z91.81	History of falling
V46.11	Dependence on respirator, status	Z99.11	Dependence on respirator [ventilator] status
338.21	Chronic pain due to trauma	G89.21	Chronic pain due to trauma
338.22	Chronic post-thoracotomy pain	G89.22	Chronic post-thoracotomy pain
338.28	Other chronic postoperative pain	G89.28	Other chronic postprocedural pain
338.29	Other chronic pain	G89.29	Other chronic pain
338.3	Neoplasm related pain (acute) (chronic)	G89.3	Neoplasm related pain (acute) (chronic)
342.01	Flaccid hemiplegia and hemiparesis affecting dominant side	G81.01	Flaccid hemiplegia affecting right dominant side G81.02 Flaccid hemiplegia affecting left dominant side

This category is to be used when hemiplegia is reported without further specification, or is stated to be old or long-standing but of unspecified cause. The category is also for use in multiple coding to identify these types of hemiplegia resulting from any cause. Excludes: congenital, hemiplegia due to late effect of cerebrovascular accident (438.XX), infantile NOS

| 342.02 | Flaccid hemiplegia and hemiparesis affecting nondominant side | G81.03 | Flaccid hemiplegia affecting right nondominant side G81.04 Flaccid hemiplegia affecting left nondominant side |

This category is to be used when hemiplegia is reported without further specification, or is stated to be old or long-standing but of unspecified cause. The category is also for use in multiple coding to identify these types of hemiplegia resulting from any cause. Excludes: congenital, hemiplegia due to late effect of cerebrovascular accident (438.xx), infantile NOS

| 342.11 | Spastic hemiplegia and hemiparesis affecting dominant side | G81.11 | Spastic hemiplegia affecting right dominant side G81.12 Spastic hemiplegia affecting left dominant side |

This category is to be used when hemiplegia is reported without further specification, or is stated to be old or long-standing but of unspecified cause. The category is also for use in multiple coding to identify these types of hemiplegia resulting from any cause. Excludes: congenital, hemiplegia due to late effect of cerebrovascular accident (438.xx), infantile NOS

| 342.12 | Spastic hemiplegia and hemiparesis affecting nondominant side | G81.13 | Spastic hemiplegia affecting right nondominant side G81.14 Spastic hemiplegia affecting left nondominant side |

This category is to be used when hemiplegia is reported without further specification, or is stated to be old or long-standing but of unspecified cause. The category is also for use in multiple coding to identify these types of hemiplegia resulting from any cause. Excludes: congenital, hemiplegia due to late effect of cerebrovascular accident (438.xx), infantile NOS

| 342.81 | Other specified hemiplegia and hemiparesis affecting dominant side | G81.91 | Hemiplegia, unspecified affecting right dominant side G81.92 Hemiplegia, unspecified affecting left dominant side |

This category is to be used when hemiplegia is reported without further specification, or is stated to be old or long-standing but of unspecified cause. The category is also for use in multiple coding to identify these types of hemiplegia resulting from any cause. Excludes: congenital, hemiplegia due to late effect of cerebrovascular accident (438.xx), infantile NOS

| 342.82 | Other specified hemiplegia and hemiparesis affecting nondominant side | G81.93 | Hemiplegia, unspecified affecting right nondominant side G81.94 Hemiplegia, unspecified affecting left nondominant side |

This category is to be used when hemiplegia is reported without further specification, or is stated to be old or long-standing but of unspecified cause. The category is also for use in multiple coding to identify these types of hemiplegia resulting from any cause. Excludes: congenital, hemiplegia due to late effect of cerebrovascular accident (438.xx), infantile NOS

| 344.31 | Monoplegia of lower limb affecting dominant side | G83.11 | Monoplegia of lower limb affecting right dominant side G83.12 Monoplegia of lower limb affecting left dominant side |

This category is to be used when the condition is reported without further specification, or is stated to be old or long-standing but of unspecified cause. The category is also for use in multiple coding to identify these conditions resulting from any cause.

| 344.32 | Monoplegia of lower limb affecting nondominant side | G83.13 | Monoplegia of lower limb affecting right nondominant side G83.14 Monoplegia of lower limb affecting left nondominant side |

This category is to be used when the condition is reported without further specification, or is stated to be old or long-standing but of unspecified cause. The category is also for use in multiple coding to identify these conditions resulting from any cause.

| 344.41 | Monoplegia of upper limb affecting dominant side | G83.21 | Monoplegia of upper limb affecting right dominant side G83.22 Monoplegia of upper limb affecting left dominant side |

This category is to be used when the condition is reported without further specification, or is stated to be old or long-standing but of unspecified cause. The category is also for use in multiple coding to identify these conditions resulting from any cause.

| 344.42 | Monoplegia of upper limb affecting nondominant side | G83.23 | Monoplegia of upper limb affecting right nondominant side G83.24 Monoplegia of upper limb affecting left nondominant side |

This category is to be used when the condition is reported without further specification, or is stated to be old or long-standing but of unspecified cause. The category is also for use in multiple coding to identify these conditions resulting from any cause.

719.7	Difficulty in walking	R26.2	Difficulty in walking, not elsewhere classified
723.1	Cervicalgia	M54.2	Cervicalgia
724.1	Pain in thoracic spine	M54.6	Pain in thoracic spine
724.2	Lumbago	M54.5	Low back pain
724.5	Backache, unspecified	M54.9	Dorsalgia, unspecified
728.85	Spasm of muscle	M62.838	Other muscle spasm

(Continued)

728.87	Muscle weakness (generalized)	M62.81	Muscle weakness (generalized)
729.5	Pain in limb	M79.609	Pain in unspecified limb
729.81	Swelling of limb	M79.89	Other specified soft tissue disorders
735.0	Hallux valgus (acquired)	M20.10	Hallux valgus (acquired), unspecified foot
735.1	Hallux varus (acquired)	M20.30	Hallux varus (acquired), unspecified foot
735.2	Hallux rigidus	M20.20	Hallux rigidus, unspecified foot
735.3	Hallux malleus	M20.40	Other hammer toe(s) (acquired), unspecified foot
735.4	Other hammer toe (acquired)	M20.40	Other hammer toe(s) (acquired), unspecified foot
735.5	Claw toe (acquired)	M20.5X9	Other deformities of toe(s) (acquired), unspecified foot
735.8	Other acquired deformities of toe	M20.5X9	Other deformities of toe(s) (acquired), unspecified foot
735.9	Unspecified acquired deformity of toe	M20.60	Acquired deformities of toe(s), unspecified, unspecified foot
736.00	Unspecified deformity of forearm, excluding fingers	M21.939	Unspecified acquired deformity of unspecified forearm
736.01	Cubitus valgus (acquired)	M21.029	Valgus deformity, not elsewhere classified, unspecified elbow
736.02	Cubitus varus (acquired)	M21.129	Varus deformity, not elsewhere classified, unspecified elbow
736.03	Valgus deformity of wrist (acquired)	M21.839	Other specified acquired deformities of unspecified forearm
736.04	Varus deformity of wrist (acquired)	M21.839	Other specified acquired deformities of unspecified forearm
736.05	Wrist drop (acquired)	M21.339	Wrist drop, unspecified wrist
736.06	Claw hand (acquired)	M21.519	Acquired clawhand, unspecified hand
736.07	Club hand, acquired	M21.529	Acquired clubhand, unspecified hand
736.09	Other acquired deformities of forearm, excluding fingers	M21.839	Other specified acquired deformities of unspecified forearm
736.1	Mallet finger	M20.019	Mallet finger of unspecified finger(s)
736.21	Boutonniere deformity	M20.029	Boutonnière deformity of unspecified finger(s)
736.22	Swan-neck deformity	M20.039	Swan-neck deformity of unspecified finger(s)
736.29	Other acquired deformities of finger	M20.099	Other deformity of finger(s), unspecified finger(s)
736.31	Coxa valga (acquired)	M21.059	Valgus deformity, not elsewhere classified, unspecified hip
736.32	Coxa vara (acquired)	M21.159	Varus deformity, not elsewhere classified, unspecified

(Continued)

736.39	Other acquired deformities of hip	M21.859	Other specified acquired deformities of unspecified thigh
736.41	Genu valgum (acquired)	M21.069	Valgus deformity, not elsewhere classified, unspecified knee
736.42	Genu varum (acquired)	M21.169	Varus deformity, not elsewhere classified, unspecified knee
736.5	Genu recurvatum (acquired)	M21.869	Other specified acquired deformities of unspecified lower leg
736.6	Other acquired deformities of knee	M21.869	Other specified acquired deformities of unspecified lower leg
736.71	Acquired equinovarus deformity	M21.549	Acquired clubfoot, unspecified foot
736.72	Equinus deformity of foot, acquired	M21.6X9	Other acquired deformities of unspecified foot
736.73	Cavus deformity of foot, acquired	M21.6X9	Other acquired deformities of unspecified foot
736.74	Claw foot, acquired	M21.539	Acquired clawfoot, unspecified foot
736.75	Cavovarus deformity of foot, acquired	M21.6X9	Other acquired deformities of unspecified foot
736.76	Other acquired calcaneus deformity	M21.6X9	Other acquired deformities of unspecified foot
736.9	Acquired deformity of limb, site unspecified	M21.90	Unspecified acquired deformity of unspecified limb
736.81	Unequal leg length (acquired)	M21.759	Unequal limb length (acquired), unspecified femur
737.10	Kyphosis (acquired) (postural)	M40.00	Postural kyphosis, site unspecified
737.20	Lordosis (acquired) (postural)	M40.40	Postural lordosis, site unspecified
737.30	Scoliosis [and kyphoscoliosis], idiopathic	M41.20	Other idiopathic scoliosis, site unspecified
738.6	Acquired deformity of pelvis	M95.5	Acquired deformity of pelvis
780.4	Dizziness and giddiness	R42	Dizziness and giddiness
780.96	Generalized pain	R52	Pain, unspecified
781.0	Abnormal involuntary movements	R25.9	Unspecified abnormal involuntary movements
781.2	Abnormality of gait	R26.9	Unspecified abnormalities of gait and mobility
781.3	Lack of coordination	R27.9	Unspecified lack of coordination
781.8	Neurologic neglect syndrome	R41.4	Neurologic neglect syndrome
781.92	Abnormal posture	R29.3	Abnormal posture
782.0	Disturbance of skin sensation	R20.9	Unspecified disturbances of skin sensation
782.3	Edema	R60.9	Edema, unspecified
783.21	Loss of weight	R63.4	Abnormal weight loss
783.22	Underweight	R63.6	Underweight
783.3	Feeding difficulties and mismanagement	R63.3	Feeding difficulties

(Continued)

784.0	Headache	R51	Headache
784.99	Other symptoms involving head and neck	R06.89	Other abnormalities of breathing
786.2	Cough	R05	Cough
788.31	Urge incontinence	N39.41	Urge incontinence
788.32	Stress incontinence, male	N39.3	Stress incontinence (female) (male)
788.33	Mixed incontinence (male) (female)	N39.46	Mixed incontinence
788.34	Incontinence without sensory awareness	N39.42	Incontinence without sensory awareness
788.35	Post-void dribbling	N39.43	Post-void dribbling
788.36	Nocturnal enuresis	N39.44	Nocturnal enuresis
788.37	Continuous leakage	N39.45	Continuous leakage
788.38	Overflow incontinence	N39.490	Overflow incontinence
788.39	Other urinary incontinence	N39.498	Other specified urinary incontinence

Algorithm Step 4: Complexities and Co-morbidities.

All codes assigned in step 4 must be MD diagnosed in the medical record. DO NOT TRY TO CODE YOURSELF.

Complexities and co-morbidities are not the diagnoses therapy is treating and are instead diagnoses that may impact treatment; therefore, these diagnoses are only added in step four of the algorithm and should not be placed as primary diagnoses. Instead, comorbidities and complexities should be assigned as the last diagnoses; therefore, they should only be assigned on the treatment line and should be added last. It is also imperative that the evaluation documentation support the impact of the complexity or co-morbidity. For example, a patient with long standing RA and significant hand acquired deformities and weakness may be in therapy for a recent LE fracture and the RA and related deficits is significantly impacting the patient's ability to use an ambulation AD. The documentation needs to note the hand weakness and deformities. Often we see cardiopulmonary complexities listed in the diagnoses but the evaluation documentation does not address the impact. It is recommended that vital signs and functional activity tolerance be documented.

APPENDIX B

Clarifications on Coding

1. I have a complicated patient that has new amputations below the elbow on one arm and a middle finger on the other arm but also has old healed below knee amputations. How do I code the aftercare for the healing amputations as well as the impact of the old healed below knee amputations?

Aftercare for healing amputations requires two codes. First code V54.89 and then code the site of the amputation (V49.6X for upper extremity and V49.7X for lower extremity. In this case code V54.89, V49.62 and V49.65

V54.89	Other orthopedic aftercare	Z47.89	Encounter for other orthopedic aftercare
V49.62	Other finger(s) amputation status	Z89.029	Acquired absence of unspecified finger(s)
V49.65	Below elbow amputation status	Z89.219	Acquired absence of unspecified upper limb below elbow

Late effects of healed amputations only require one code, 905.9. In this case code 905.9 for the healed below knee amputations that are impacting care.

2. I noticed that all of the surgical aftercare codes (V58.42-V58.44 and V58.71-V58.78) have acute ICD-9 codes. Why are the acute codes listed?

V58.42	Aftercare following surgery for neoplasm	Z48.3	Aftercare following surgery for neoplasm
V58.43	Aftercare following surgery for injury and trauma	Z48.89	Encounter for other specified surgical aftercare
V58.44	Aftercare following organ transplant	Z48.298	Encounter for aftercare following other organ transplant
V58.71	Aftercare following surgery of the sense organs, NEC	Z48.810	Encounter for surgical aftercare following surgery on the sense organs
V58.72	Aftercare following surgery of the nervous system, NEC	Z48.811	Encounter for surgical aftercare following surgery on the nervous system
V58.73	Aftercare following surgery of the circulatory system, NEC	Z48.812	Encounter for surgical aftercare following surgery on the circulatory system
V58.74	Aftercare following surgery of the respiratory system, NEC	Z48.813	Encounter for surgical aftercare following surgery on the respiratory system
V58.75	Aftercare following surgery of the teeth, oral cavity and digestive system, NEC	Z48.814	Encounter for surgical aftercare following surgery on the teeth or oral cavity
V58.76	Aftercare following surgery of the genitourinary system, NEC	Z48.816	Encounter for surgical aftercare following surgery on the genitourinary system
V58.77	Aftercare following surgery of the skin and subcutaneous tissue, NEC	Z48.817	Encounter for surgical aftercare following surgery on the skin and subcutaneous tissue
V58.78	Aftercare following surgery of the musculoskeletal system, NEC	Z48.89	Encounter for other specified surgical aftercare

The acute ICD-9 codes are the acute diagnoses that are the conditions classifiable under the surgical code to assist you in choosing the correct aftercare surgical code. For example: if the patient's hospital discharge summary reports the patient had a carotid endarterectomy for carotid artery occlusion (433.10) the acute condition, 433.10, is a condition classifiable to V58.73, aftercare following surgery of the circulatory system (ICD-9: 390-459).

433.10	Occlusion and stenosis of carotid artery without mention of cerebral infarction	I65.29	Occlusion and stenosis of unspecified carotid artery
V58.73	Aftercare following surgery of the circulatory system, NEC	Z48.812	Encounter for surgical aftercare following surgery on the circulatory system

1. My patient had an inguinal hernia (ICD-9: 550.90) repair and is now receiving therapy. How do I code the surgical aftercare?

The diagnosis for which surgery was done was 550.90 falls into the digestive system so the correct aftercare code is V58.75, aftercare following surgery of the teeth, oral cavity, and digestive system. The acute ICD-9 codes have been included after the surgical aftercare codes to assist you in choosing the correct surgical aftercare code.

550.90	Inguinal hernia, without mention of obstruction or gangrene, unilateral or unspecified (not specified as recurrent)	K40.90	Unilateral inguinal hernia, without obstruction or gangrene, not specified as recurrent
V58.75	Aftercare following surgery of the teeth, oral cavity and digestive system, NEC	Z48.814	Encounter for surgical aftercare following surgery on the teeth or oral cavity

1. My patient had surgery for a traumatic tibia fracture. Do I code v58.43, aftercare following surgery for injury or trauma, V58.78, aftercare following surgery of the musculoskeletal system, or V54.16, aftercare for healing traumatic fracture of lower leg?

V58.43	Aftercare following surgery for injury and trauma	Z48.89	Encounter for other specified surgical aftercare
V58.78	Aftercare following surgery of the musculoskeletal system, NEC	Z48.89	Encounter for other specified surgical aftercare
V54.16	Aftercare for healing traumatic fracture of lower leg	S82.009D	Unspecified fracture of unspecified patella, subsequent encounter for closed fracture with routine healing

Code V54.16, aftercare for healing traumatic fracture of lower leg in this scenario.

ICD-9 code V58.43, aftercare following surgery for injury or trauma excludes aftercare for healing traumatic fractures, V54.10-V54.19

V54.10	Aftercare for healing traumatic fracture of arm, unspecified	S52.90XD	Unspecified fracture of unspecified forearm, subsequent encounter for closed fracture with routine healing
V54.11	Aftercare for healing traumatic fracture of upper arm	S42.116D	Nondisplaced fracture of body of scapula, unspecified shoulder, subsequent encounter for fracture with routine healing
V54.12	Aftercare for healing traumatic fracture of lower arm	S52.009E	Unspecified fracture of upper end of unspecified ulna, subsequent encounter for closed fracture with routine healing
V54.13	Aftercare for healing traumatic fracture of hip	S32.309D	Unspecified fracture of unspecified ilium, subsequent encounter for fracture with routine healing

(Continued)

V54.14	Aftercare for healing traumatic fracture of leg, unspecified	S82.90XD	Unspecified fracture of unspecified lower leg, subsequent encounter for closed fracture with routine healing
V54.15	Aftercare for healing traumatic fracture of upper leg	S72.23XD	Displaced subtrochanteric fracture of unspecified femur, subsequent encounter for closed fracture with routine healing
V54.16	Aftercare for healing traumatic fracture of lower leg	S82.009D	Unspecified fracture of unspecified patella, subsequent encounter for closed fracture with routine healing
V54.17	Aftercare for healing traumatic fracture of vertebrae	S12.001D	Unspecified nondisplaced fracture of first cervical vertebra, subsequent encounter for fracture with routine healing
V54.19	Aftercare for healing traumatic fracture of other bone	S32.19XD	Other fracture of sacrum, subsequent encounter for fracture with routine healing

ICD-9 code V58.78, aftercare following surgery of the musculoskeletal system excludes aftercare for healing traumatic fractures, healing pathologic fractures, aftercare for joint replacements, V54.01-V54.9

V54.01	Encounter for removal of internal fixation device	Z47.2	Encounter for removal of internal fixation device
V54.02	Encounter for lengthening/adjustment of growth rod	Z51.89	Encounter for other specified aftercare
V54.09	Other aftercare involving internal fixation device	Z51.89	Encounter for other specified aftercare
V54.10	Aftercare for healing traumatic fracture of arm, unspecified	S52.90XD	Unspecified fracture of unspecified forearm, subsequent encounter for closed fracture with routine healing
V54.11	Aftercare for healing traumatic fracture of upper arm	S42.116D	Nondisplaced fracture of body of scapula, unspecified shoulder, subsequent encounter for fracture with routine healing
V54.12	Aftercare for healing traumatic fracture of lower arm	S52.009E	Unspecified fracture of upper end of unspecified ulna, subsequent encounter for closed fracture with routine healing
V54.9	Unspecified orthopedic aftercare	Z51.89	Encounter for other specified aftercare

1. What code do I use for late effects of a subdural hemorrhage that are impacting my current treatment?

In order to correctly code late effects of any type of brain hemorrhage, it is imperative to know if the cause of the was traumatic (ICD-9: 850-854) or non-traumatic (430-437).

If the cause was traumatic (TBI ICD-9 850-854), code 907.0, Late effect of intracranial injury without mention of skull fracture.

907.0	Late effect of intracranial injury with-out mention of skull fracture	S06.9X9S	Unspecified intracranial injury with loss of consciousness of unspecified duration, sequela

If the cause was non-traumatic (ICD-9: 430-437), code the appropriate late effect of cerebrovascular disease code from the 438.XX series.

    1. How do I code late effects of a burn that have caused contracture in a hand impacting ADLs?

First code the residual condition such as contracture or scar and then the appropriate late effect code of burn (906.5-906.8).

906.5	Late effect of burn of eye, face, head, and neck	T20.00XS	Burn of unspecified degree of head, face, and neck, unspecified site, sequela
906.6	Late effect of burn of wrist and hand	T23.009S	Burn of unspecified degree of unspecified hand, unspecified site, sequela
906.7	Late effect of burn of other extremities	T22.00XS	Burn of unspecified degree of shoulder and upper limb, except wrist and hand, unspecified site, sequela
906.8	Late effect of burns of other specified sites	T21.00XS	Burn of unspecified degree of trunk, unspecified site, sequela

In this case first code the contracture of the hand, 718.44 and then code

718.44	Contracture of joint, hand	M24.549	Contracture, unspecified hand

906.6, late effect of burn of wrist and hand.

906.6	Late effect of burn of wrist and hand	T23.009S	Burn of unspecified degree of unspecified hand, unspecified site, sequela

1. How do I code dysphagia that is related to a CVA?

This requires two codes. First code 438.82, late effects of cerebrovascular disease, dysphagia and also code the phase of dysphagia(787.21-787.29). Be sure to code the phase of dysphagia to the highest level of specificity.

438.82	Other late effects of cerebrovascular disease, dysphagia	I69.991	Dysphagia following unspecified cerebrovascular disease
787.21	Dysphagia, oral phase	R13.11	Dysphagia, oral phase
787.22	Dysphagia, oropharyngeal phase	R13.12	Dysphagia, oropharyngeal phase
787.23	Dysphagia, pharyngeal phase	R13.13	Dysphagia, pharyngeal phase
787.24	Dysphagia, pharyngoesophageal phase	R13.14	Dysphagia, pharyngoesophageal phase
787.29	Other dysphagia	R13.19	Other dysphagia

1. When is it appropriate to use 438.89, late effects of cerebrovascular disease, other late effects?

438.89	Other late effects of cerebrovascular disease	I69.898	Other sequelae of other cerebrovascular disease

It is appropriate to code 438.89 when the patient has late effects of one of the causal conditions listed in 430-437 AND none of the other more specific 438 codes describe the late effect. ICD-9 code 438.89 CANNOT stand alone and instead REQUIRES a second code to describe the "other" late effect. Often the second code is not documented resulting in incorrect coding.

It is often used incorrectly as a catch all term. For example, it is often used with weakness when instead the more specific code is actually a hemiplegia code (438.2X).

1. Is there a code for self-feeding decline?

Yes, you can code 783.3, feeding difficulties and mismanagement.

783.3	Feeding difficulties and mismanagement	R63.3	Feeding difficulties

2. Can v15.88, history of fall be a primary diagnosis? Yes

V15.88	History of fall	Z91.81	History of falling

3. Can I code728.87, generalized weakness if I documented strength on the eval to be WFL?

728.87	Muscle weakness (generalized)	M62.81	Muscle weakness (generalized)

No, there must be a documented strength deficit to support the code.

4. What is the difference between 781.2, abnormal gait, and 719.7, difficulty walking?

| 781.2 | Abnormality of gait | R26.9 | Unspecified abnormalities of gait and mobility |
| 719.7 | Difficulty in walking | R26.2 | Difficulty in walking, not elsewhere classified |

ICD-9 code 781.2 includes ataxic, paralytic, spastic, and staggering gait. All other gait issues should be reported with 719.7, difficulty walking.

5. What is the difference between the three symbolic dysfunction codes?

The description of the three codes are as follows and the correct code should be chosen based on highest level of specificity:

784.60	Symbolic dysfunction, unspecified	R48.9	Unspecified symbolic dysfunctions
784.61	Alexia and dyslexia	R48.0	Dyslexia and alexia
784.69	Other symbolic dysfunction	R48.8	Other symbolic dysfunctions

6. Can the new cognition codes only be used for patients with a TBI?

No, the new cognition codes can be used for all neurological conditions with some exceptions including late effects of cerebrovascular disease (438). The codes are:

799.51	Attention or concentration deficit	R41.840	Attention and concentration deficit
799.52	Cognitive communication deficit	R41.841	Cognitive communication deficit
799.53	Visuospatial deficit	R41.842	Visuospatial deficit
799.54	Psychomotor deficit	R41.843	Psychomotor deficit
799.55	Frontal lobe and executive function deficit	R41.844	Frontal lobe and executive function deficit
799.59	Other signs and symptoms involving cognition	R41.89	Other symptoms and signs involving cognitive functions and awareness

APPENDIX C

General Equivalency Mappings of ICD-9 codes to ICD-10

Medicare is establishing the following limited coverage for electrical stimulation			
ICD-9	ICD-9 Description	ICD-10	ICD-10 Description
274.00	Gouty arthropathy	M10.00	Idiopathic gout, unspecified site
333.83	Spasmodic torticollis	G24.3	Spasmodic torticollis
337.20-337.22	Reflex sympathetic dystrophy	G90.59	Complex regional pain syndrome I of other specified site
342.00-342.02	Hemiplegia and hemiparesis	G81.00	Flaccid hemiplegia affecting unspecified side
342.90-342.92	Hemiplegia, unspecified	G81.90	Hemiplegia, unspecified affecting unspecified side
344.60-344.61	Cauda equina syndrome	G83.4	Cauda equina syndrome
353.0-353.6	Nerve root and plexus disorders	G54.0	Brachial plexus disorders
354.0-354.5	Mononeuritis of lover limb and unspecified site	G58.7	Mononeuritis multiplex
457.0	Post mastectomy lymphedema syndrome	I97.2	Postmastectomy lymphedema syndrome
524.60-524.63	Temporomandibular joint disorders, unspecified	M26.60	Temporomandibular joint disorder, unspecified

(Continued)

711.50-711.59	Arthropathy associated with infections	M01.X0	Direct infection of unspecified joint in infectious and parasitic diseases classified elsewhere
712.10-712.19	Crystal arthropathies	M11.80	Other specified crystal arthropathies, unspecified site
713.0-713.8	Arthropathies associated with other disorders classified elsewhere	M14.80	Arthropathies in other specified diseases classified elsewhere, unspecified site
714.0-714.2	Rheumatoid arthritis and other inflammatory polyarthropathies	M05.60	Rheumatoid arthritis of unspecified site with involvement of other organs and systems
715.00	Osteoarthritis and allied disorders	M15.0	Primary generalized (osteo)arthritis
716.00-716.09	Other and unspecified arthropathies	M12.10	Kaschin-Beck disease, unspecified site
718.20-718.29	Pathological dislocation	M24.30	Pathological dislocation of unspecified joint, not elsewhere classified
718.30-718.39	Recurrent dislocation of joint	M24.40	Recurrent dislocation, unspecified joint
718.40-718.49	Contracture of joint	M24.50	Contracture, unspecified joint
719.00-719.09	Other and unspecified disorders of joint	M25.40	Effusion, unspecified joint
720.0-720.2	Ankylosing spondylitis and other inflammatory spondylopathies	M45.9	Ankylosing spondylitis of unspecified sites in spine
722.0	Intervertebral disc disorder	M50.20	Other cervical disc displacement, unspecified cervical region
723.0	Other disorders of cervical region	M48.02	Spinal stenosis, cervical region
724.01-724.02	Other and unspecified disorders of the back	M48.04	Spinal stenosis, thoracic region
726.0	Peripheral enthesopathies and allied syndromes	M75.00	Adhesive capsulitis of unspecified shoulder
727.00-727.06	Other disorders of synovium, tendon, and bursa	M65.9	Synovitis and tenosynovitis, unspecified
728.11	Progressive myositis ossificans	M61.10	Myositis ossificans progressiva, unspecified site
728.12	Traumatic myositis ossificans	M61.00	Myositis ossificans traumatica, unspecified site
728.2	Muscular wasting and disuse atrophy, not elsewhere classified	M62.50	Muscle wasting and atrophy, not elsewhere classified, unspecified site
728.6	Other disorders of cervical region	M72.0	Palmar fascial fibromatosis [Dupuytren]

(Continued)

728.71	Plantar fascial fibromatosis	M72.2	Plantar fascial fibromatosis
728.83	Rupture of muscle, non-traumatic	M62.10	Other rupture of muscle (nontraumatic), unspecified site
728.85	Spasm of muscle	M62.40	Contracture of muscle, unspecified site
729.1	Myalgia and myositis, unspecified	M60.9	Myositis, unspecified
729.4	Fasciitis, unspecified	M72.9	Fibroblastic disorder, unspecified
729.5 729.81-729.82	Pain in limb 729.81-729.82	M79.609	Pain in unspecified limb
729.81	Swelling of limb	M79.89	Other specified soft tissue disorders
729.82	Cramp of limb	R25.2	Cramp and spasm
782.3	Edema	R60.9	Edema, unspecified
816.00-816.03	Fracture of one or more phalanges of hand	S62.609A	Fracture of unspecified phalanx of unspecified finger, initial encounter for closed fracture
817.0-817.1	Multiple fractures of hand bones Fracture of neck of femur	S62.90XA	Unspecified fracture of unspecified wrist and hand, initial encounter for closed fracture
820.00-820.03	Closed fracture of intracapsular section of neck of femur, unspecified	S72.019A	Unspecified intracapsular fracture of unspecified femur, initial encounter for closed fracture
821.00-821.01	Fracture of other and unspecified parts of the femur	S72.90XA	Unspecified fracture of unspecified femur, initial encounter for closed fracture
822.0-822.1	Fracture of the patella	S82.009A	Unspecified fracture of unspecified patella, initial encounter for closed fracture
823.00-823.02	Fracture of tibia and fibula	S82.101A	Unspecified fracture of upper end of right tibia, initial encounter for closed
824.0-824.9	Fracture of the ankle	S82.899B	Other fracture of unspecified lower leg, initial encounter for open fracture type I or II
825.0-825.1	Fracture of one or more tarsal and metatarsal bones	S92.009A	Unspecified fracture of unspecified calcaneus, initial encounter for closed fracture
826.0-826.1	Fracture of one or more phalanges of foot	S92.403A	Displaced unspecified fracture of unspecified great toe, initial encounter for closed fracture
830.0	Dislocation of jaw	S03.0XXA	Dislocation of jaw, initial encounter
831.00-831.04	Dislocation of shoulder	S43.006A	Unspecified dislocation of unspecified shoulder joint, initial encounter
832.00-832.04	Dislocation of elbow	S53.006A	Unspecified dislocation of unspecified radial head, initial encounter

(Continued)

833.00-833.05	Dislocation of wrist	S63.006A	Unspecified dislocation of unspecified wrist and hand, initial encounter
834.00-834.02	Dislocation of finger	S63.259A	Unspecified dislocation of unspecified finger, initial encounter
835.10-835.13	Dislocation of hip	S73.006A	Unspecified dislocation of unspecified hip, initial encounter
836.0-836.4	Dislocation of knee	S83.249A	Other tear of medial meniscus, current injury, unspecified knee, initial encounter
836.50-836.54	Dislocation of knee	S83.219A	Bucket-handle tear of medial meniscus, current injury, unspecified knee, initial encounter
837.0-837.1	Dislocation of ankle	S93.06XA	Dislocation of unspecified ankle joint, initial encounter
838.00-838.06	Dislocation of foot	S93.306A	Unspecified dislocation of unspecified foot, initial encounter
840.0-840.6	Sprains and strains of shoulder and upper arm	S43.50XA	Sprain of unspecified acromioclavicular joint, initial encounter
841.0-841.3	Sprains and strains of elbow and forearm	S53.439A	Radial collateral ligament sprain of unspecified elbow, initial encounter
845.00-845.03	Sprains and strains of ankle and foot	S93.409A	Sprain of unspecified ligament of unspecified ankle, initial encounter
846.0-846.3	Sprains and strains of sacroiliac region	S96.919A	Strain of unspecified muscle and tendon at ankle and foot level, unspecified foot, initial encounter
847.0-847.4	Sprains and strains of other and unspecified parts of back	S13.4XXA	Sprain of ligaments of cervical spine, initial encounter
848.0-848.3	Other and ill-defined sprains and strains	S03.1XXA	Dislocation of septal cartilage of nose, initial encounter
848.40-848.42	Sprain of septal cartilage of nose	S23.429A	Unspecified sprain of sternum, initial encounter
923.00-923.03	Contusion of upper limb	S40.019A	Contusion of unspecified shoulder, initial encounter
924.00-924.01	Contusion of lower limb and other and unspecified sites	S70.10XA	Contusion of unspecified thigh, initial encounter
924.10-924.11 924.20-924.21 924.3-924.4	Contusion of lower leg	S80.10XA	Contusion of unspecified lower leg, initial encounter
926.0	Crushing injury of the trunk	S38.001A	Crushing injury of unspecified external genital organs, male, initial encounter
927.00-927.03	Crushing injury of upper limb	S47.9XXA	Crushing injury of shoulder and upper arm, unspecified arm, initial encounter
928.00-928.01	Crushing injury of lower limb	S77.10XA	Crushing injury of unspecified thigh, initial encounter

(Continued)

928.10-928.11 928.20-928.21	Crushing injury of lower leg	S87.80XA	Crushing injury of unspecified lower leg, initial encounter
953.0-953.5	Injury to nerve roots and spinal plexus	S14.2XXA	Injury of nerve root of cervical spine, initial encounter
955.0-955.9	Injury to peripheral nerve(s) of pelvic girdle and upper limb	S44.30XA	Injury of axillary nerve, unspecified arm, initial encounter
956.0-956.5	Injury to peripheral nerve(s) of pelvic girdle and lower limb	S74.00XA	Injury of sciatic nerve at hip and thigh level, unspecified leg, initial encounter
956.8	Injury to multiple nerves of pelvic girdle and lower limb	S84.809A	Injury of other nerves at lower leg level, unspecified leg, initial encounter
997.61	Late amputation stump complication	T87.30	Neuroma of amputation stump, unspecified extremity
V43.60-V43.66	Organ or tissue replaced by joint	Z96.60	Presence of unspecified orthopedic joint implant
V43.7	Organ or tissue replaced by limb	Z97.10	Presence of artificial limb (complete) (partial), unspecified
V45.4	Arthrodesis status	Z98.1	Arthrodesis status
V49.60-V49.67	Upper limb amputation status	Z89.209	Acquired absence of unspecified upper limb, unspecified level
V49.70-V49.77	Lower limb amputation status	Z89.9	Acquired absence of limb, unspecified
V54.01	Encounter for removal of internal fixation device	Z47.2	Encounter for removal of internal fixation device
V54.09	Other aftercare involving internal fixation device	Z51.89	Encounter for other specified aftercare

Medicare is establishing the following limited coverage for paraffin bath:

ICD-9	ICD-9 Description	ICD-10	ICD-10 Description
274.00	Gouty arthropathy	M10.00	Idiopathic gout, unspecified site
337.21-337.22	Reflex sympathetic dystrophy 3	G90.519	Complex regional pain syndrome I of unspecified upper limb
354.0-354.5	Mononeuritis of upper limb and mononeuritis multiplex	G56.00	Carpal tunnel syndrome, unspecified upper limb
355.3-355.6	Mononeuritis of lower limb and unspecified site	G57.30	Lesion of lateral popliteal nerve, unspecified lower limb
711.14	Arthropathy associated with Reiter's disease and non-specific urethritis, hand	M02.349	Reiter's disease, unspecified hand
711.17	Arthropathy associated with Reiter's disease and non-specific urethritis, ankle and foot	M02.379	Reiter's disease, unspecified ankle and foot
712.14	Crystal arthropathies	M11.849	Other specified crystal arthropathies, unspecified hand

(Continued)

714.0-714.2	Rheumatoid arthritis and other inflammatory polyarthropathies	M06.9	Rheumatoid arthritis, unspecified

Medicare is establishing the following limited coverage for whirlpool, and Hubbard tank:

ICD-9	ICD-9 Description	ICD-10	ICD-10 Description
274.00	Gouty arthropathy	M10.00	Idiopathic gout, unspecified site
337.20-337.22	Reflex sympathetic dystrophy	G90.59	Complex regional pain syndrome I of other specified site
353.0-353.6	Nerve root and plexus disorders	G54.0	Brachial plexus disorders
454.0-454.2	Varicose veins	I83.009	Varicose veins of unspecified lower extremity with ulcer of unspecified site
457.0	Postmastectomy lymphedema syndrome	I97.2	Postmastectomy lymphedema syndrome
682.3-682.7	Cellulitis	L03.119	Cellulitis of unspecified part of limb
695.81	Extensive exfoliative dermatitis	L00	Staphylococcal scalded skin syndrome
713.0-713.8	Arthropathies associated with other disorders classified elsewhere	M14.80	Arthropathies in other specified diseases classified elsewhere, unspecified site
714.0-714.2	Rheumatoid arthritis and other inflammatory polyarthropathies	M06.9	Rheumatoid arthritis, unspecified
715.00	Osteoarthritis and allied disorders	M15.0	Primary generalized (osteo)arthritis
716.00-716.09	Other and unspecified arthropathies	M12.10	Kaschin-Beck disease, unspecified site
718.20-718.29	Pathological dislocation	M24.30	Pathological dislocation of unspecified joint, not elsewhere classified
718.30-718.39	Recurrent dislocation of joint	M24.40	Recurrent dislocation, unspecified joint
718.40-718.49	Contracture of joint	M24.50	Contracture, unspecified joint
719.00-719.09	Other and unspecified disorders of joint	M25.40	Effusion, unspecified joint
720.0-720.2	Ankylosing spondylitis and other inflammatory spondylopathies	M45.9	Ankylosing spondylitis of unspecified sites in spine
728.2	Muscular wasting and disuse atrophy, not elsewhere classified	M62.50	Muscle wasting and atrophy, not elsewhere classified, unspecified site
728.6	Contracture of palmar fascia	M72.0	Palmar fascial fibromatosis [Dupuytren]
728.71	Plantar fascial fibromatosis	M72.2	Plantar fascial fibromatosis
728.83	Rupture of muscle, non-traumatic	M62.10	Other rupture of muscle (nontraumatic), unspecified site
728.85	Spasm of muscle	M62.40	Contracture of muscle, unspecified site
729.1	Myalgia and myositis, unspecified	M60.9	Myositis, unspecified

(Continued)

729.4-729.5 729.81-729.82 808.0-808.3	Fracture of pelvis	M72.9	Fibroblastic disorder, unspecified
808.41-808.43	Closed fracture of ilium	S32.309A	Unspecified fracture of unspecified ilium, initial encounter for closed fracture
809.0-809.1	Ill-defined fractures of bones of trunk	S22.9XXA	Fracture of bony thorax, part unspecified, initial encounter for closed fracture
810.00-810.03	Fracture of clavicle	S42.009A	Fracture of unspecified part of unspecified clavicle, initial encounter for closed fracture
810.10-810.13 811.00-811.03	Fracture of scapula	S42.009B	Fracture of unspecified part of unspecified clavicle, initial encounter for open fracture
812.00-812.03	Fracture of humerus	S42.209A	Unspecified fracture of upper end of unspecified humerus, initial encounter for closed fracture
813.00-813.08	Fracture of radius and ulna	S52.90XA	Unspecified fracture of unspecified forearm, initial encounter for closed fracture
814.00-814.09	Fracture of carpal bone(s)	S62.109A	Fracture of unspecified carpal bone, unspecified wrist, initial encounter for closed fracture
815.00-815.04	Fracture of metacarpal bone(s)	S62.309A	Unspecified fracture of unspecified metacarpal bone, initial encounter for closed fracture
816.00-816.03	Fracture of one or more phalanges of hand	S62.609A	Fracture of unspecified phalanx of unspecified finger, initial encounter for closed fracture
817.0-817.1	Multiple fractures of hand bones	S62.90XA	Unspecified fracture of unspecified wrist and hand, initial encounter for closed fracture
820.00-820.03	Fracture of neck of femur	S72.019A	Unspecified intracapsular fracture of unspecified femur, initial encounter for closed fracture
821.00-821.01	Fracture of other and unspecified parts of the femur	S72.90XA	Unspecified fracture of unspecified femur, initial encounter for closed fracture
822.0-822.1	Fracture of the patella	S82.009A	Unspecified fracture of unspecified patella, initial encounter for closed fracture
823.00-823.02	Fracture of the tibia and fibula	S82.109A	Unspecified fracture of upper end of unspecified tibia, initial encounter for closed fracture
824.0-824.9	Fracture of the ankle	S82.53XA	Displaced fracture of medial malleolus of unspecified tibia, initial encounter for closed fracture

(Continued)

825.0-825.1	Fracture of one or more tarsal and metatarsal bones	S92.009A	Unspecified fracture of unspecified calcaneus, initial encounter for closed fracture
825.39 826.0-826.1	Fracture of one or more phalanges of foot	S92.209B	Fracture of unspecified tarsal bone(s) of unspecified foot, initial encounter for open fracture
831.00-831.04	Dislocation of shoulder	S43.006A	Unspecified dislocation of unspecified shoulder joint, initial encounter
831.19 832.00-832.01	Dislocation of elbow	S41.009A	Unspecified open wound of unspecified shoulder, initial encounter
832.19 833.00-833.05	Dislocation of wrist	S53.096A	Other dislocation of unspecified radial head, initial encounter
834.00-834.02	Dislocation of finger	S63.259A	Unspecified dislocation of unspecified finger, initial encounter
835.00-835.03	Dislocation of hip	S73.006A	Unspecified dislocation of unspecified hip, initial encounter
836.0-836.4	Dislocation of knee	S83.249A	Other tear of medial meniscus, current injury, unspecified knee, initial encounter
836.69 837.0-837.1	Dislocation of ankle	S83.196A	Other dislocation of unspecified knee, initial encounter
838.00-838.06	Dislocation of foot	S93.306A	Unspecified dislocation of unspecified foot, initial encounter
840.0-840.6	Sprains and strains of shoulder and upper arm	S43.50XA	Sprain of unspecified acromioclavicular joint, initial encounter
841.0-841.3	Sprains and strains of elbow and forearm	S53.439A	Radial collateral ligament sprain of unspecified elbow, initial encounter
842.00-842.02	Sprains and strains of wrist and hand	S63.509A	Unspecified sprain of unspecified wrist, initial encounter
843.0-843.1	Sprains and strains of hip and thighs	S53.439A	Radial collateral ligament sprain of unspecified elbow, initial encounter
844.0-844.3	Sprains and strains of knee and leg	S83.429A	Sprain of lateral collateral ligament of unspecified knee, initial encounter
845.00-845.03	Sprains and strains of ankle and foot	S93.429A	Prain of deltoid ligament of unspecified ankle, initial encounter
846.0-846.3	Sprains and strains of sacroiliac region	S33.8XXA	Sprain of other parts of lumbar spine and pelvis, initial encounter
847.0-847.4	Sprain of neck	S13.4XXA	sprain of ligaments of cervical spine, initial encounter
848.0-848.3	Sprain of septal cartilage of nose	S03.1XXA	Dislocation of septal cartilage of nose, initial encounter

(Continued)

880.00-880.03	Open wound of shoulder region, without mention of complication	S41.009A	Unspecified open wound of unspecified shoulder, initial encounter
881.00-881.02	Open wound of forearm, without mention of complication	S51.809A	Unspecified open wound of unspecified forearm, initial encounter
882.0-882.2	Unspecified open wound of unspecified forearm, initial encounter	S61.409A	Unspecified open wound of unspecified hand, initial encounter
883.0-883.2	Unspecified open wound of unspecified hand, initial encounter	S61.209A	Unspecified open wound of unspecified finger without damage to nail, initial encounter
884.0-884.2	Multiple and unspecified open wound of upper limb, without mention of complication	S41.009A	Unspecified open wound of unspecified shoulder, initial encounter
890.0-890.2	Open wound of hip and thigh, without mention of complication	S71.009A	Unspecified open wound, unspecified hip, initial encounter
891.0-891.2	Open wound of knee, leg [except thigh], and ankle, without mention of complication	S81.009A	Unspecified open wound, unspecified knee, initial encounter
892.0-892.2	Open wound of foot except toe(s) alone, without mention of complication	S91.309A	Unspecified open wound, unspecified foot, initial encounter
893.0-893.2	Open wound of toe(s), without mention of complication	S91.109A	Unspecified open wound of unspecified toe(s) without damage to nail, initial encounter
923.00-923.03	Contusion of shoulder region	S40.019A	Contusion of unspecified shoulder, initial encounter
924.00-924.01	Contusion of thigh	S70.10XA	Contusion of unspecified thigh, initial encounter
926.0	Crushing injury of external genitalia	S38.001A	Crushing injury of unspecified external genital organs, male, initial encounter
927.00-927.03	Crushing injury of shoulder region	S47.9XXA	Crushing injury of shoulder and upper arm, unspecified arm, initial encounter
928.00-928.01	Crushing injury of thigh	S77.10XA	Crushing injury of unspecified thigh, initial encounter
942.00-942.25	Burn of unspecified degree of trunk, unspecified site	T21.00XA	Burn of unspecified degree of trunk, unspecified site, initial encounter
943.00-943.26	Burn of unspecified degree of upper limb, except wrist and hand, unspecified site	T22.00XA	Corrosion of unspecified degree of shoulder and upper limb, except wrist and hand, unspecified site, initial encounter
944.00-944.28	Burn of unspecified degree of hand, unspecified site	T23.009A	Burn of unspecified degree of unspecified hand, unspecified site, initial encounter

(Continued)

946.0-946.5	Burns of multiple specified sites, unspecified degree	T30.0	Burn of unspecified body region, unspecified degree
948.00	Burn [any degree] involving less than 10 percent of body surface with third degree burn, less than 10 percent or unspecified	T31.0	Burns involving less than 10% of body surface
953.0-953.5	Injury to cervical nerve root	S14.2XXA	Injury of nerve root of cervical spine, initial encounter
955.0-955.9	Injury to axillary nerve	S44.30XA	Injury of axillary nerve, unspecified arm, initial encounter
956.0-956.5	Injury of axillary nerve, unspecified arm, initial encounter	S74.00XA	Injury of sciatic nerve at hip and thigh level, unspecified leg, initial encounter
997.61	Injury to sciatic nerve	T87.30	Neuroma of amputation stump, unspecified extremity
V43.60-V43.66	Unspecified joint replacement	Z96.60	Presence of unspecified orthopedic joint implant
V43.7 -V45.4	Limb replaced by other means	Z97.10	Presence of artificial limb (complete) (partial), unspecified
V49.60-V49.67	Unspecified level upper limb amputation status	Z89.209	Acquired absence of unspecified upper limb, unspecified level

Medicare is establishing limited coverage for diathermy:

ICD-9	ICD-9 Description	ICD-10	ICD-10 Description
274.00	Gouty arthropathy, unspecified	M10.00	Idiopathic gout, unspecified site
711.00-711.09	Pyogenic arthritis, site unspecified	M00.10	Pneumococcal arthritis, unspecified joint
712.10-712.19	Chondrocalcinosis, due to dicalcium phosphate crystals, site unspecified	M11.80	Other specified crystal arthropathies, unspecified site
713.0-713.8	Arthropathy associated with other endocrine and metabolic disorders	M14.80	Arthropathies in other specified diseases classified elsewhere, unspecified site
714.0-714.2	Rheumatoid arthritis	M06.9	Rheumatoid arthritis, unspecified
716.00-716.09	Kaschin-Beck disease, site unspecified	M12.10	Kaschin-Beck disease, unspecified site
719.00-719.09	Effusion of joint, site unspecified	M25.40	Effusion, unspecified joint
720.0-720.2	Ankylosing spondylitis	M45.9	Ankylosing spondylitis of unspecified sites in spine
722.0	Displacement of cervical intervertebral disc without myelopathy	M50.20	Other cervical disc displacement, unspecified cervical region
727.00-727.06	Synovitis and tenosynovitis, unspecified	M65.9	Synovitis and tenosynovitis, unspecified

(Continued)

728.0	Infective myositis	M60.009	Infective myositis, unspecified site
814.00-814.09	Closed fracture of carpal bone, unspecified	S62.109A	Fracture of unspecified carpal bone, unspecified wrist, initial encounter for closed fracture
815.00-815.04	Closed fracture of carpal bone, unspecified	S62.309A	Unspecified fracture of unspecified metacarpal bone, initial encounter for closed fracture
816.00-816.03	Closed fracture of phalanx or phalanges of hand, unspecified	S62.509A	Fracture of unspecified phalanx of unspecified thumb, initial encounter for closed fracture
817.0-817.1	Multiple closed fractures of hand bones	S62.90XA	Unspecified fracture of unspecified wrist and hand, initial encounter for closed fracture
820.00-820.03	Closed fracture of intracapsular section of neck of femur, unspecified	S72.019A	Unspecified intracapsular fracture of unspecified femur, initial encounter for closed fracture
821.00-821.01	Closed fracture of unspecified part of femur	S72.90XA	Unspecified fracture of unspecified femur, initial encounter for closed fracture
822.0-822.1	Closed fracture of patella	S82.009A	Unspecified fracture of unspecified patella, initial encounter for closed fracture
823.00-823.02	Closed fracture of upper end of tibia alone	S82.109A	Unspecified fracture of upper end of unspecified tibia, initial encounter for closed fracture
824.0-824.9	Fracture of medial malleolus, closed	S82.53XA	Displaced fracture of medial malleolus of unspecified tibia, initial encounter for closed fracture
825.0-825.1	Fracture of calcaneus, closed	S92.009A	Unspecified fracture of unspecified calcaneus, initial encounter for closed fracture
845.00-845.03	Sprain of ankle, unspecified site	S93.409A	Sprain of unspecified ligament of unspecified ankle, initial encounter
846.0-846.3	Sprain of lumbosacral (joint) (ligament)	S33.8XXA	Sprain of other parts of lumbar spine and pelvis, initial encounter
847.0-847.4	Sprain of neck	S13.4XXA	Sprain of ligaments of cervical spine, initial encounter
848.0-848.3	Sprain of septal cartilage of nose	S03.1XXA	Dislocation of septal cartilage of nose, initial encounter
923.00-923.03	Contusion of shoulder region	40.019A	Contusion of unspecified shoulder, initial encounter
924.00-924.01	Contusion of thigh	S70.10XA	Contusion of unspecified thigh, initial encounter

(Continued)

926.0	Crushing injury of external genitalia	S38.001A	Crushing injury of unspecified external genital organs, male, initial encounter
927.00-927.03	Crushing injury of shoulder region	S47.9XXA	Crushing injury of shoulder and upper arm, unspecified arm, initial encounter
928.00-928.01	Crushing injury of thigh	S77.10XA	Crushing injury of unspecified thigh, initial encounter
928.10-928.11	Crushing injury of lower leg	S87.80XA	Crushing injury of unspecified lower leg, initial encounter
942.20-942.25	Burn of unspecified degree of trunk, unspecified site	T21.00XA	Burn of unspecified degree of trunk, unspecified site, initial encounter
943.00-943.26	Burn of unspecified degree of upper limb, except wrist and hand, unspecified site	T22.00XA	Burn of unspecified degree of shoulder and upper limb, except wrist and hand, unspecified site, initial encounter
944.00-944.28	Burn of unspecified degree of hand, unspecified site	T23.009A	Burn of unspecified degree of unspecified hand, unspecified site, initial encounter
945.00-945.26	Burn of unspecified degree of lower limb [leg], unspecified site	T24.009A	Burn of unspecified degree of unspecified site of unspecified lower limb, except ankle and foot, initial encounter
946.0-946.5	Burns of multiple specified sites, unspecified degree	T30.0	Burn of unspecified body region, unspecified degree
948.00	Burn [any degree] involving less than 10 percent of body surface with third degree burn, less than 10 percent or unspecified	T31.0	Burns involving less than 10% of body surface
953.0-953.5	Injury to cervical nerve root	S14.2XXA	Injury of nerve root of cervical spine, initial encounter
955.0-955.9	Injury to axillary nerve	44.30XA	Injury of axillary nerve, unspecified arm, initial encounter
956.0-956.5	Injury to sciatic nerve	S74.00XA	Injury of sciatic nerve at hip and thigh level, unspecified leg, initial encounter
997.61	Neuroma of amputation stump	T87.30	Neuroma of amputation stump, unspecified extremity

Mediacre is establishing the following limited coverage for ultrasound:

ICD-9	ICD-9 Description	ICD-10	ICD-10 Description
274.00	Gouty arthropathy, unspecified	M10.00	Idiopathic gout, unspecified site
274.9	Gout, unspecified	M10.9	Gout, unspecified
333.83	Spasmodic torticollis	G24.3	Spasmodic torticollis
337.00-337.22	Idiopathic peripheral autonomic neuropathy, unspecified	G90.09	Other idiopathic peripheral autonomic neuropathy
353.1-353.6	Lumbosacral plexus lesions	G54.1	Lumbosacral plexus disorders

(Continued)

353.8 354.0-354.5	Other nerve root and plexus disorders	G54.8	Other nerve root and plexus disorders
355.0-355.6	Lesion of sciatic nerve	G57.00	Lesion of sciatic nerve, unspecified lower limb
457.0	Postmastectomy lymphedema syndrome	I97.2	Postmastectomy lymphedema syndrome
711.00-711.09	Pyogenic arthritis, site unspecified	M00.10	Pneumococcal arthritis, unspecified joint
720.0-720.2	Ankylosing spondylitis	M45.9	Ankylosing spondylitis of unspecified sites in spine
722.0	Displacement of cervical intervertebral disc without myelopathy	M50.20	Other cervical disc displacement, unspecified cervical region
723.0	Other cervical disc displacement, unspecified cervical region	M48.02	Spinal stenosis, cervical region
724.79	Other disorders of coccyx	M53.3	Sacrococcygeal disorders, not elsewhere classified
726.0	Adhesive capsulitis of shoulder	M75.00	Adhesive capsulitis of unspecified shoulder
727.00-727.06	Synovitis and tenosynovitis, unspecified	M65.9	Synovitis and tenosynovitis, unspecified
728.11	Progressive myositis ossificans	M61.10	Myositis ossificans progressiva, unspecified site
728.12	Traumatic myositis ossificans	M61.00	Myositis ossificans traumatica, unspecified site
728.2	Muscular wasting and disuse atrophy, not elsewhere classified	M62.50	Muscle wasting and atrophy, not elsewhere classified, unspecified site
728.6	Contracture of palmar fascia	M72.0	Palmar fascial fibromatosis [Dupuytren]
728.71	Palmar fascial fibromatosis [Dupuytren]	M72.2	Plantar fascial fibromatosis
728.83	Rupture of muscle, nontraumatic	M62.10	Other rupture of muscle (nontraumatic), unspecified site
728.85	Spasm of muscle	M62.40	Contracture of muscle, unspecified site
729.0	Rheumatism, unspecified and fibrositis	M79.0	Rheumatism, unspecified
729.4	Fasciitis, unspecified	M72.9	Fibroblastic disorder, unspecified
729.5	Pain in limb	M79.609	Pain in unspecified limb
782.3	Edema	R60.0	Localized edema
808.0-808.3	Closed fracture of acetabulum	S32.409A	Unspecified fracture of unspecified acetabulum, initial encounter for closed fracture

(Continued)

809.0-809.1	Fracture of bones of trunk, closed	S22.9XXA	Fracture of bony thorax, part unspecified, initial encounter for closed fracture
810.00-810.03	Closed fracture of clavicle, unspecified part	S42.009A	Fracture of unspecified part of unspecified clavicle, initial encounter for closed fracture
811.00-811.03	Closed fracture of scapula, unspecified part	S42.109A	Fracture of unspecified part of scapula, unspecified shoulder, initial encounter for closed fracture
812.00-812.03	Closed fracture of unspecified part of upper end of humerus	S42.209A	Unspecified fracture of upper end of unspecified humerus, initial encounter for closed fracture
840.0-840.6	Acromioclavicular (joint) (ligament) sprain	S43.50XA	Sprain of unspecified acromioclavicular joint, initial encounter
841.0-841.3	Radial collateral ligament sprain	S53.439A	Radial collateral ligament sprain of unspecified elbow, initial encounter
842.00-842.02	Sprain of wrist, unspecified site	S63.509A	Unspecified sprain of unspecified wrist, initial encounter
843.0-843.1	Iliofemoral (ligament) sprain	S73.119A	Iliofemoral ligament sprain of unspecified hip, initial encounter
845.00-845.03	Sprain of ankle, unspecified site	S93.409A	Sprain of unspecified ligament of unspecified ankle, initial encounter
846.0-846.3	Sprain of lumbosacral (joint) (ligament)	S33.8XXA	Sprain of other parts of lumbar spine and pelvis, initial encounter
847.0-847.4	Sprain of neck	S13.4XXA	Sprain of ligaments of cervical spine, initial encounter
848.0-848.3	Sprain of septal cartilage of nose	S03.1XXA	Dislocation of septal cartilage of nose, initial encounter
923.00-923.03	Contusion of shoulder region	S40.019A	Contusion of unspecified shoulder, initial encounter
924.00-924.01	Contusion of thigh	S70.10XA	Contusion of unspecified thigh, initial encounter
926.0	Crushing injury of external genitalia	S38.001A	Crushing injury of unspecified external genital organs, male, initial encounter

Medicare is establishing the following limited coverage for therapeutic exercise:

ICD-9	ICD-9 Description	ICD-10	ICD-10 Description
274.00	Gouty arthropathy	M10.00	Idiopathic gout, unspecified site
274.9	Gout, unspecified	M10.9	Gout, unspecified
332.0-332.1	Paralysis agitans	G20	Parkinson's disease
333.83	Spasmodic torticollis	G24.3	Spasmodic torticollis

(Continued)

333.90-333.91	Unspecified extrapyramidal disease and abnormal movement disorder	G25.9	Extrapyramidal and movement disorder, unspecified
334.0	Friedreich's ataxia	G11.1	Early-onset cerebellar ataxia
335.0	Werdnig-Hoffmann disease	G12.0 I	Infantile spinal muscular atrophy, type I [Werdnig-Hoffman]
457.0	Postmastectomy lymphedema syndrome	I97.2	Postmastectomy lymphedema syndrome
524.60-524.63	Temporomandibular joint disorders, unspecified	M26.60	Temporomandibular joint disorder, unspecified
681.00-681.01	Cellulitis and abscess of finger, unspecified	L03.019	Cellulitis of unspecified finger
682.3-682.7	Cellulitis and abscess of upper arm and forearm	L03.119	Cellulitis of unspecified part of limb
711.00-711.09	Arthropathy associated with Reiter's disease and nonspecific urethritis, site unspecified	M00.10	Pneumococcal arthritis, unspecified joint
711.10-711.19	Arthropathy associated with Reiter's disease and non-specific urethritis	M02.30	Reiter's disease, unspecified site
711.20-711.29	Arthropathy in Behcet's syndrome, site unspecified	M35.2	Behçet's disease
711.30-711.39	Postdysenteric arthropathy, site unspecified	M02.10	Postdysenteric arthropathy, unspecified site
711.40-711.49	Arthropathy associated with other bacterial diseases, site unspecified	M01.X0	Direct infection of unspecified joint in infectious and parasitic diseases classified elsewhere
711.50-711.59	Arthropathy associated with other viral diseases, site unspecified	M01.X0	Direct infection of unspecified joint in infectious and parasitic diseases classified elsewhere
711.60-711.69	Arthropathy associated with mycoses, site unspecified	M01.X0	Direct infection of unspecified joint in infectious and parasitic diseases classified elsewhere
711.70-711.79	Arthropathy associated with Reiter's disease and nonspecific urethritis, site unspecified	M01.X0	Direct infection of unspecified joint in infectious and parasitic diseases classified elsewhere
711.80-711.89	Arthropathy associated with other infectious and parasitic diseases, site unspecified	M01.X0	Direct infection of unspecified joint in infectious and parasitic diseases classified elsewhere
712.10-712.19	Chondrocalcinosis, due to dicalcium phosphate crystals, site unspecified	M11.80	Other specified crystal arthropathies, unspecified site

(Continued)

713.0-713.8	Arthropathies associated with other disorders classified elsewhere	M14.80	Arthropathies in other specified diseases classified elsewhere, unspecified site
714.0-714.2	Rheumatoid arthritis and other inflammatory polyarthropathies	M05.60	Rheumatoid arthritis of unspecified site with involvement of other organs and systems
723.0	Other disorders of cervical region	M48.02	Spinal stenosis, cervical region
724.01-724.02	Other and unspecified disorders of the back	M48.04	Spinal stenosis, thoracic region
726.0	Peripheral enthesopathies and allied syndromes	M75.00	Adhesive capsulitis of unspecified shoulder
727.00-727.06	Other disorders of synovium, tendon, and bursa	M65.9	Synovitis and tenosynovitis, unspecified
728.11	Progressive myositis ossificans	M61.10	Myositis ossificans progressiva, unspecified site
728.12	Traumatic myositis ossificans	M61.00	Myositis ossificans traumatica, unspecified site
728.2	Muscular wasting and disuse atrophy, not elsewhere classified	M62.50	Muscle wasting and atrophy, not elsewhere classified, unspecified site
728.6	Other disorders of cervical region	M72.0	Palmar fascial fibromatosis [Dupuytren]
728.71	Plantar fascial fibromatosis	M72.2	Plantar fascial fibromatosis
728.83	Rupture of muscle, non-traumatic	M62.10	Other rupture of muscle (nontraumatic), unspecified site
728.85	Spasm of muscle	M62.40	Contracture of muscle, unspecified site
729.1	Myalgia and myositis, unspecified	M60.9	Myositis, unspecified
729.4	Fasciitis, unspecified	M72.9	Fibroblastic disorder, unspecified
729.5	Pain in limb	M79.609	Pain in unspecified limb
729.5 729.81-729.82	Pain in limb	M79.609	Pain in unspecified limb
781.0	Abnormal involuntary movements	R25.9	Unspecified abnormal involuntary movements
781.2	Abnormality of gait	R26.9	Unspecified abnormalities of gait and mobility
781.3	Lack of coordination	R27.9	Unspecified lack of coordination
781.9	Other symptoms involving nervous and musculoskeletal systems	R29.898	Other symptoms and signs involving the musculoskeletal system
782.3	Edema	R60.9	Edema, unspecified
799.4	Cachexia	R64	Cachexia

(Continued)

—— *Starting your Own Practice from Scratch* ——

805.00-805.08	Fracture of vertebral column without mention of spinal cord injury	S12.9XXA	Fracture of neck, unspecified, initial encounter
806.00-806.09	Cervical fracture, closed	S12.000A	Unspecified displaced fracture of first cervical vertebra, initial encounter for closed fracture
806.10-806.19	Cervical fracture, open	S12.001B	Unspecified nondisplaced fracture of first cervical vertebra, initial encounter for open fracture
806.20-806.29	Dorsal (thoracic) fracture, closed	S22.019A	Unspecified fracture of first thoracic vertebra, initial encounter for closed fracture
806.30-806.39	Dorsal (thoracic) fracture, open	S22.019B	Unspecified fracture of first thoracic vertebra, initial encounter for open fracture
806.4-806.5	Lumbar fracture, open or closed	S34.119A	Complete lesion of unspecified level of lumbar spinal cord, initial encounter
806.60-806.62	Sacrum and coccyx, fracture, closed	S32.10XA	Unspecified fracture of sacrum, initial encounter for closed fracture
806.70-806.72	Sacrum and coccyx, fracture, open	S32.10XB	Unspecified fracture of sacrum, initial encounter for open fracture
806.8-806.9	Unspecified fracture, open or closed	S14.109A	Unspecified injury at unspecified level of cervical spinal cord, initial encounter
808.0-808.3	Fracture of pelvis	S32.409A	Unspecified fracture of unspecified acetabulum, initial encounter for closed fracture
809.0-809.1	Ill-defined fractures of bones of trunk	S22.9XXA	Fracture of bony thorax, part unspecified, initial encounter for closed fracture
821.00-821.01	Fracture of other and unspecified parts of the femur	S72.90XA	Unspecified fracture of unspecified femur, initial encounter for closed fracture
822.0-822.1	Fracture of the patella	S82.009A	Unspecified fracture of unspecified patella, initial encounter for closed fracture
823.00-823.02	Fracture of tibia and fibula	S82.109A	Unspecified fracture of upper end of unspecified tibia, initial encounter for closed fracture
824.0-824.9	Fracture of the ankle	S82.53XA	Displaced fracture of medial malleolus of unspecified tibia, initial encounter for closed fracture
825.0-825.1	Fracture of one or more tarsal and metatarsal bones	S92.009A	Unspecified fracture of unspecified calcaneus, initial encounter for closed fracture
826.0-826.1	Fracture of one or more phalanges of foot	S92.406A	Displaced unspecified fracture of unspecified great toe, initial encounter for closed fracture

(Continued)

827.0-827.1	Other, multiple, and ill-defined fractures of lower limb	T14.8	Other injury of unspecified body region
830.0-830.1	Dislocation of jaw	S03.0XXA	Dislocation of jaw, initial encounter
831.00-831.04	Dislocation of shoulder	S43.006A	Unspecified dislocation of unspecified shoulder joint, initial encounter
832.00-832.04	Dislocation of elbow	S53.006A	Unspecified dislocation of unspecified radial head, initial encounter
833.00-833.05	Dislocation of wrist	S63.0006A	Unspecified dislocation of unspecified wrist and hand, initial encounter
834.00-834.02	Dislocation of finger	S63.259A	Unspecified dislocation of unspecified finger, initial encounter
835.00-835.03	Dislocation of hip	S73.006A	Unspecified dislocation of unspecified hip, initial encounter
836.0-836.4	Dislocation of knee	S83.219A	Bucket-handle tear of medial meniscus, current injury, unspecified knee, initial encounter
837.0-837.1	Dislocation of ankle	S93.06XA	Dislocation of unspecified ankle joint, initial encounter
838.00-838.06	Dislocation of foot	S93.306A	Unspecified dislocation of unspecified foot, initial encounter
840.0-840.6	Sprains and strains of shoulder and upper arm	S43.50XA	Sprain of unspecified acromioclavicular joint, initial encounter
841.0-841.3	Sprains and strains of elbow and forearm	S53.439A	Radial collateral ligament sprain of unspecified elbow, initial encounter
842.00-842.02	Sprains and strains of wrist and hand	S63.509A	Unspecified sprain of unspecified wrist, initial encounter
843.0-843.1	Sprains and strains of hip and thighs	S73.119A	Iliofemoral ligament sprain of unspecified hip, initial encounter
844.0-844.3	Sprains and strains of knee and leg	S83.429A	Sprain of lateral collateral ligament of unspecified knee, initial encounter
845.00-845.03	Sprains and strains of ankle and foot	S96.919A	Strain of unspecified muscle and tendon at ankle and foot level, unspecified foot, initial encounter
846.0-846.3	Sprains and strains of sacroiliac region	S33.8XXA	Sprain of other parts of lumbar spine and pelvis, initial encounter
847.0-847.4	Sprains and strains of other and unspecified parts of back	S13.8XXA	Sprain of joints and ligaments of other parts of neck, initial encounter
848.0-848.3	Other and ill-defined sprains and strains	S03.1XXA	Dislocation of septal cartilage of nose, initial encounter
923.00-923.03	Contusion of upper limb	S40.019A	Contusion of unspecified shoulder, initial encounter

(Continued)

924.00-924.10	Contusion of lower limb and other and unspecified sites	S70.10XA	Contusion of unspecified thigh, initial encounter
926.0	Crushing injury of the trunk	S38.001A	Crushing injury of unspecified external genital organs, male, initial encounter
927.00-927.03	Crushing injury of upper limb	S47.99XXA	Crushing injury of shoulder and upper arm, unspecified arm, initial encounter
928.00-928.01	Crushing injury of lower limb	S77.10XA	Crushing injury of unspecified thigh, initial encounter
952.00-952.09	Spinal cord injury without evidence of spinal bone injury, cervical dorsal (thoracic)	S14.101A	Unspecified injury at C1 level of cervical spinal cord, initial encounter
952.10-952.19	Lumbar	S24.102A	Unspecified injury at T2-T6 level of thoracic spinal cord, initial encounter
952.2	Sacral	S34.109A	Unspecified injury to unspecified level of lumbar spinal cord, initial encounter
952.3	Cauda equina	S34.139A	Unspecified injury to sacral spinal cord, initial encounter
952.4	Multiple sites of spinal cord	S34.3XXA	Injury of cauda equina, initial encounter
953.0-953.5	Injury to nerve roots and spinal plexus	S14.2XXA	Injury of nerve root of cervical spine, initial encounter
955.0-955.9	Injury to peripheral nerve(s) of pelvic girdle and upper limb	S44.30XA	Injury of axillary nerve, unspecified arm, initial encounter
956.0-956.6	Injury to peripheral nerve(s) of pelvic girdle and lower limb	S74.00XA	Injury of sciatic nerve at hip and thigh level, unspecified leg, initial encounter
997.61	Late amputation stump complication	T87.30	Neuroma of amputation stump, unspecified extremity
V54.01	Aftercare involving removal of fracture plate or other internal fixation device	Z47.2	Encounter for removal of internal fixation device
V54.89	Other orthopedic aftercare	Z47.89	Encounter for other orthopedic aftercare

Medicare is establishing the following limited coverage for neuromuscular re-education:

ICD-9	ICD-9 Description	ICD-10	ICD-10 Description
274.00	Gouty arthropathy	M10.00	Idiopathic gout, unspecified site
274.9	Gout, unspecified	M10.9	Gout, unspecified
332.0-332.1	Parkinsonism	G20	Parkinson's disease
333.0	Other degenerative diseases of the basal ganglia	G23.8	Other specified degenerative diseases of basal ganglia
333.83	Spasmodic torticollis	G24.3	Spasmodic torticollis

(Continued)

334.9	Unspecified extrapyramidal diseases and abnormal movement disorders	G11.9	Hereditary ataxia, unspecified
333.91	Stiff-man syndrome	G25.82	Stiff-man syndrome
334.0-334.4	Spinocerebellar disease	G11.1	Early-onset cerebellar ataxia
335.0	Anterior horn cell disease	G12.0	Infantile spinal muscular atrophy, type I [Werdnig-Hoffman]
336.0-336.3	Other diseases of spinal cord	G95.0	Syringomyelia and syringobulbia
337.20-337.22	Reflex sympathetic dystrophy	G90.59	Complex regional pain syndrome I of other specified site
337.29 340	Multiple sclerosis	G90.59	Complex regional pain syndrome I of other specified site
341.1	Other demyelinating disease of central nervous system	G37.0	Diffuse sclerosis of central nervous system
711.00-711.09 711.10-711.19 711.20-711.29 711.30-711.39 711.40-711.49	Hereditary and idiopathic peripheral neuropathy	M00.9	Pyogenic arthritis, unspecified
369.20	Moderate or severe vision impairment, both eyes Edema Arthropathy associated with infections	H54.2	Low vision, both eyes
342.00	Hemiplegia and hemiparesis	G81.00	Flaccid hemiplegia affecting unspecified side
369.24	Moderate or severe vision impairment	H54.10	Blindness, one eye, low vision other eye, unspecified eyes
369.06	Profound vision impairment	H54.10	Blindness, one eye, low vision other eye, unspecified eyes
359.0	Muscular dystrophies	G71.2	Congenital myopathies
357.9	Inflammatory and toxic neuropathy Myoneural disorders	G61.9	Inflammatory polyneuropathy, unspecified
344.1	Locked in state	G82.20	Paraplegia, unspecified
353.8	Nerve root/plexus disorders	G54.8	Other nerve root and plexus disorders
342.91	Hemiplegia (affecting non-dominant site), unspecified Quadriplegia	G81.91	Hemiplegia, unspecified affecting right dominant side
828.0	Monoplegia of lower limb Upper limb Cauda equine	T07	Unspecified multiple injuries
348.1	Other specific paralytic syndromes Anoxic brain damage Bell's Palsy	G93.1	Anoxic brain damage, not elsewhere classified
727.00-727.06	Other disorders of synovium, tendon, and bursa	M65.9	Synovitis and tenosynovitis, unspecified

(Continued)

—— *Starting your Own Practice from Scratch* ——

728.11	Progressive myositis ossificans	M61.10	Myositis ossificans progressiva, unspecified site
728.12	Traumatic myositis ossificans	M61.00	Myositis ossificans traumatica, unspecified site
728.2	Muscular wasting and disuse atrophy, not elsewhere classified	M62.50	Muscle wasting and atrophy, not elsewhere classified, unspecified site
728.6	Contracture of palmar fascia	M72.0	Palmar fascial fibromatosis [Dupuytren]
728.71	Plantar fascial fibromatosis	M72.2	Plantar fascial fibromatosis
728.83	Rupture of muscle, non-traumatic	M62.10	Other rupture of muscle (nontraumatic), unspecified site
728.85	Spasm of muscle	M62.838	Other muscle spasm
729.1	Myalgia and myositis, unspecified	M60.9	Myositis, unspecified
729.4	Fasciitis, unspecified	M72.9	Fibroblastic disorder, unspecified
729.5	Pain in limb	M79.609	Pain in unspecified limb
729.81-729.82	Swelling of limb, cramp	M79.89	Other specified soft tissue disorders
781.0	Abnormal involuntary movement	R25.9	Unspecified abnormal involuntary movements
781.2	Abnormality of gait	R26.9	Unspecified abnormalities of gait and mobility
781.3	Lack of coordination	R27.9	Unspecified lack of coordination
782.3	Edema	R60.9	Edema, unspecified
809.0	Ill-defined fractures of bones of trunk	S22.9XXA	Fracture of bony thorax, part unspecified, initial encounter for closed fracture
810.00-810.03	Fracture of clavicle	S42.009A	Fracture of unspecified part of unspecified clavicle, initial encounter for closed fracture
811.01-811.03	Fracture of scapula	S42.123A	Displaced fracture of acromial process, unspecified shoulder, initial encounter for closed fracture
812.00-812.03	Fracture of humerus	S42.209A	Unspecified fracture of upper end of unspecified humerus, initial encounter for closed fracture
840.0-840.6	Sprains and strains of shoulder and upper arm	S43.50XA	Sprain of unspecified acromioclavicular joint, initial encounter
841.0-841.3	Sprains and strains of elbow and forearm	S53.439A	Radial collateral ligament sprain of unspecified elbow, initial encounter
842.00-842.02	Sprains and strains of wrist and hand	S63.509A	Unspecified sprain of unspecified wrist, initial encounter
842.09	842.10-842.13	S63.599A	Other specified sprain of unspecified wrist, initial encounter

(Continued)

843.0-843.1	Sprains and strains of hip and thighs	S73.119A	Iliofemoral ligament sprain of unspecified hip, initial encounter
844.0-844.3	Sprains and strains of knee and leg	S83.429A	Sprain of lateral collateral ligament of unspecified knee, initial encounter
845.00-845.03	Sprains and strains of ankle and foot	S93.429A	Sprain of deltoid ligament of unspecified ankle, initial encounter
846.0-846.3	Sprains and strains of sacroiliac region	S33.8XXA	Sprain of other parts of lumbar spine and pelvis, initial encounter
847.0-847.4	Sprains and strains of other and unspecified parts of back	S13.4XXA	Sprain of ligaments of cervical spine, initial encounter
848.0-848.3	Other and ill-defined sprains and strains	S03.1XXA	Dislocation of septal cartilage of nose, initial encounter
923.00-923.03	Contusion of upper limb	S40.019A	Contusion of unspecified shoulder, initial encounter
924.00-924.01	Contusion of lower limb and other and unspecified sites	S70.10XA	Contusion of unspecified thigh, initial encounter
926.0	Crushing injury of the trunk	S38.001A	Crushing injury of unspecified external genital organs, male, initial encounter
926.11-926.12	Crushing injury of back	S38.1XXA	Crushing injury of abdomen, lower back, and pelvis, initial encounter
956.0-956.5	Injury to peripheral nerve(s) of pelvic girdle and lower limb	S74.00XA	Injury of sciatic nerve at hip and thigh level, unspecified leg, initial encounter
997.61	Late amputation stump complication	T87.30	Neuroma of amputation stump, unspecified extremity
V43.60-V43.66	Organ or tissue replaced by joint	Z96.60	Presence of unspecified orthopedic joint implant
V43.69	Organ or tissue replaced by limb	Z96.698	Presence of other orthopedic joint implants
V45.4XXA	Arthrodesis status	E824.8	Other motor vehicle nontraffic accident while boarding and alighting injuring other specified person
V49.60-V49.67	Upper limb amputation status	Z89.209	Acquired absence of unspecified upper limb, unspecified level
V49.70-V49.77	Lower limb amputation status	Z89.9	Acquired absence of limb, unspecified
V54.09	Aftercare involving removal of fracture plate or other internal fixation device	Z51.89	Encounter for other specified aftercare
V54.89	Other orthopedic aftercare	Z47.89	Encounter for other orthopedic aftercare

(Continued)

Medicare is establishing the following limited coverage for aquatic therapy:

ICD-9	ICD-9 Description	ICD-10	ICD-10 Description
340	Multiple sclerosis	G35	Multiple sclerosis
342.00-342.02	Hemiplegia and hemiparesis	G81.00	Flaccid hemiplegia affecting unspecified side
711.00-711.09	Arthropathy associated with infections	M00.10	Pneumococcal arthritis, unspecified joint
712.10-712.19	Crystal arthropathies	M11.80	Other specified crystal arthropathies, unspecified site
713.0-713.8	Arthropathies associated with other disorders classified elsewhere	M14.80	Arthropathies in other specified diseases classified elsewhere, unspecified site
714.0-714.2	Rheumatoid arthritis and other inflammatory polyarthropathies	M06.9	Rheumatoid arthritis, unspecified
715.00	Osteoarthritis and allied disorders	M15.0	Primary generalized (osteo)arthritis
716.00-716.09	Other and unspecified arthropathies	M12.10	Kaschin-Beck disease, unspecified site
718.20-718.29	Pathological dislocation	M24.30	Pathological dislocation of unspecified joint, not elsewhere classified
718.30-718.39	Recurrent dislocation of joint	M24.40	Recurrent dislocation, unspecified joint
718.40-718.49	Contracture of joint	M24.50	Contracture, unspecified joint
719.00-719.09	Other and unspecified disorders of joint	M25.40	Effusion, unspecified joint
720.0-720.2	Ankylosing spondylitis and other inflammatory spondylopathies	M45.9	Ankylosing spondylitis of unspecified sites in spine
722.0	Intervertebral disc disorder	M50.20	Other cervical disc displacement, unspecified cervical region
723.0-723.5	Other disorders of cervical region	M48.02	Spinal stenosis, cervical region
724.01-724.02	Other and unspecified disorders of the back	M48.04	Spinal stenosis, thoracic region
726.0	Peripheral enthesopathies and allied syndromes	M75.00	Adhesive capsulitis of unspecified shoulder
727.00-727.06	Other disorders of synovium, tendon, and bursa	M65.9	Synovitis and tenosynovitis, unspecified
728.11	Progressive myositis ossificans	M61.10	Myositis ossificans progressiva, unspecified site
728.12	Traumatic myositis ossificans	M61.00	Myositis ossificans traumatica, unspecified site

(Continued)

728.2	Muscular wasting and disuse atrophy, not elsewhere classified	M62.50	Muscle wasting and atrophy, not elsewhere classified, unspecified site
728.6	Contracture of palmar fascia	M72.0	Palmar fascial fibromatosis [Dupuytren]
728.71	Plantar fascial fibromatosis	M72.2	Plantar fascial fibromatosis
728.83	Rupture of muscle, non-traumatic	M62.10	Other rupture of muscle (nontraumatic), unspecified site
728.85	Spasm of muscle	M62.40	Contracture of muscle, unspecified site
729.1	Myalgia and myositis, unspecified	M60.9	Myositis, unspecified
729.4	Fasciitis, unspecified	M72.9	Fibroblastic disorder, unspecified
729.5	Pain in limb	M79.609	Pain in unspecified limb
729.81-729.82	Swelling of limb, cramp	M79.89	Other specified soft tissue disorders
781.2	Abnormality of gait	R26.9	Unspecified abnormalities of gait and mobility
781.3	Lack of coordination	R27.9	Unspecified lack of coordination

Medicare is establishing the following limited coverage for gait training:

ICD-9	ICD-9 Description	ICD-10	ICD-10 Description
358.2	Inflammatory and toxic neuropathy Myoneural disorders	G70.1	Toxic myoneural disorders
359.0	Muscular dystrophies	G71.2	Congenital myopathies
369.08	Profound vision impairment	H54.10	Blindness, one eye, low vision other eye, unspecified eyes
369.24	Moderate or severe vision impairment	H54.10	Blindness, one eye, low vision other eye, unspecified eyes
369.20	Moderate or severe vision impairment, both eyes	H54.2	Low vision, both eyes
436	Acute, ill-defined, cerebrovascular disease Other acquired deformities of foot Reduction deformities of lower limb Other anomalies of lower limb, including pelvic girdle	I67.89	Other cerebrovascular disease
781.0	Abnormal involuntary movements Abnormality of gait Lack of coordination Other symptoms involving nervous and musculoskeletal systems	R25.9	Unspecified abnormal involuntary movements
V42.89	Organ or tissue replaced by joint; hip, knee, ankle Lower limb amputation status Orthotic training	Z94.89	Other transplanted organ and tissue status

(Continued)

Medicare is establishing the following limited coverage for massage:

ICD-9	ICD-9 Description	ICD-10	ICD-10 Description
480.8-480.9 481	Pneumococcal pneumonia (streptococcus pneumoniae pneumonia)	J12.89	Other viral pneumonia
482.0-482.2	Other bacterial pneumonia	J15.0	Pneumonia due to Klebsiella pneumoniae
482.30-482.32	Pneumonia due to streptococcus	J15.4	Pneumonia due to other streptococci
482.40	Pneumonia due to staphylo-coccus	J15.20	Pneumonia due to staphylococcus, un-specified
482.81-482.83	Pneumonia due to other speci-fied bacteria	J15.20	Pneumonia due to staphylococcus, un-specified
483.0	Pneumonia due to other speci-fied organism	J15.7	Pneumonia due to Mycoplasma pneumo-niae
484.1	Pneumonia in infectious diseases classified elsewhere	B25.0	Cytomegaloviral pneumonitis
485	Bronchopneumonia, organism unspecified	J18.0	Bronchopneumonia, unspecified organism
486	Pneumonia, organism unspec-ified	J18.9	Pneumonia, unspecified organism
487.0-487.1	Influenza	J11.00	Influenza due to unidentified influenza virus with unspecified type of pneumonia
490	Bronchitis, not specified as acute or chronic	J40	Bronchitis, not specified as acute or chronic
491.0-491.1	Chronic bronchitis	J41.0	Simple chronic bronchitis
494.0	Bronchiectasis	J47.9	Bronchiectasis, uncomplicated
495.0-495.9	Extrinsic allergic alveolitis	J67.0	Farmer's lung
496	Chronic airway obstruction, not elsewhere classified	J44.9	Chronic obstructive pulmonary disease, unspecified
500	Coal workers' pneumoconiosis	J60	Coalworker's pneumoconiosis
501	Asbestosis	J61	Pneumoconiosis due to asbestos and other mineral fibers
502	Pneumoconiosis due to other silica or silicates	J62.8	Pneumoconiosis due to other dust con-taining silica
503	Pneumoconiosis due to other inorganic dust	J63.6	Pneumoconiosis due to other specified inorganic dusts
504	Pneumonopathy due to inhala-tion of other dust	J66.8	Airway disease due to other specific organic dusts
505	Pneumoconiosis, unspecified	J64	Unspecified pneumoconiosis
506.9	Respiratory conditions due to chemical fumes and vapors	J68.9	Unspecified respiratory condition due to chemicals, gases, fumes and vapors

(Continued)

507.0-507.1	Pneumonitis due to solids and liquids	J69.0	Pneumonitis due to inhalation of food and vomit
508.0-508.1	Respiratory conditions due to other and unspecified external agents	J70.0	Acute pulmonary manifestations due to radiation
513.0-513.1	Abscess of lung and mediastinum	J85.1	Abscess of lung with pneumonia
514	Pulmonary congestion and hypostasis	J18.2	Hypostatic pneumonia, unspecified organism
515	Postinflammatory pulmonary fibrosis	J84.10	Pulmonary fibrosis, unspecified
516.1-516.3	Other alveolar and parietoalveolar pneumonopathies	J84.03	Idiopathic pulmonary hemosiderosis
517.1-517.2	Lung involvement in conditions classified elsewhere	J17	Pneumonia in diseases classified elsewhere
524.60 524.63	Temporomandibular joint disorders, unspecified	M26.60	Temporomandibular joint disorder, unspecified
724.1	Pain in thoracic spine	M54.6	Pain in thoracic spine
724.2	Lumbago	M54.5	Low back pain
724.5	Backache, unspecified	M54.9	Dorsalgia, unspecified
726.2	Peripheral enthesopathies and allied syndromes	M75.40	Impingement syndrome of unspecified shoulder
727.81	Contracture of tendon (sheath)	M67.00	Short Achilles tendon (acquired), unspecified ankle
728.6	Contracture of palmar fascia	M72.0	Palmar fascial fibromatosis [Dupuytren]
728.71	Plantar fascial fibromatosis	M72.2	Plantar fascial fibromatosis
728.79	Other fibromatosis	M72.4	Pseudosarcomatous fibromatosis
728.85	Spasm of muscle	M62.40	Contracture of muscle, unspecified site
729.5	Pain in limb	M79.609	Pain in unspecified limb
729.81	Swelling of limb	M79.89	Other specified soft tissue disorders
729.82	Cramp	R25.2	Cramp and spasm
754.1	Certain congenital musculoskeletal deformities of sternocleidomastoid muscle	Q68.0	Congenital deformity of sternocleidomastoid muscle
840.0-840.6	Sprains and strains of shoulder and upper arm	S43.50XA	Sprain of unspecified acromioclavicular joint, initial encounter
841.0-841.3	Sprains and strains of elbow and forearm	S53.439A	Radial collateral ligament sprain of unspecified elbow, initial encounter
842.00-842.02	Sprains and strains of wrist and hand	S63.509A	Unspecified sprain of unspecified wrist, initial encounter

(Continued)

843.0-843.1	Sprains and strains of hip and thighs	S73.119A	Iliofemoral ligament sprain of unspecified hip, initial encounter
844.0-844.3	Sprains and strains of knee and leg	S83.429A	Sprain of lateral collateral ligament of unspecified knee, initial encounter
845.00-845.03	Sprains and strains of ankle and foot	S93.409A	Sprain of unspecified ligament of unspecified ankle, initial encounter
846.0-846.3	Sprains and strains of sacroiliac region	S33.8XXA	Sprain of other parts of lumbar spine and pelvis, initial encounter
847.0-847.4	Sprains and strains of other and unspecified parts of back	S13.4XXA	Sprain of ligaments of cervical spine, initial encounter
848.0-848.3	Other and ill-defined sprains and strains	S03.1XXA	Dislocation of septal cartilage of nose, initial encounter

Medicare is establishing the following limited coverage for manual therapy:

For Manual Traction:

ICD-9	ICD-9 Description	ICD-10	ICD-10 Description
333.83	Spasmodic torticollis Cervical root lesions, NEC Lumbosacral root lesions, NEC Intervertebral disc disorders	G24.3	Spasmodic torticollis
723.1	Cervicalgia Torticollis, unspecified	M54.2	Cervicalgia
724.01	Spinal stenosis, lumbar region Lumbago Sciatica Thoracic or lumbosacral neuritis or radiculitis,	M48.04	Spinal stenosis, thoracic region
848.8	Sprains and strains, neck Sprains and strains, lumbar Injury to cervical root Injury to lumbar root Injury to sacral root	S03.9XXA	Sprain of joints and ligaments of unspecified parts of head, initial encounter
729.90	Myofascial Release/Soft Tissue Mobilization, One or More Regions :	M79.9	Soft tissue disorder, unspecified
333.6	Idiopathic torsion dystonia Symptomatic torsion dystonia Spasmodic torticollis Organic writers' cramp	G24.1	Genetic torsion dystonia
337.20	Reflex sympathetic dystrophy	G90.59	Complex regional pain syndrome I of other specified site

(Continued)

457.0	Postmastectomy lymphedema syndrome Scar conditions and fibrosis of skin Systemic sclerosis Dermatomyositis Polymyositis Other specified diffuse diseases of connective	I97.2	Postmastectomy lymphedema syndrome
714.2	Rheumatoid arthritis and other inflammatory	M05.30	Rheumatoid heart disease with rheumatoid arthritis of unspecified site
718.34	Pathological dislocation Recurrent dislocation of joint Contracture of joint Other and unspecified disorders of joint	M24.443	Recurrent dislocation, unspecified hand
720.1	Ankylosing spondylitis Spinal enthesopathy Cervicalgia Cervicocranial syndrome	M46.00	Spinal enthesopathy, site unspecified
723.5	Torticollis, unspecified Pain in thoracic spine Lumbago	M43.6	Torticollis
726.8	Peripheral enthesopathies and allied syndromes	M77.8	Other enthesopathies, not elsewhere classified
727.81	Contracture of tendon (sheath) Plantar fascial fibromatosis	M67.00	Short Achilles tendon (acquired), unspecified ankle
729.4	Fasciitis, unspecified Pain in limb Swelling of limb Cramp Certain congenital musculoskeletal deformities of	M72.9	Fibroblastic disorder, unspecified
754.1	sternocleidomastoid muscle	Q68.0	Congenital deformity of sternocleidomastoid muscle
840.9	Edema Headache Sprains and strains of shoulder and upper arm	S46.919A	Strain of unspecified muscle, fascia and tendon at shoulder and upper arm level, unspecified arm, initial encounter
841.8	Sprains and strains of elbow and forearm	S53.499A	Other sprain of unspecified elbow, initial encounter
842.09	Sprains and strains of wrist and hand Sprains and strains of hip and thighs Sprains and strains of knee and let Sprains and strains of ankle and foot	S63.599A	Other specified sprain of unspecified wrist, initial encounter
846.9	Sprains and strains of sacroiliac region Sprains and strains of other and unspecified parts	S33.9XXA	Sprain of unspecified parts of lumbar spine and pelvis, initial encounter
848.8	Other and ill-defined sprains and strains	S03.9XXA	Sprain of joints and ligaments of unspecified parts of head, initial encounter
724.4	Manipulation (Cervical, Thoracic, Lumbosacral, Sacroiliac, Hand, Wrist), One Area and Each Additional Area	M54.16	Radiculopathy, lumbar region

(Continued)

710.8	Other specified diffuse diseases of connective Rheumatoid arthritis and other inflammatory	M35.5	Multifocal fibrosclerosis
718.20	Pathological dislocation	M24.30	Pathological dislocation of unspecified joint, not elsewhere classified
718.33	Recurrent dislocation of joint	M24.439	Recurrent dislocation, unspecified wrist
718.40	Contracture of joint	M24.50	Contracture, unspecified joint
719.80	Other and unspecified disorders of joint	M25.80	Other specified joint disorders, unspecified joint
720.0	Ankylosing spondylitis	M45.9	Ankylosing spondylitis of unspecified sites in spine
720.1	Spinal enthesopathy	M46.00	Spinal enthesopathy, site unspecified
723.1	Cervicalgia	M54.2	Cervicalgia
723.2	Cervicocranial syndrome	M53.0	Cervicocranial syndrome
723.5	Torticollis, unspecified	M43.6	Torticollis
724.02	Spinal stenosis, lumbar region	M48.06	Spinal stenosis, lumbar region
724.1	Pain in thoracic spine	M54.6	Pain in thoracic spine
724.2	Lumbago	M54.5	Low back pain
726.8	Peripheral enthesopathies and allied syndromes	M77.8	Other enthesopathies, not elsewhere classified
840.9	Sprains and strains of shoulder and upper arm	S46.919A	Strain of unspecified muscle, fascia and tendon at shoulder and upper arm level, unspecified arm, initial encounte
841.8	Sprains and strains of elbow and forearm	S53.499A	Other sprain of unspecified elbow, initial encounter
842.19	Sprains and strains of wrist and hand	S63.8X9A	Sprain of other part of unspecified wrist and hand, initial encounter
843.8	Sprains and strains of hip and thighs	S73.199A	Other sprain of unspecified hip, initial encounter
844.9	Sprains and strains of knee and leg	S86.919A	Strain of unspecified muscle(s) and tendon(s) at lower leg level, unspecified leg, initial encounter
845.09	Sprains and strains of ankle and foot	S93.499A	Sprain of other ligament of unspecified ankle, initial encounter
846.9	Sprains and strains of sacroiliac region	S33.9XXA	Sprain of unspecified parts of lumbar spine and pelvis, initial encounter
848.9	Sprains and strains of other and unspecified parts	T14.90	Injury, unspecified
848.8	Other and ill-defined sprains and strains	S29.019A	Strain of muscle and tendon of unspecified wall of thorax, initial encounter

(Continued)

826.1	Joint Mobilization, One or More Areas Covered for:	S92.403B	Displaced unspecified fracture of unspecified great toe, initial encounter for open fracture
713.1	Arthropathy associated with infections	M02.00	Arthropathy following intestinal bypass, unspecified site
712.80	Crystal arthropathies	M11.80	Other specified crystal arthropathies, unspecified site
V82.2	Arthropathies associated with other disorders Rheumatoid arthritis and other inflammatory	Z13.89	Encounter for screening for other disorder
715.00	Osteoarthritis and allied disorders	M15.0	Primary generalized (osteo)arthritis
716.00-716.09	Other and unspecified arthropathies	M12.10	Kaschin-Beck disease, unspecified site
718.40-718.9	Contracture of joint	M24.50	Contracture, unspecified joint
719.00-719.09	Other and unspecified disorders of joint	M25.40	Effusion, unspecified joint
720.0-720.2	Ankylosing spondylitis and other inflammatory spondylopathies	M45.9	Ankylosing spondylitis of unspecified sites in spine
726.19	Peripheral enthesopathies and allied syndromes	M75.80	Other shoulder lesions, unspecified shoulder
727.00	Synovitis and tenosynovitis, unspecified	M65.9	Synovitis and tenosynovitis, unspecified
727.04	Radial styloid tenosynovitis	M65.4	Radial styloid tenosynovitis [de Quervain]
727.06	Tenosynovitis of foot and ankle other internal fixation device	M65.879	Other synovitis and tenosynovitis, unspecified ankle and foot
V54.89	Other orthopedic aftercare	Z47.89	Encounter for other orthopedic aftercare

Medicare is establishing the following limited coverage for orthotics:

ICD-9	ICD-9 Description	ICD-10	ICD-10 Description
952.00-952.09	bone injury	S14.101A	Unspecified injury at C1 level of cervical spinal cord, initial encounter
956.0-956.3	lower limb	S74.00XA	Injury of sciatic nerve at hip and thigh level, unspecified leg, initial encounter
726.70	Enthesopathy of ankle and tarsus, unspecified Other acquired deformities of ankle and foot	M76.899	Other specified enthesopathies of unspecified lower limb, excluding foot
952.4	Spinal cord injury without evidence of spinal	S34.3XXA	Injury of cauda equina, initial encounter
907.5	Injury to peripheral nerve(s) of pelvic girdle and	S74.90XS	Injury of unspecified nerve at hip and thigh level, unspecified leg, sequela
V49.1	Mechanical problems with limbs	R68.89	$Other general symptoms and signs

(Continued)

| V49.2 | Motor problems with limbs Upper limb amputation status Lower limb amputation status | R68.89 | Other general symptoms and signs |
| V53.7 | Fitting and adjustment of ortho- pedic device | Z46.89 | Encounter for fitting and adjustment of other specified devices |

Medicare is establishing the following limited coverage for prosthetic training:

ICD-9	ICD-9 Description	ICD-10	ICD-10 Description
885.1	Traumatic amputation of thumb (complete)	S68.019A	Complete traumatic metacarpophalangeal amputation of unspecified thumb, initial encounter
886.1	Traumatic amputation of fingers (complete)	S68.119A	Complete traumatic metacarpophalangeal amputation of unspecified finger, initial encounter
887.1	Traumatic amputation of arm and hand	S58.119A	Complete traumatic amputation at level between elbow and wrist, unspecified arm, initial encounter
896.1	Traumatic amputation of foot (complete)	S98.019A	Complete traumatic amputation of unspecified foot at ankle level, initial encounter
897.5	Traumatic amputation of leg(s) (complete)	S78.919A	Complete traumatic amputation of un- specified hip and thigh, level unspecified, initial encounter
V49.60	Upper limb amputation status	Z89.209	Acquired absence of unspecified upper limb, unspecified level
V49.70	Lower limb amputation status Fitting and adjustment of artifi- cial arm (complete)	Z89.9	Acquired absence of limb, unspecified
V52.1	Fitting and adjustment of artificial leg (complete) Other specified prosthetic device Fitting and adjustment of other orthopedic device	Z44.109	Encounter for fitting and adjustment of unspecified artificial leg, unspecified leg

Medicare is establishing the following limited coverage for therapeutic activities:

ICD-9	ICD-9 Description	ICD-10	ICD-10 Description
274.00	Gouty arthropathy Gout, un- specified	M10.00	Idiopathic gout, unspecified site
333.90	Parkinsonism Spasmodic torticollis Unspecified extrapy- ramidal diseases and abnormal movement disorders	G25.9	Extrapyramidal and movement disorder, unspecified
369.20	Moderate or severe vision impairment	H54.2	Low vision, both eyes

(Continued)

369.10	Moderate or severe vision impairment, both eyes Acute, but ill-defined cerebrovascular disease	H54.10	Blindness, one eye, low vision other eye, unspecified eyes
711.88	Arthropathy associated with infections	M01.X8	Direct infection of vertebrae in infectious and parasitic diseases classified elsewhere
712.80	Crystal arthropathies	M11.80	Other specified crystal arthropathies, unspecified site
713.0	Arthropathies associated with other disorders	M14.80	Arthropathies in other specified diseases classified elsewhere, unspecified site
714.31	Rheumatoid arthritis and other inflammatory	M08.3	Juvenile rheumatoid polyarthritis (sero-negative)
721.8	Osteoarthritis and allied disor-ders	M48.9	Spondylopathy, unspecified
716.00-716.09	Other and unspecified arthrop-athies	M12.10	Kaschin-Beck disease, unspecified site
718.20-718.29	Pathological dislocation	M24.30	Pathological dislocation of unspecified joint, not elsewhere classified
718.30-728.39	Recurrent dislocation of joint	M24.40	Recurrent dislocation, unspecified joint
718.40-718.49	Contracture of joint	M24.50	Contracture, unspecified joint
719.00-719.09	Other and unspecified disorders of joint	M25.40	Effusion, unspecified joint
720.0-720.2	Ankylosing spondylitis and oth-er inflammatory spondylopathies	M45.9	Ankylosing spondylitis of unspecified sites in spine
722.0	Intervertebral disc disorder	M50.20	Other cervical disc displacement, unspeci-fied cervical region
722.91	Other disorders of cervical region	M50.80	Other cervical disc disorders, unspecified cervical region
724.9	Other and unspecified disorders of the back	M53.9	Dorsopathy, unspecified
726.8	Peripheral enthesopathies and allied syndromes	M77.8	Other enthesopathies, not elsewhere classified
727.89	Other disorders of synovium, tendon, and bursa	M67.88	Other specified disorders of synovium and tendon, other site
728.11	Progressive myositis ossificans	M61.10	Myositis ossificans progressiva, unspeci-fied site
728.12	Traumatic myositis ossificans	M61.00	Myositis ossificans traumatica, unspecified site
728.2	Muscular wasting and disuse atrophy	M62.50	Muscle wasting and atrophy, not else-where classified, unspecified site
728.6	Contracture of palmar fascia	M72.0	Palmar fascial fibromatosis [Dupuytren]

(Continued)

728.71	Plantar fascial fibromatosis	M72.2	Plantar fascial fibromatosis
728.83	Rupture of muscle, non-traumatic	M62.10	Other rupture of muscle (nontraumatic), unspecified site
728.85	Spasm of muscle	M62.40	Contracture of muscle, unspecified site
729.1	Myalgia and myositis, unspecified musculoskeletal systems	M79.1	Myalgia
782.3	Edema	R60.9	Edema, unspecified
799.3	Debility, unspecified	R53.81	Other malaise
799.4	Cachexia	R64	Cachexia
805.00–805.08	Fracture of vertebral column without mention of spinal cord injury,	S12.9XXA	Fracture of neck, unspecified, initial encounter
805.8	Fracture of vertebral column without mention of spinal cord injury, dorsal, lumbar, sacrum, and coccyx, unspecified, open/closed fracture of rib(s), sternum, larynx, and trachea Fracture of pelvis	S32.009A	Unspecified fracture of unspecified lumbar vertebra, initial encounter for closed fracture
803.89	Fracture of other and unspecified parts of the	S02.91XB	Unspecified fracture of skull, initial encounter for open fracture
823.22	Fracture of the patella Fracture of tibia and fibula	S82.201A	Unspecified fracture of shaft of right tibia, initial encounter for closed fracture
824.8	Fracture of the ankle Fracture of one or more tarsal and metatarsal	S82.899A	Other fracture of unspecified lower leg, initial encounter for closed fracture
826.1	Fracture of one or more phalanges of foot Other, multiple, an ill-defined fractures of lower	S92.403B	Displaced unspecified fracture of unspecified great toe, initial encounter for open fracture
830.0	Dislocation of jaw	S03.0XXA	Dislocation of jaw, initial encounter
831.00	Dislocation of shoulder	S43.006A	Unspecified dislocation of unspecified shoulder joint, initial encounter
832.00	Dislocation of elbow	S53.006A	Unspecified dislocation of unspecified radial head, initial encounter
833.09	Dislocation of wrist	S63.096A	Other dislocation of unspecified wrist and hand, initial encounter
834.00	Dislocation of finger	S63.259A	Unspecified dislocation of unspecified finger, initial encounter
835.01	Dislocation of hip	S73.016A	Posterior dislocation of unspecified hip, initial encounter
836.50	Dislocation of knee	S83.106A	Unspecified dislocation of unspecified knee, initial encounter

(Continued)

837.0	Dislocation of ankle	S93.06XA	Dislocation of unspecified ankle joint, initial encounter
838.00	Dislocation of foot	S93.306A	Unspecified dislocation of unspecified foot, initial encounter
840.8	Sprains and strains of shoulder and upper arm	S46.019A	Strain of muscle(s) and tendon(s) of the rotator cuff of unspecified shoulder, initial encounter
841.8	Sprains and strains of elbow and forearm	S53.499A	Other sprain of unspecified elbow, initial encounter
842.19	Sprains and strains of wrist and hand	S63.8X9A	Sprain of other part of unspecified wrist and hand, initial encounter
843.9	Sprains and strains of hip and thighs	S76.919A	Strain of unspecified muscles, fascia and tendons at thigh level, unspecified thigh, initial encounter
844.9	Sprains and strains of knee and leg	S86.919A	Strain of unspecified muscle(s) and tendon(s) at lower leg level, unspecified leg, initial encounter
845.09	Sprains and strains of ankle and foot	S93.499A	Sprain of other ligament of unspecified ankle, initial encounter
846.9	Sprains and strains of sacroiliac region	S33.9XXA	Sprain of unspecified parts of lumbar spine and pelvis, initial encounter
848.8	Sprains and strains of other and unspecified parts	S39.011A	Strain of muscle, fascia and tendon of abdomen, initial encounter
848.0-848.3	Other and ill-defined sprains and strains	S03.1XXA	Dislocation of septal cartilage of nose, initial encounter
851.00-851.06	Cerebral laceration and contusion	S06.330A	Contusion and laceration of cerebrum, unspecified, without loss of consciousness, initial encounter
923.00-923.03	Contusion of upper limb	S40.019A	Contusion of unspecified shoulder, initial encounter
924.00-924.01	Contusion of lower limb and other and unspecified sites	S70.10XA	Contusion of unspecified thigh, initial encounter
926.0	Crushing injury of the trunk	S38.001A	Crushing injury of unspecified external genital organs, male, initial encounter
955.0-955.9	Injury of upper limb	S44.30XA	Injury of axillary nerve, unspecified arm, initial encounter
956.0-956.5	Injury of lower limb	S74.00XA	Injury of sciatic nerve at hip and thigh level, unspecified leg, initial encounter
927.9	Crushing injury of upper limb	S47.9XXA	Crushing injury of shoulder and upper arm, unspecified arm, initial encounter
928.9	Crushing injury of lower limb	S77.20XA	Crushing injury of unspecified hip with thigh, initial encounter

(Continued)

952.4	Spinal cord injury without evidence of spinal	S34.3XXA	Injury of cauda equina, initial encounter
953.8	Injury to nerve roots and spinal plexus	S34.21XA	Injury of nerve root of lumbar spine, initial encounter
907.5	Late effect of injury to peripheral nerve of pelvic girdle and lower limb	S74.90XS	Injury of unspecified nerve at hip and thigh level, unspecified leg, sequela
956.5	Injury to other specified nerve(s) of pelvic girdle and lower limb	S74.8X9A	Injury of other nerves at hip and thigh level, unspecified leg, initial encounter
905.9	Late amputation stump complication Organ or tissue replaced by joint	S48.919S	Complete traumatic amputation of unspecified shoulder and upper arm, level unspecified, sequela
V49.70	Arthrodesis status Upper limb amputation status Lower limb amputation status	Z89.9	Acquired absence of limb, unspecified
V54.09	Aftercare involving removal of fracture plate or other internal fixation device	Z51.89	Encounter for other specified aftercare
V54.89	Other orthopedic aftercare	Z47.89	Encounter for other orthopedic aftercare

Medicare is establishing the following limited coverage for wheelchair management:

ICD-9	ICD-9 Description	ICD-10	ICD-10 Description
334.0–334.4	Spinocerebellar disease	G11.1	Early-onset cerebellar ataxia
335.0	Anterior horn cell disease	G12.0	Infantile spinal muscular atrophy, type I [Werdnig-Hoffman]
335.10–335.11	Spinal muscular atrophy, unspecified	G12.9	Spinal muscular atrophy, unspecified
733.15	Fracture of other and unspecified parts of the femur	M84.453A	Pathological fracture, unspecified femur, initial encounter for fracture
851.00–851.06	Cerebral laceration and contusion	S06.330A	Contusion and laceration of cerebrum, unspecified, without loss of consciousness, initial encounter
851.99			Traumatic amputation of leg(s) (complete) (partial) Crushing injury to hip and thigh Crushing injury to knee and lower leg Lower limb amputation status Fitting and adjustment of wheelchair

Medicare is establishing the following limited coverage for orthotic/prosthetic use:

ICD-9	ICD-9 Description	ICD-10	ICD-10 Description
524.60–524.63	Temporomandibular joint disorders, unspecified	M26.60	Temporomandibular joint disorder, unspecified
V49.0–V49.5	Problems with limbs and other problems	R68.89	Other general symptoms and signs

(Continued)

V52.0	Fitting and adjustment of prosthetic device and implant, artificial arm (complete) (partial)	Z44.009	Encounter for fitting and adjustment of unspecified artificial arm, unspecified arm
V52.1	Fitting and adjustment of prosthetic device and implant, artificial leg (complete) (partial)	Z44.009	Encounter for fitting and adjustment of unspecified artificial leg, unspecified leg
Other PT/OT/SP codes:			
338.21	Chronic pain due to trauma, Excludes: causalgia (355.9, 355.71, 354.4), chronic pain syndrome, myofascial pain syndrome, neoplasm related chronic pain, reflex sympathetic dystrophy (337.20-337.29)	G89.21	hronic pain due to trauma
338.22	Chronic post-thoracotomy pain, Excludes: causalgia (355.9, 355.71, 354 4), chronic pain syndrome, myofascial pain syndrome, neoplasm related chronic pain, reflex sympathetic dystrophy (337.20-337.29)	G89.22	Chronic post-thoracotomy pain
338.28	Other chronic postoperative pain, Excludes: causalgia (355.9, 355.71, 354.4), chronic pain syndrome, myofascial pain syndrome, neoplasm related chronic pain, reflex sympathetic dystrophy (337.20-337.29)	G89.28	Other chronic postprocedural pain
338.29	Other chronic pain, Excludes: causalgia (355.9, 355.71, 354.4), chronic pain syndrome, myofascial pain syndrome, neoplasm related chronic pain, reflex sympathetic dystrophy (337.20-337.29)	G89.29	Other chronic pain
338.3	Neoplasm related pain, cancer assoc. pain, pain d/t malignancy, tumor assoc. pain	G89.3	Neoplasm related pain (acute) (chronic)

(Continued)

342.01	Flaccid hemiplegia, dominant side; this category is to be used when hemiplegia is reported without further specification, or is stated to be old or long-standing but of unspecified cause. The category is also for use in multiple coding to identify these types of hemiplegia resulting from any cause. Excludes: congenital, hemiplegia due to late effect of cerebrovascular accident (438.XX), infantile NOS	G81.01	Flaccid hemiplegia affecting right dominant side
342.02	Flaccid hemiplegia, nondominant side; this category is to be used when hemiplegia is reported without further specification, or is stated to be old or long-standing but of unspecified cause. The category is also for use in multiple coding to identify these types of hemiplegia resulting from any cause. Excludes: congenital, hemiplegia due to late effect of cerebrovascular accident (438.xx), infantile NOS	G81.03	Flaccid hemiplegia affecting right non-dominant side
342.11	Spastic hemiplegia, dominant side; this category is to be used when hemiplegia is reported without further specification, or is stated to be old or long-standing but of unspecified cause. The category is also for use in multiple coding to identify these types of hemiplegia resulting from any cause. Excludes: congenital, hemiplegia due to late effect of cerebrovascular accident (438.xx), infantile NOS	G81.11	Spastic hemiplegia affecting right dominant side
342.12	Spastic hemiplegia, nondominant side; this category is to be used when hemiplegia is reported without further specification, or is stated to be old or long-standing but of unspecified cause. The category is also for use in multiple coding to identify these types of hemiplegia resulting from any cause. Excludes: congenital, hemiplegia due to late effect of cerebrovascular accident (438.xx), infantile NOS	G81.13	Spastic hemiplegia affecting right non-dominant side

(Continued)

342.81	Other specified hemiplegia, dominant side; this category is to be used when hemiplegia is reported without further specification, or is stated to be old or long-standing but of unspecified cause. The category is also for use in multiple coding to identify these types of hemiplegia resulting from any cause. Excludes: congenital, hemiplegia due to late effect of cerebrovascular accident (438.xx), infantile NOS	G81.91	Hemiplegia, unspecified affecting right dominant side
342.82	Other specified hemiplegia, nondominant side; this category is to be used when hemiplegia is reported without further specification, or is stated to be old or long-standing but of unspecified cause. The category is also for use in multiple coding to identify these types of hemiplegia resulting from any cause. Excludes: congenital, hemiplegia due to late effect of cerebrovascular accident (438.xx), infantile NOS	G81.93	Hemiplegia, unspecified affecting right nondominant side
344.31	Monoplegia of lower limb, affecting dominant side; this category is to be used when the condition is reported without further specification, or is stated to be old or long-standing but of unspecified cause. The category is also for use in multiple coding to identify these conditions resulting from any cause.	G83.11	Monoplegia of lower limb affecting right dominant side
344.32	Monoplegia of lower limb, affecting nondominant side; this category is to be used when the condition is reported without further specification, or is stated to be old or long-standing but of unspecified cause. The category is also for use in multiple coding to identify these conditions resulting from any cause.	G83.13	Monoplegia of lower limb affecting right nondominant side

(Continued)

344.41	Monoplegia of upper limb, affecting dominant side; this category is to be used when the condition is reported without further specification, or is stated to be old or long-standing but of unspecified cause. The category is also for use in multiple coding to identify these conditions resulting from any cause.	G83.21	Monoplegia of upper limb affecting right dominant side
344.42	Monoplegia of upper limb, affecting nondominant side; this category is to be used when the condition is reported without further specification, or is stated to be old or long-standing but of unspecified cause. The category is also for use in multiple coding to identify these conditions resulting from any cause.	G83.23	Monoplegia of upper limb affecting right nondominant side
438.20	Hemiplegia affecting dominant side	I69.959	Hemiplegia and hemiparesis following unspecified cerebrovascular disease affecting unspecified side
438.22	Hemiplegia affecting nondominant side	I69.953	Hemiplegia and hemiparesis following unspecified cerebrovascular disease affecting right non-dominant side
438.31	Monoplegia of upper limb affecting dominant side	I69.931	Monoplegia of upper limb following unspecified cerebrovascular disease affecting right dominant side
438.32	Monoplegia of upper limb affecting nondominant side	I69.991	Dysphagia following unspecified cerebrovascular disease
438.81	Apraxia	I69.990	Apraxia following unspecified cerebrovascular disease
438.82	Dysphagia (use 787.2x code as treatment code to describe TYPE of dysphagia)	I69.991	Dysphagia following unspecified cerebrovascular disease
438.83	Facial Weakness	I69.992	Facial weakness following unspecified cerebrovascular disease
438.84	Ataxia	I69.993	Ataxia following unspecified cerebrovascular disease
438.85	Vertigo	I69.998	Other sequelae following unspecified cerebrovascular disease

(Continued)

438.89	Other late effects of cerebrovascular disease (This can be used as Med diagnosis and should be used with additional code to identify the late effect) Ex: 438.89/438.20 Pressure Ulcer. This should be coded FIRST: 707.01 Elbow	I69.898	Other sequelae of other cerebrovascular disease
625.6	Stress Incontinence, Female	N39.3	Stress incontinence (female) (male)
707.02	Upper Back	L89.119	Pressure ulcer of right upper back, unspecified stage
707.03	Lower back (includes sacrum, coccyx)	L89.139	Pressure ulcer of right lower back, unspecified stage
707.04	Hip	L89.209	Pressure ulcer of unspecified hip, unspecified stage
707.05	Buttock	L89.309	Pressure ulcer of unspecified buttock, unspecified stage
707.06	Ankle	L89.509	Pressure ulcer of unspecified ankle, unspecified stage
707.07	Heel	L89.609	Pressure ulcer of unspecified heel, unspecified stage
707.09	Other site (includes head)	L89.899	Pressure ulcer of other site, unspecified stage
707.23	Pressure Ulcer Stage III	N/A	Not Available
707.24	Pressure Ulcer Stage IV	N/A	Not Available
707.25	Pressure Ulcer, Unstageable (assing only if ulcer is covered by eschar)	N/A	Not Available
718.40	(contractures) with fifth digit	M24.50	Contracture, unspecified joint
718.4X	Contracture of joint, Requires fifth digit of 1-9	M24.50	Contracture, unspecified joint
719.00	(fusion of joints) with fifth digit	M25.40	Effusion, unspecified joint
719.4X	Pain in joint, Requires fifth digit of 1-9	M25.50	Pain in unspecified joint
719.5X	Stiffness in joint, not elsewhere classified, Requires fifth digit of 1-9	M25.60	Stiffness of unspecified joint, not elsewhere classified
719.7	Difficulty in walking (use this code when dealing with joint or musculoskeletal issues)	R26.2	Difficulty in walking, not elsewhere classified
719.0X	Effusion of joint, Includes: hydrarthrosis; swelling of joint, with or without pain Requires fifth digit of 1-9	M25.40	Effusion, unspecified joint

(Continued)

722.91	Cervical Region, Other and un-specified disc disorder (Calcification of intervertebral cartilage or disc; Discitis)	M50.80	Other cervical disc disorders, unspecified cervical region
722.92	Thoracic Region , Other and un-specified disc disorder (Calcification of intervertebral cartilage or disc; Discitis)	M51.84	Other intervertebral disc disorders, thoracic region
722.93	Lumbar Region, Other and un-specified disc disorder (Calcification of intervertebral cartilage or disc; Discitis)	M51.86	Other intervertebral disc disorders, lumbar region
723.0	Spinal Stenosis of cervical region	M48.02	Spinal stenosis, cervical region
723.1	Cervicalgia (pain in neck)	M54.2	Cervicalgia
723.5	Torticollis, unspecified (contracture of neck)	M43.6	Torticollis
724.01	Spinal stenosis, thoracic region	M43.6	Torticollis
724.02	Spinal stenosis, lumbar region	M48.06	Spinal stenosis, lumbar region
724.1	Pain in thoracic region	M54.6	Pain in thoracic spine
724.2	Lumbago	M54.5	Low back pain
724.3	Sciatica	M54.30	Sciatica, unspecified side
724.5	Backache unspecified	M54.9	Dorsalgia, unspecified
728.85	Spasm of muscle	M62.838	Other muscle spasm
728.87	Muscle weakness (generalized) Excludes: generalized weakness (780.79)	M62.81	Muscle weakness (generalized)
728.9	Unspecified disorder of muscle, ligament, and fascia (evaluation or doc MUST describe disorder)	M62..9	Disorder of muscle, unspecified
729.5	(pain in limb) with fifth digit – this one is also used for pain in extremities not related to a joint.	M79.609	Pain in unspecified limb
729.81	Swelling of limb	M79.89	Other specified soft tissue disorders
733.00	Osteoporosis unspecified	M81.0	Age-related osteoporosis without current pathological fracture
735.0	Acquired deformity of toes, hallux valgus	M20.10	Hallux valgus (acquired), unspecified foot
735.1	Acquired deformity of toes, hallux varus	M20.30	Hallux varus (acquired), unspecified foot
735.2	Acquired deformity of toes, hallux rigidus	M20.20	Hallux rigidus, unspecified foot
735.3	Acquired deformity of toes, hallux malleus	M20.40	Other hammer toe(s) (acquired), unspecified foot

(Continued)

735.4	Acquired deformity of toes, other hammer toe	M20.40	Other hammer toe(s) (acquired), unspecified foot
735.5	Acquired deformity of toes, claw toe	M20.5X9	Other deformities of toe(s) (acquired), unspecified foot
735.8	Acquired deformity of toes, other deformity of toes	M20.5X9	Other deformities of toe(s) (acquired), unspecified foot
735.9	Acquired deformity of toes, unspecified deformity	M20.60	Acquired deformities of toe(s), unspecified, unspecified foot
736.00	Acquired deformity of forearm, unspecified deformity	M21.939	Unspecified acquired deformity of unspecified forearm
736.01	Acquired deformity of forearm, cubitus valgus	M21.029	Valgus deformity, not elsewhere classified, unspecified elbow
736.02	Acquired deformity of forearm, cubitus varus	M21.129	Varus deformity, not elsewhere classified, unspecified elbow
736.03	Acquired deformity of forearm, valgus deformity of wrist	M21.839	Other specified acquired deformities of unspecified forearm
736.04	Acquired deformity of forearm, varus deformity of wrist	M21.839	Other specified acquired deformities of unspecified forearm
736.05	Acquired deformity of forearm, wrist drop	M21.339	Wrist drop, unspecified wrist
736.06	Acquired deformity of forearm, claw hand	M21.519	Acquired clawhand, unspecified hand
736.07	Acquired deformity of forearm, club hand	M21.529	Acquired clubhand, unspecified hand
736.09	Acquired deformity of forearm, other	M21.839	Other specified acquired deformities of unspecified forearm
736.1	Mallet finger	M20.019	Mallet finger of unspecified finger(s)
736.21	Acquired deformity of finger, Boutonniere deformity	M20.029	Boutonnière deformity of unspecified finger(s)
736.22	Acquired deformity of finger, Swan-neck deformity	M20.039	Swan-neck deformity of unspecified finger(s)
736.29	Acquired deformity of finger, other	M20.099	Other deformity of finger(s), unspecified finger(s)
736.31	Acquired deformity of hip, coxa valga	M21.059	Valgus deformity, not elsewhere classified, unspecified hip
736.32	Acquired deformity of hip, coxa vara	M21.159	Varus deformity, not elsewhere classified, unspecified
736.39	Acquired deformity of hip, other	M21.859	Other specified acquired deformities of unspecified thigh
736.41	Acquired deformity of knee, Genu valgum	M21.069	Valgus deformity, not elsewhere classified, unspecified knee
736.42	Acquired deformity of knee, Genu varum	M21.169	Varus deformity, not elsewhere classified, unspecified knee

(Continued)

736.5	Acquired deformity of knee, Genu recurvatum	M21.869	Other specified acquired deformities of unspecified lower leg
736.6	Acquired deformity of knee, Other	M21.869	Other specified acquired deformities of unspecified lower leg
736.71	Acquired deformity of ankle and foot, equinovarus (club foot) Excludes: clubfoot not specified as acquired (754.5-754.7)	M21.549	Acquired clubfoot, unspecified foot
736.72	Acquired deformity of ankle and foot, equinus deformity	M21.6X9	Other acquired deformities of unspecified foot
736.73	Acquired deformity of ankle and foot, cavus deformity Excludes: with claw foot (736.74)	M21.6X9	Other acquired deformities of unspecified foot
736.74	Acquired deformity of ankle and foot, claw foot	M21.539	Acquired clawfoot, unspecified foot
736.75	Acquired deformity of ankle and foot, cavovarus deformity	M21.6X9	Other acquired deformities of unspecified foot
736.76	Acquired deformity of ankle and foot, other calcaneus deformity	M21.6X9	Other acquired deformities of unspecified foot
736.79	Acquired deformity of ankle and foot, other, Includes: pes not elsewhere classified, talipes not elsewhere classified	M21.6X9	Other acquired deformities of unspecified foot
736.81	Acquired unequal leg length	M21.759	Unequal limb length (acquired), unspecified femur
736.89	Acquired deformity, other, Includes: arm or leg not elsewhere classified, shoulder	M21.80	Other specified acquired deformities of unspecified limb
737.10	Kyphosis (acquired) (postural) 737.20 Lordosis (acquired) (postural)	M40.00	Postural kyphosis, site unspecified
737.20	Acquired lordosis	M40.40	Postural lordosis, site unspecified
737.30	Scoliosis (and kyphoscoliosis), idiopathic	M41.20	Other idiopathic scoliosis, site unspecified
738.6	Acquired deformity of pelvis Includes: pelvic obliquity	M95.5	Acquired deformity of pelvis
780.4	Dizziness and giddiness	R42	Dizziness and giddiness
780.93	Memory loss, Excludes: memory loss due to intracranial injuries (850.0-854.19), skull fractures (800-801.99, 803-804.99, mild memory disturbance due to organic brain damage (310.8), transient global amnesia (437.7)	R41.2	Retrograde amnesia
780.96	Generalized pain	R52	Pain, unspecified

(Continued)

781.0	Abnormal involuntary movements, Includes: abnormal head movements, fasciculation, spasms, tremor Excludes: abnormal reflex (796.1), chorea (333.5), infantile spasms (345.60-345.61), spastic paralysis (342.1, 343.0-344.9), specified movement disorders classifiable to 333, that of non-organic origin	R25.9	Unspecified abnormal involuntary movements
781.2	Abnormality of gait, used with neurological conditions; Includes: ataxic, paralytic, spastic, staggering	R26.9	Unspecified abnormalities of gait and mobility
781.3	Lack of coordination, Includes: ataxia, muscular incoordination	R27.0	Ataxia, unspecified
781.8	Neurologic neglect syndrome, Includes: asomatognosia, hemi-akinesia, hemi-inattention, hemispatial neglect, left sided neglect, sensory extinction, sensory neglect, visuospatial neglect	R41.4	Neurologic neglect syndrome
781.92	Abnormal posture	R29.3	Abnormal posture
782.0	Disturbance of skin sensation, Includes: anesthesia of skin, burning or prickling sensation, hyperesthesia, hypoesthesia, numbness, paresthesia, tingling	R20.0	Anesthesia of skin
782.3	Edema, Includes: anasarca, dropsy, localized edema	R60.0	Localized edema
783.21	Loss of weight	R63.4	Abnormal weight loss
783.22	Underweight	R63.6	Underweight
783.3	Feeding difficulties and mismanagement	R63.3	Feeding difficulties
784.0	Headache	R51	Headache
784.3	Aphasia, Excludes: aphasia due to late effects of cerebrovascular disease (438.11), developmental aphasia (315.31)	R47.01	Aphasia
784.41	Aphonia (loss of voice)	R49.1	Aphonia
784.42	Dysphonia (hoarseness)	R49.0	Dysphonia
784.51	Dysarthria, Excludes: dysarthria due to late effects of cerebrovascular disease	R47.1	Dysarthria and anarthria

(Continued)

784.52	Fluency disorder in conditions classified elsewhere; Excludes: adult onset fluency disorder (307.0), childhood onset fluency disorder (315.35), fluency disorder due to late effect CVA (438.14); Must code underlying disorder first	R47.82	Fluency disorder in conditions classified elsewhere
784.59	Includes: dysphasia, slurred speech, speech disturbance NOS	R47.89	Other speech disturbances
784.60	Symbolic dysfunction, unspecified	R48.9	Unspecified symbolic dysfunctions
784.61	Alexia and dyslexia, Includes: alexia (with agraphia)	R48.0	Dyslexia and alexia
784.69	Other symbolic dysfunction, Includes: acalculia, agnosia, agraphia, apraxia	R48.8	Other symbolic dysfunctions
784.99	Other symptoms involving head and neck (incl. choking sensation)	R06.89	Other abnormalities of breathing
786.2	Cough	R05	Cough
788.31	Urge incontinence	N39.41	Urge incontinence
788.32	Stress incontinence	N39.3	Stress incontinence (female) (male)
788.33	Mixed incontinence (stress and urge)	N39.46	Mixed incontinence
788.34	Incontinence without sensory awareness	N39.42	Incontinence without sensory awareness
788.35	Post-void dribbling	N39.43	Post-void dribbling
788.36	Nocturnal enuresis	N39.44	Nocturnal enuresis
788.37	Continuous leakage	N39.45	Continuous leakage
788.38	Overflow incontinence	N39.490	Overflow incontinence
788.39	Other urinary incontinence	N39.498	Other specified urinary incontinence
788.41	Urinary frequency	R35.0	Frequency of micturition
788.43	Nocturia	R35.1	Nocturia
799.3	Debility (To be used as a medical diagnosis only)	R53.81	Other malaise
799.51	Attention or concentration deficit	R41.840	Attention and concentration deficit
799.52	Cognitive communication deficit	R41.841	Cognitive communication deficit
799.53	Visuospatial deficit	R41.842	Visuospatial deficit
799.54	Psychomotor deficit	R41.843	Psychomotor deficit

(Continued)

799.55	Frontal lobe and executive function deficit	R41.844	Frontal lobe and executive function deficit
799.59	Other signs and symptoms involving cognition	R41.89	Other symptoms and signs involving cognitive functions and awareness
905.5	codes: Late effects of of musculoskeletal and connective	M84.40XS	Pathological fracture, unspecified site, sequela
V13.51	Personal history of pathological fracture (healed) Excludes: Personal history of traumatic fracture (V15.51); if providing aftercare for healing pathological fracture, assign appropriate V54.2X code	Z87.311	Personal history of (healed) other pathological fracture
V13.52	Personal history of stress fracture (healed), Excludes: Personal history of traumatic fracture (V15.51)	Z87.312	Personal history of (healed) stress fracture
V15.51	Personal history of traumatic fracture (healed), Excludes: Personal history pathologic (V13.51) and stress (V13.52) fracture; if providing aftercare for healing traumatic fracture, assign V54-1X; if providing care for late effect of healed traumatic fracture, assign 905.X; cannot be coded as primary diagnosis	Z87.81	Personal history of (healed) traumatic fracture
V15.52	Personal history of traumatic brain injury; If providing care for late effect of TBI, assign 907.0; if providing care for late effect of nontraumatic brain hemorrhage, assign 438.XX; cannot be coded as primary diagnosis	Z87.820	Personal history of traumatic brain injury
V15.88	Fall May be coded as primary diagnosis	Z91.81	History of falling
V46.11	Dependence on respirator; cannot be coded as primary diagnosis	Z99.11	Dependence on respirator [ventilator] status

Appendix D

Examination

Upon meeting the Satisfactory Completion Statement, you may receive a certificate of completion at the end of this course.

Contact ceu@rehabsurge.com to find out if this distance-learning course is an approved course from your board. Save your course outline and contact your own board or organization for specific filing requirements.

In order to obtain continuing education hours, you must have read the book, have completed the exam and survey. Please include a $120.00 exam fee for your exam. Mail the exam answer sheet and survey sheet to:

Rehabsurge, Inc.
PO Box 287
Baldwin, NY 11510

Allow 2–4 weeks to receive your certificate.

You can also take the exam online at www.rehabsurge.com. Register and pay the exam fee of $120.00. After you passed the exam with a score of 70%, you will be able to print your certificate immediately. See rehabsurge.com for more details.

Exam Questions

Please encircle the correct answer.

1. The first step in starting a business is defining your practice. All of the following are examples except:

    a. Being the only facility that offers hand therapy in your area

    b. Offering sports, hand therapy and hydrotherapy

    c. Assessing if there is a market for wellness in your area, since your practice focuses on wellness

    d. Choosing the best slogan for your practice and printing it on all your corporate identity products

2. Which type of business identity is owned by a single identity? Only one is personally liable for all debts that might be incurred by the business.

    a. Sole proprietorship

    b. Partnership

    c. S-corporation

    d. C-corporation

3. How can you decrease your overhead?

    a. Sell vitamins

    b. Decrease patient visits

    c. Decrease office hours

    d. Increase your fees

4. Which type of insurance provides protection to the building you are using as well as your equipment?

    a. Liability

    b. Malpractice

    c. Casualty

    d. Property

5. Which system is used as a standard means to categorize medical services, supplies and equipment?

    a. CPT

    b. CMS

    c. HCPCS

    d. HIPAA

6. All of the following are discussed in this book as important areas, a facility should have except:

    a. New Patient Area

    b. Billing Area

    c. Treatment Area

    d. Rest Area

7. What is an example of an internal marketing action?

    a. Have your facility's name and contact details placed in the local Yellow pages

    b. Hold public speaking engagements

    c. Hold free health screenings

    d. Have a family and friends voucher

8. Which technique is used to make your website rise in search index position?

    a. Search Engine Optimization

    b. Social Bookmarking

    c. Video Marketing

    d. Blogging

9. Which act governs the privacy of individual protected health information?

    a. OSHA

    b. HIPAA

    c. OIG

    d. DOL

10. What is the penalty for violating HIPAA laws when the offense is committed with intent to sell, transfer or use individually identifiable health information for commercial advantage, personal gain or malicious harm?

   a. Fined not more than $500,000

   b. Imprisoned not more than 10 years

   c. Fined not more than $50, 000

   d. Imprisoned not more than 5 years

11. Which type of expense are paid every month and do not fluctuate even if time passes by?

   a. Utilities

   b. Rent

   c. Subscription fees

   d. Business meals

12. What is a concise enumeration and explanation of the requirements, duties and responsibilities of the person who hold the position?

   a. Employee manual

   b. Employee eligibility

   c. Job Description

   d. Terms of Employment

13. As you study your competition, you notice that they are open 5 days/week. They offer 3 services-PT, OT and chiropractic. They are a high volume clinic who serves the no-fault population. In order for your business to succeed, all of the following can be done except:

   a. Focus on wellness

   b. Be open on hours they are closed

   c. Hire more PTs

   d. Focus on third party payers and managed care plans

14. Which type of expense includes construction cost of premises, rental fees, rates and connection of utilities?

   a. Premises

   b. Staffing

   c. Sales

   d. Marketing

15. All of the following are suitable days to hold your grand opening day except:

    a. Sunday

    b. Tuesday

    c. Wednesday

    d. Thursday

16. All of the following are good advice in choosing a business name except:

    a. It should be limited to the services you offer

    b. It should be original

    c. It should be legally available

    d. It should be capable of representing you for many years to come

17. In choosing a location, all of the following are very important except:

    a. In a mall where there is ample parking

    b. In the vicinity of businesses that attract similar clients

    c. Easily reached on foot, close to major train and bus stations

    d. Has a low crime rate

18. This refers to helpful ways of modifying a patient's home environment when she is afflicted with a lasting disability:

    a. Prevention advice

    b. Rehabilitation advice

    c. Providing of daily equipment

    d. Adaptation techniques

19. This type of insurance protect your establishment from liability resulting from negligence that may inflict injury on other individuals:

    a. Unemployment

    b. Health

    c. Liability

    d. Casualty

20. Which type of code is made up of 5 digits and its primary purpose is for billing transaction between patients and their attending physicians and other healthcare practitioners?

    a. Common Procedure Coding System

    b. Current Procedure Terminology

    c. Correct Coding Initiative

    d. Functional Independence Measure

ANSWER SHEET

Name:_____

Address:_____

Profession:_____

License Number:_____

Date:_____

E-mail Address (optional):_____

Exam:

1. a b c d

2. a b c d

3. a b c d

4. a b c d

5. a b c d

6. a b c d

7. a b c d

8. a b c d

9. a b c d

10. a b c d

11. a b c d

12. a b c d

13. a b c d

14. a b c d

15. a b c d

16. a b c d

17. a b c d

18. a b c d

19. a b c d

20. a b c d

Please mail $120.00 and completed form to:

CEU Certificate Request

Rehabsurge, Inc.
PO Box 287
Baldwin, NY 11510.
Contact Us at:
Phone: +1 (516) 515-1267
Email: ceu@rehabsurge.com

Alternatively, you can take the exam online at www.rehabsurge.com

You will receive your certificate instantly.

It is the learner's responsibility to comply with all state and national regulatory board's rules and regulations. This includes but is not limited to:

- verifying and complying with applicable continuing education requirements;

- verifying and complying with all applicable standards of practice;

- verifying and complying with all licensure requirements;

- any other rules or laws identified in the learners state or regulatory board that is not mentioned here.

It is the learner's responsibility to complete ALL coursework in order to receive credit. This includes but is not limited to:

- Reading all course materials fully;

- Completing all course activities to meet the criteria set forth by the instructor;

- Completing and passing all applicable tests and quizzes. All learner's MUST take a comprehensive online exam where they MUST get at least 70%. Getting 70% is a requirement to pass.

IMPORTANT: Rehabsurge reserves the right to deny continuing education credits or withdraw credits issued at any time if: Coursework is found to be incomplete; It is determined that a user falsified, copied, and/or engaged in any flagrant attempt to manipulate, modify, or alter the coursework just to receive credit; and/or It is determined that the coursework was not completed by the user.

If any of the conditions above are determined, Rehabsurge reserves the right to notify any applicable state and national boards along with supporting documentation.

PROGRAM EVALUATION FORM

Rehabsurge, Inc. works to develop new programs based on your comments and suggestions, making your feedback on the program very important to us. We would appreciate you taking a few moments to evaluate this program.

Course Start Date:_____ Course End Date: _____

Course Start Time:_____ Course End Time:_____

Identity Verification: Name:_____

Profession:_____ License Number:_____State: _____

Please initial to indicate that you are the individual who read the book and completed the test. Initial here:_____

May we use your comments and suggestions in upcoming marketing materials? Yes   No

Would you take another seminar from Rehabsurge, Inc.?   Yes   No

The educational level required to read the book is: Beginner   Intermediate   Advanced

The course is:	(5-Yes/Excellent)			(1-No/Poor)	
Relevant to my profession	5	4	3	2	1
Valuable to my profession	5	4	3	2	1
Content matched stated objectives	5	4	3	2	1
Complete coverage of materials	5	4	3	2	1
Teaching ability	5	4	3	2	1
Organization of material	5	4	3	2	1
Effective	5	4	3	2	1

Please rate the objectives. After reading the material, how well do you feel you are able to meet?

Objective 1	5	4	3	2	1
Objective 2	5	4	3	2	1
Objective 3	5	4	3	2	1
Objective 4	5	4	3	2	1
Objective 5	5	4	3	2	1

What was the most beneficial part of the program? What was the least beneficial part of the program?

_____ _____

_____ _____

_____

What would you like to see added to the program? In what ways might we make this program experience better for you?_____

_____ _____

_____

If you have any general comments on this topic or program please explain. _____

_____ _____

_____ _____

_____

Please tell us what other programs or topics might interest you?_____

_____ _____

_____ _____

_____

Thank you for participating and taking the time to join us today!

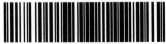

Made in the USA
Lexington, KY
28 September 2018